CHILD PSYCHIATRY
CASE STUDIES

64 CASE STUDIES
RELATED TO
CHILD PSYCHIATRY,
PSYCHOLOGY AND DEVELOPMENT

By

R. DEAN CODDINGTON, M.D.
Professor, Departments of Psychiatry and Pediatrics
Ohio State University College of Medicine;
Director, Division of Child Psychiatry

L. EUGENE ARNOLD, M.Ed., M.D.
Assistant Professor,
Departments of Psychiatry and Pediatrics,
Ohio State University College of Medicine,
Director, Child Psychiatry Outpatient Department

DAVID R. LEAVERTON, M.D.
Assistant Professor
Departments of Psychiatry and Pediatrics,
Ohio State University College of Medicine;
Head, Pediatric Liaison Program

MARJORIE ROWE, Ph.D.
Assistant Professor
Department of Psychiatry,
Ohio State University College
Psychoanalyst,
Division of Child Psyc

D1297527

MEDICAL EXAMINATION PUBLISHING COMPANY, INC.
65-36 Fresh Meadow Lane
Flushing, N.Y. 11365

Library of Congress
Catalog Card Number
74-168269

ISBN 0-87488-029-7

August, 1973

FOREWORD

"Child Psychiatry Case Studies" presents a selection of patients who have been instructive to the authors. They were important to us in our own professional growth, and we felt that these children, their families, and their problems might also be instructive to our readers. They present challenging diagnostic and therapeutic problems, with which we have sometimes dealt successfully and sometimes unsuccessfully. For the most part, we have chosen children whom we knew well and with whom we had extensive contact; some of them have been followed for as long as ten years.

Although we have attempted to include examples of the major diagnostic categories, we have not been entirely comprehensive. The distribution parallels rather closely that of the usual child psychiatric population, with only a smattering of rare cases.

In our discussions, we have tried to be pragmatic rather than erudite. We have attempted to aid readers in understanding children through examples. The references appended to each case study are intended to sample the literature, not exhaust it.

The studies are randomly ordered and self-contained. The index will guide those with special interests to the appropriate cases. Occasionally, we direct the reader to a similar or contrasting case elsewhere in the book. The questions are mainly intended to provoke thought, rather than to test for well-established facts. We consider some of the questions to have more than one correct answer. Sometimes, these will be of approximately equal merit; sometimes, one answer will be "best," even though others are also correct. Occasionally, the reader may disagree with our choice of the best answer. If, in the process, he is thinking critically about the pertinent issues, our purpose will have been achieved.

Our aim was to present child psychiatry and child psychology as a dynamic, deductive process rather than a static body of facts. This is the way we see it: an exciting, challenging field which daily presents new permutations of pathogenic and therapeutic elements. If we occasionally leave the reader with a feeling of uncertainty, it is because " 'that's the way it is,' said Pooh." No two children are alike, no truly matched controls are obtainable, and any one of our cases might have been treated in another way. But we have given you our best judgment and the reasons for it — as well as we knew how.

R. Dean Coddington
L. Eugene Arnold
David R. Leaverton
Marjorie Rowe

ACKNOWLEDGMENT

The authors wish to pay tribute to the efforts of many without whom this book would not have been written. Mary Cantrell, Marcia Norman, Sharon Clark, Jerrie Shea, and Bertina Povenmire typed and retyped the manuscript and gave welcomed editorial advice when our writing was unclear.

We would also like to thank our families, students, and colleagues, who put up with us during our preoccupation with the writing.

DEDICATION

This book is dedicated to:

The children and families who have taught us so much.

CHILD PSYCHIATRY CASE STUDIES

TABLE OF CONTENTS

CASE STUDY #1

A 7-Year-Old Almost Drives His Beloved Teacher Out of Teaching

A seven year-old white Protestant rural first-grade boy was referred to the clinic in March by the school psychologist because of behavior problems and underachievement.

His mother described him as always active and intense, "sometimes very hateful and other times very loving." His gestational, birth, and developmental history was otherwise unremarkable.

He presented as a likable, bright, well-developed, stocky boy who quickly made rapport and kept himself busy drawing pictures. He fiddled with his fingers and on the finger twitch test* could hold them still for only 5 seconds. One of his three wishes was to do better in school. He verbalized frustration and disappointment in not being able to control himself better. He reported hitting himself in the face to stop his impulsive acts. Even this did not help, and he felt like giving up. His Bender Gestalt (Fig. 1.1) showed borderline impairment of visualmotor coordination, with a Koppitz error score of 8 (age norm 5.3).

He was the oldest of three boys whose mother was obese, anxious, but pleasant. She had remarried shortly before the birth of the seven-month-old baby, a result of a between-marriage liaison with a larceny fugitive. She indicated a willingness to talk with someone about her own feelings and problems, which she felt had improved with her present happy marriage.

Additional information from the school revealed that the boy was restless, overactive, disruptive, inattentive, impulsive, immature, attention-demanding, and unable to follow group directions, requiring one-to-one attention.

QUESTION A:
THE BEST INITIAL DIAGNOSTIC IMPRESSION IS:
1. Adjustment reaction of childhood in an intelligent boy who is reacting to a chaotic early life and a troubled mother
2. Learning disability with underachievement, frustration, and consequent misbehavior
3. Hearing loss and maternal deprivation
4. Hyperkinetic syndrome (minimal brain dysfunction) aggravated by chaotic early life in an intelligent boy with a troubled mother
5. Passive-aggressive personality with mental retardation

The best answer is four. This boy presents an almost classical picture of hyperkinetic syndrome, which appears the primary problem. One is incompletely correct, not presenting the whole picture. Two may be a subsidiary part of the problem; many hyperkinetic children have learning disabilities. See case 28 for an overactive, aggressive boy who was not truly "hyperkinetic," and case 32 for a hyperkinetic boy masquerading with an unusual problem.

QUESTION B:
THE BEST INTERVENTION AT THIS POINT IS:
1. A trial of stimulant medication with weekly reports from the teacher to monitor progress and adjust dosage
2. Family therapy
3. Parent counseling and school consultation, with a behavior modification program
4. A trial of a stimulant and counseling for the mother
5. Play therapy, parent guidance, and school consultation

*In the finger twitch test, the child sits on the edge of a seat with elbows on knees, hands and head hanging down, and tries to hold still. (Barcai, 1971)

CASE STUDY #1

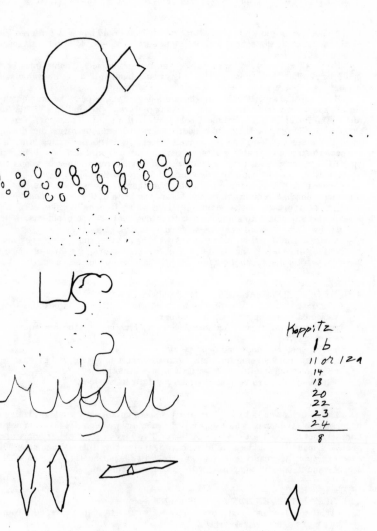

Koppitz
1 b
11 or 12 a
14
18
20
22
23
24
‾‾‾
8

7 yr. 2 mo

FIGURE 1.1

CASE STUDY #1

Any therapeutic program for an obviously hyperkinetic child should include a trial of stimulant medication, though this should not be seen as the only intervention. The best single answer is four, but an even better answer would be a combination of one and three. However, see cases 48 and 60 for apparently hyperkinetic children who did not benefit from stimulants.

With supportive psychotherapy for his mother and with 2.5 mg d-amphetamine (Dexedrine) twice a day, the boy made a good school adjustment and was promoted to the second grade. His mother, who was very concerned about his having to take medicine, about the family's financial difficulties, and about the distance she had to drive from their small town, decided to terminate the clinic visits and stop the medication at the end of the school year.

When school resumed in the autumn, the medication was not restarted. His school behavior and achievement gradually deteriorated despite heroic efforts by a young, dedicated teacher, to whom he was very attached. In fact, he begged her to get married and let him live with her. By November his classroom hyperactivity, misbehavior, and inability to follow directions had become so intolerable that his mother restarted the d-amphetamine. The previously effective 5 mg per day did nothing, but 7.5 mg per day seemed to help his behavior, his ability to sit still, and his academic achievement. However, this dose caused abdominal pain severe enough that he refused to take the drug, and his mother did not insist on it.

QUESTION C:
THE ABDOMINAL COMPLAINT:
1. May be "negative placebo effect" resulting from the mother's anxiety about drugs
2. Must be psychosomatic, because stimulants do not have gastrointestinal side effects
3. Is an indication for switching to methylphenidate (Ritalin), which is well known to have fewer side effects
4. Is a common side effect of amphetamine
5. Warrants a thorough pediatric examination

Since the abdominal complaints abated by the time they were reported, pediatric examination appeared unnecessary. Abdominal complaints have been reported as a side effect of stimulants. Though not common, they seem to be more of a problem with methylphenidate than with d-amphetamine (Weiss, 1971), in contrast to anorexia, which is reported by some authors to be worse with d-amphetamine. The best answer is one. In view of his mother's reservations about the medicine and his teacher's report of many somatic complaints, including tummy aches, prior to restarting the medicine, some of the abdominal complaint was probably "negative placebo effect."

On return to the clinic, his mother appeared more anxious than ever and felt that the boy's problems were her fault because of her feelings about her former paramour. At first she had claimed that the present marriage was very stable and satisfactory. However, at this time she volunteered that she was unhappy and was worried about her former paramour coming to town and killing both her and her husband for her "unfaithfulness." Her feelings for him, both of fear and love, were in many ways more real to her than her feelings for her present husband. They constituted a continuing irritation to the marriage. She had begun "protecting" the boys from her husband's discipline, with consequent deterioration in the stepfather-son relationship and manipulation by the patient. She related much of this to her feelings of inadequacy as a wife and mother, which in turn she related to her own mothering.

She resumed psychotherapy and the boy tried an allergen-free diet. His teacher was advised by telephone about his management, and a teacher consultant furnished by the school system cooperated in setting up a behavior modification

CASE STUDY #1

program in the classroom. During this time he showed some improvement, temporally associated with the allergen-free diet. However, severe problems still remained, and his mother did not feel that she could afford to continue the diet. In January he produced the Bender Gestalt shown in Fig. 1.2, which showed no improvement over the previous year. In fact, his Koppitz error score had risen to 10 (age norm 3.9) because of increased emotional stress. At this point he was included in a 3-month double-blind cross-over comparison of placebo, dextro-amphetamine, and levo-amphetamine, mainly to clarify the reality of the gastro-intestinal side effects which had necessitated the previous discontinuation of medicine.

He complained of no abdominal pain on any of the drug conditions, even though the doses of amphetamine used ranged up to 30 mg per day in contrast to his previous 7.5 mg per day. On the first drug condition, placebo, his behavior continued to deteriorate, and his teacher stated that she was planning to quit teaching, considering herself a failure. She related this decision solely to her experience with the patient, having been very pleased with all the other children in this, her first class. With both of the active drugs, his behavior and classroom achievement dramatically improved. With dextroamphetamine, however, he seemed overly calm and withdrawn, not very spontaneous. With levoamphetamine, he showed equal improvement in behavior and performance, but preserved his natural spontaneity and outgoing manner. Therefore, he continued taking levo-amphetamine as a maintenance drug. His teacher decided to continue teaching.

During this time, continuing efforts had been made to work with the parents. The stepfather consented to come in on two occasions. The first time, during the placebo period, the marital problems appeared insoluble, and the mother began seriously considering divorce. On the second occasion, about a month after the patient started showing improvement on one of the active drugs, the marital atmosphere had completely changed, with both parties being much more understanding and forgiving. Both parents attributed the improvement in their relationship to the boy's improvement, which allowed the stepfather to resume a good relationship with him and removed him as a focus of their disagreement.

QUESTION D:
HYPERACTIVITY, MISBEHAVIOR AND UNDERACHIEVEMENT:
1. Are never caused by family turmoil and/or parental psychopathology
2. Can cause family turmoil and aggravate parental psychopathology
3. Can be locked into a vicious cycle with family turmoil and parental psychopathology
4. Should always be treated with drugs
5. Often, but not always respond well to stimulants such as amphetamine or methylphenidate
6. Occur only in firstborns

This case beautifully illustrates the aggravation of parental psychopathology by a child's hyperkinetic behavior syndrome which in turn is more likely to manifest itself under the stress of maternal anxiety and marital discord. Children with brain dysfunction are more likely to show their symptoms under stress than in stable, well-structured, secure situations. This phenomenon seems to substantiate the half-truth that adult caretakers are responsible for the behavior of children. In this case, it is interesting that not only did this belief tap the mother's insecurity so that she tended to blame herself for the boy's problems, but it also tapped the insecurity of an otherwise competent, dedicated first-year teacher, who saw herself as a bad teacher because of her inability to handle this boy's problems. Both of these adults were made more anxious and less efficient in their efforts to deal with the situation. Note that this vicious circle was broken up by pharmacological intervention, which facilitated the effectiveness of the psychosocial efforts. Nevertheless, this does not mean such symptoms should always

CASE STUDY #1

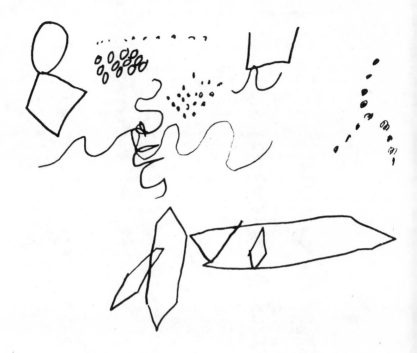

Koppitz score
2
10
11
14
15
16
18
21 a
21 b
24
10

8 yr.

before med

FIGURE 1.2

CASE STUDY #1

be treated with drugs; they may sometimes occur outside the hyperkinetic syndrome. The correct answers are two, three, and five.

QUESTION E:
THE LEVOAMPHETAMINE EVENTUALLY USED AS MAINTENANCE MEDICATION IN THIS CASE:
1. Is the drug of choice for hyperkinetic children
2. Is a research drug and cannot be used without an FDA investigational drug permit
3. Constitutes half of the racemic mixture of amphetamine marketed as Benzedrine, and as such has been used for decades in the treatment of hyperkinetic children
4. Has recently been found useful for some hyperkinetic children, especially the more aggressive ones, when dextroamphetamine is considered unsatisfactory because of side effects
5. Is probably primarily anti-dopaminergic, compared to dextroamphetamine which is probably both anti-dopaminergic and antinorepinephrinergic

The stimulants of choice for the first trial with hyperkinetic children appear at this writing to be methylphenidate (Ritalin), dextroamphetamine (Dexedrine), and racemic (dl) amphetamine (Benzedrine). Other useful ones include desoxyephedrine (Desoxyn), imipramine (Tofranil), and levoamphetamine (Cydril). The latter is commercially available in 7 mg tablets of levoamphetamine succinate, equivalent in amphetamine base to 5 mg amphetamine sulfate. Three and four are correct. Five would be correct if all the "anti's" were removed.

QUESTION F:
WHICH OF THE FOLLOWING ARE LIKELY REASONS FOR THE FACT THAT THOUGH 5 mg PER DAY OF DEXTROAMPHETAMINE WAS SUFFICIENT TO ALLEVIATE THIS BOY'S SYMPTOMS IN APRIL AND MAY, THE SAME DOSE WAS NOT SATISFACTORY IN NOVEMBER?:
1. Tolerance developed
2. The boy's body mass increased in the interim, requiring a larger dose
3. A different batch or brand of the drug had a different potency
4. He was under more stress in November
5. Teachers are tired in the spring and grateful for any relief from such a troublesome boy

This boy, in fact, had grown considerably during the summer, and in the autumn had the additional stress of the deteriorating family situation and harder academic work which he had not faced the previous year. Two and four are correct. Though tolerance is not usually considered a serious problem for this use of amphetamine, it has been reported. However, in this case it is effectively ruled out by the fact that the patient had not been taking the medicine in the interim. The tablets given him in November were from the prescription dispensed in April, so there can be no question of a different batch or brand.

QUESTION G:
THE HYPERKINETIC SYNDROME, OR MINIMAL BRAIN DYSFUNCTION:
1. Is a rather rare condition which should be diagnosed only after other likely causes of the presenting problem are ruled out
2. Is a constellation of symptoms affecting almost one percent of elementary school age children
3. Often coexists with other problems such as neuroses, adjustment reaction, or special symptom disturbance
4. Is more likely to cause problems at home than at school

CASE STUDY #1

5. Is equally likely to cause problems either at home or at school or both
6. Sometimes masquerades as "lack of motivation," cruelty, "orneriness," clowning, or dependency
7. Is a clearcut etiological diagnosis with a well-established cause

Minimal brain dysfunction is actually a diagnostic waste basket of psychosocial and psychoneurological deficits apparently expressed through approximately the same common behavioral pathways. It is a fairly common group of conditions afflicting about 4% of elementary school children, and accounting for close to half of the under-12 referrals to some child guidance clinics. Therefore it warrants a high index of diagnostic suspicion, even in the presence of other obvious problems. This is particularly so in the case of school referrals, since hyperkinetic children are more likely to have trouble in school than at home, although they may have behavior problems both places. Three and six are correct.

QUESTION H:
THE ALLERGEN-FREE DIET TRIED FOR THIS BOY:
1. Has been reported helpful in some hyperkinetic children with a history of food intolerance or allergy
2. Was used as a means to convince the mother the boy needed medicine
3. Has no theoretical basis for its effectiveness
4. Probably helped through "placebo effect" because of the mother's expectation that such an expensive remedy should help
5. Was actually a disguised behavior modification program with aversive deprivation of favorite foods for misbehavior

Though allergen-free diets have been facetiously suspected of operating via answers four and five, there seems convincing evidence of their real efficacy for some children (Weiss, G. et al.). One hypothetical explanation is that a high allergen-induced histamine level causes, or at least exacerbates, the hyperkinesis. We cannot completely rule out four as a correct answer in this case, but one is more certain, and therefore the best answer.

REFERENCES:
1. Arnold, L. E., 1973: The art of medicating hyperkinetic children. Clinical Pediatrics 12:35-41

2. Arnold, L. E. and P. H. Wender, In press, 1973: Levoamphetamine's changing place in the treatment of children with behavior disorders. Excerpta Medica, 1973

3. Arnold, L. E., In press, 1973: Is this label necessary? Journal of School Health, October, 1973

4. Arnold, L. E., Wender, P. H., McClosky, K. R. and S. H. Snyder, 1972: Levoamphetamine and dextroamphetamine: Comparative efficacy in the hyperkinetic syndrome; Assessment by target symptoms. Archives of Gen Psychiatry 27:816-822

5. Barcai, A., 1971: Predicting the response of children with learning disabilities and behavior problems to dextroamphetamine sulfate: The clinical interview and the finger twitch test. Pediatrics 47:73-79

6. Connors, K., 1971: Recent drug studies with hyperkinetic children, J Learning Disabilities 4:476-483

CASE STUDY #1

7. Eisenberg, L. , 1972: The hyperkinetic child and stimulant drugs. New England Journal of Medicine 287:249-250

8. Koppitz, E. , 1963: The Bender Gestalt Test for Young Children, Grune and Stratton, New York

9. Lauffer, M. and E. Denhoff, 1957: Hyperkinetic behavior syndrome in children. J Pediatrics 50:463-473

10. Safer, D. , Allen, R. and E. Barr, 1972: Depression of growth in hyperactive children on stimulant drugs. New England Journal of Medicine 287:217-220

11. Weiss, G. , Minde, K. and V. Douglas, 1971: Comparison of the effects of chlorpromazine, dextroamphetamine and methylphenidate on the behavior and intellectual functioning of the hyperactive child. Canadian Med J 104:20-25

12. Weiss, J. M. and H. S. Kaufman, 1971: A subtle organic component in some cases of mental illness. Archives of Gen Psychiatry 25:74-78

13. Wender, P. H. , 1971: Minimal Brain Dysfunction in Children, John Wiley and Sons, New York

CASE STUDY #2

"The Individual Delinquent"

Larry, a 15 year-old Caucasian boy, was admitted to a psychiatric hospital by order of the Juvenile Court. The chief complaints were destructiveness, fighting, poor peer relations, truancy, and generally anti-social behavior.

This young man had never adjusted well to life. His problem probably dated back to infancy, when his natural father was determined to make him a "rough and tough guy." He attempted to do this by throwing the baby around, terrorizing him, and being punitive. The patient became very frightened of his father and gradually came to see the world as a rather threatening place. Because of the father's failure to support and other difficulties between the parents, they were divorced when Larry was six. The mother remarried when he was eleven, but the relationship between him and his stepfather was not especially good. The two were mutually distrustful and rather non-communicative. The mother tended to be overprotective and overindulgent, failed to encourage sufficiently the control of impulsive behavior.

At school, Larry was involved in many fights. His achievement was very poor, and he had several "social promotions." In the year prior to admission Larry resorted to delinquent behavior, such as stealing and destruction of property. He compiled a rather lengthy police record.

Two years prior to admission, the family sought help from a child guidance clinic. After five months of family therapy they were referred to a private psychiatrist. He worked with the family for two months and arranged Larry's admission to a special school. After more acting out and delinquency, he was apprehended and placed in the county detention home, whence he was referred to the psychiatric hospital adolescent unit.

Past medical history revealed severe headaches from age 7-1/2, decreasing in frequency. The physical examination at admission was completely unremarkable. Larry was a neatly dressed, clean, short-haired, straight-appearing 15 year-old who maintained good eye contact and stream of talk.

The MMPI showed difficulties in impulse control and an absence of anxiety. This fostered an initial impression of a sociopathic personality. During the projective testing, Larry's style across all tests reflected a strong fear of failure. His approach to parts of the tests that were difficult for him was to rush through them, as if in panic. It seemed as if he wanted to get them out of sight as soon as possible and then use his haste as an excuse for failing. His self-esteem was poor: he seemed convinced of his own incompetence and lack of worth. He seemed more anxious than depressed. The psychologist felt that Larry had learned to appear strong and tough as the only way to deal with a frightening world and that the degree of anxiety on projective testing tended to rule out sociopathy.

The hospital course showed a dramatic change in Larry's behavior. Upon admission he related in his usual "rough and tough" manner. He said that when he grew up, he would join the Mafia. His individual therapists, both males, were able to see through this defensive posture and give Larry some insight into its meaning. Beneath the hard exterior he was a warm, friendly boy. His warmth and concern for others was illustrated during a one-week therapeutic group living experience at camp with five other patients and three staff. In a card game Larry, another boy, and one of the authors participated in some friendly teasing. The other boy became angry and started fighting with Larry. The author pulled Larry to one side in order to stop the fight, and found himself and Larry being threatened with an upraised log by the other boy. Rather than carry on the fight, Larry concentrated on protecting the author in a rather maternalistic way. The incident subsided almost as quickly as it began.

Larry responded to the firm limits of the therapeutic milieu. He developed a very close relationship with a male group worker. On one occasion Larry had inadvertently stepped on the man's guitar, damaging it considerably. The two of them worked out a compromise whereby each would pay for half the repairs.

CASE STUDY #2

Larry had to work to earn his share, but thought that this was really fair. He remarked several times that he was amazed by the judicious handling of the incident.

During his hospitalization a male mathematics teacher taught him to add and subtract, skills he had failed to learn previously. These new skills were recognized publicly when he was given the responsibility for handling the money at a bake sale held by the teen-age patients.

QUESTION A:
"ACTING-OUT" IS AN OFTEN MISUSED TERM. ITS USE SHOULD BE CONFINED TO:
1. Specific delinquent acts
2. The expression through behavior of unconscious wishes, impulses, or feelings
3. The expression of feelings towards parents, indirectly, that is outside the home
4. Sexual promiscuity
5. "Game-playing" activity

Acting out is used to describe a patient who engages in activity which can be interpreted as a substitute for remembering past events. When the unconscious impulse is too intense to talk about, or the patient lacks the capacity for inhibition, and replaces thought with action, he is said to be acting out. The term is often erroneously used to indicate consciously mediated unacceptable behavior. Delinquent acts and sexual promiscuity are not necessarily acting out, but can be. A 13 year-old girl who has introjected and identified with her mother's wish for sexual excitement and deals with this by becoming promiscuous, is acting out her and her mother's unconscious wish. On the other hand, a girl who is promiscuous because it is approved in her subculture or just because she likes it is not necessarily acting out in the true sense. The second answer is correct.

QUESTION B:
WHICH OF THE FOLLOWING WAS A MAJOR CONTRIBUTOR TO LARRY'S DELINQUENT BEHAVIOR?:
1. Poor relationships with father and stepfather
2. Scholastic failure
3. Peer pressure
4. Genetic disposition
5. Depression

Dr. William Healey wrote The Individual Delinquent in 1909. This classical study of 1000 delinquents showed very clearly the complexities that produce delinquent behavior. Poverty, mental retardation, learning disorders, epilepsy, gang activity, broken homes, and many other factors contribute. The "Westside Story" dramatically illustrates depression as a cause of antisocial behavior, even resulting in murder. In Larry's case there was suggestive evidence of a genetic loading through his father, but Larry did not suffer from a sociopathic (psychopathic) personality disorder. His trouble was based primarily on 1. the lack of an accepting, stable father, 2. scholastic failure, 3. role casting in the "rough and tough" attitude his father taught him, and 4. pressure from peers to maintain that role because of their vicarious satisfaction. He also seemed quite depressed over his current situation. Hence, all of the answers are correct. See case 12 for another anxious delinquent.

CASE STUDY #2

QUESTION C:
LARRY'S FATHER COULD MORE APPROPRIATELY HAVE HELPED HIM DE-
VELOP MASCULINITY BY:
1. Arranging for Karate lessons
2. Consulting an endocrinologist about testosterone injections
3. Playing games which depend on chance so Larry could occasionally win
4. Talking with him, teaching him manly pursuits
5. Teaching him not to "flinch" when threatened

Answer two is completely inappropriate, of course. One and five would do no harm, but don't seem as useful as four or three, the best answer. "Manliness," from a psychological viewpoint, has to do with independence, confidence, and maturity rather than athletic prowess or stoicism, and is desirable in girls as well as boys. A child gets great satisfaction out of beating his parent in any kind of game or play. Each success enhances his feeling of self-worth and builds his confidence. He is similarly stimulated by scholastic successes. With such preparation he feels ready to tackle anything, ready to risk failure when the prospect of success is also possible. The essence of Larry's treatment was to help him experience success, first at simple tasks such as learning to add and subtract in private, then more gradually difficult tasks where failure would be subject to public ridicule, such as making change at the bake sale. At a deeper level, success in establishing sincere friendships taught him that he was valued by at least one other person. Such successes are growth-producing, independence-promoting experiences, regardless of the age at which they occur.

QUESTION D:
PROBABLY LARRY'S POOR ACADEMIC ACHIEVEMENT RESULTED PRIMARILY
FROM:
1. Truancy - if you're not there, you can't learn
2. Anxiety interfering with learning
3. Mental retardation
4. A learning disability present when he started school
5. An anti-establishment attitude of non-cooperation with the school

This boy's I.Q. was 93, so mental retardation could not explain the problem. Answers one, two, and five undoubtedly contributed to the school failure syndrome in a "snowballing" way once it was established. However, the best bet for the primary cause is answer four. Estimates of primary learning disability in juvenile delinquents range from 50% (Poremba, Holte, & Berman, 1972) to 80% (Mulligan, 1970).

It has even been argued that the disability-induced frustration and failure are the chief causes of delinquent behavior and anti-social attitudes. This, of course, is not proven. See case 49 for a discussion of the high correlation (Rutter, 1970) between learning disabilities and emotional problems. There is, in fact, a large overlap since many delinquents are emotionally disturbed and many psychiatric patients engage in delinquent acting out of their problems. Without appropriate intervention, the learning-disabled child tends to drop further behind and to lapse into a vicious cycle of psychosocial-educational maladaptation. Silver and associates (1972) seem to have demonstrated that early intervention can prevent this. Such collaboration between mental health professionals and educators is an area of prevention which will no doubt receive increasing attention.

CASE STUDY #2

REFERENCES:

1. Aichhorn, A., 1935, 1963: Wayward Youth. New York Viking Press

2. Bowlby, J., 1944: 44 Juvenile Thieves. Int J Psychoanalysis 25:107-128

3. Healy, W., 1915: The Individual Delinquent. Little Brown & Co., New York

4. Johnson, A., 1949: Sanctions for Superego Lacunae of Adolescents, in Searchlights on Delinquency. Eissler, K. R. (Ed.), Int Univ. Press, New York

5. Mulligan, W., 1970: A Study of Dyslexia and Delinquency. CANCH Publication Center, P. O. Box 1526, Vista, California, 92083

6. Poremba, C. D., Holte, A. O. and A. A. Berman, 1972: Learning Disabilities and Juvenile Delinquency Workshop; ACLD, International Conference

7. Rutter, M., Lizard, J. and K. Whitmore, 1970: Education, Health and Behavior. Longman Group Limited, Great Britain

8. Silver, A. A. and R. A. Hagin, 1972: The Profile of a First Grade Class. J Am Acad of Child Psychiatry 11:645-674

CASE STUDY #3

Stanley "Makes the Rounds" - and Finds a Home

Stanley, an 8 year-old Protestant boy, was repeating the first grade when first seen for evaluation. His mother had several complaints. Recently he had stolen a bike and some money. He had been enuretic for three years. He lied a great deal, had considerable difficulty in school, and didn't get along with his stepsisters and stepbrother.

Mother had been separated and divorced while she was pregnant with Stanley. She then married a man with four children from a previous marriage. She was an obese, red-haired, freckled-faced woman who usually appeared at the clinic untidy and unkempt. She seemed rather depressed and blamed herself a great deal. She had been deprived as a child.

Stanley's stepfather had not worked since his early 40's and was considered a "cardiac cripple" due to earlier rheumatic heart disease. He also had suffered ulcers in the past and had done a great deal of "doctoring." He was an odd-looking, mousey individual who was given to bombastic outbursts. He showed no respect for his wife and criticized her for being immature and abusive to Stanley.

The social worker reported marital conflict, usually concerning home orderliness and cleanliness or the discipline of the children.

Stanley's stepfather's four children included a 15 year-old boy, and girls aged 6, 10, and 11. The boy, Ralph, had been seen in mental health clinics for behavior disorders, school failure, immaturity, bedwetting, and delinquency of a minor nature. Two of the stepsisters had great difficulty in school. A half-sister was born one year after Stanley's treatment started.

At first Stanley was seen individually for intermittent evaluations. On a Wechsler Intelligence Scale for Children (WISC) he scored a verbal IQ of 82, a performance IQ of 79, and a full scale IQ of 79. Intelligence tests at school indicated slightly higher intellectual functioning.

Stanley had repeated dreams of himself and his favorite stepsister, two years older, both riding a black pony as pictured in one of his school books. In the dream both he and his sister had pajama pants on without tops. He stated that it was a pleasant dream but was always accompanied by enuresis. When he did not have the dream, he did not wet the bed. He usually went to bed with both pajama tops and bottoms on, but awoke with the top off. His mother confirmed that this had occurred for several years.

The family lived in an Appalachian ghetto with a very mobile population and the highest crime rate in the city. They received aid to dependent children and social security benefits in order to sustain themselves.

Stanley was seen by many different therapists in both individual and group therapy during his three years in the clinic. Just before first coming to the clinic, he was seen in another hospital where an "abnormal" EEG was found. Because of his behavior disorder and the abnormal EEG, he was given diphenyl-hydantoin and phenobarbital. Although he had never had a seizure and did not seem to benefit from this medication, it was continued for almost a year and a half by his desperate mother.

After stopping the anticonvulsants, Stanley was included in a double-blind crossover study of levoamphetamine (Cydril), dextroamphetamine (Dexedrine), and placebo. The group co-therapists spontaneously reported behavioral improvement with both active drugs and noticed increased aggressiveness during placebo, the last drug condition. Though the mother and teacher reported equivocally, the clinician felt Stanley definitely benefitted from amphetamine and gave him a prescription. However, he soon stopped taking it because of abdominal side effects, and his mother did not insist on it.

CASE STUDY #3

QUESTION A:

WHICH OF THE FOLLOWING IS THE BEST EXPLANATION OF STANLEY'S DIFFICULTIES?:

1. Stanley's symptoms are classic for lead poisoning and can be explained by pica during the second year of life
2. Stanley's problems result from the mother's early difficulties in parenting (due to immaturity at the time of her first marriage), the parents' marital difficulties, and stepfather's poor image as a breadwinner
3. Stanley's problems are due to his sibling rivalry with his stepbrother who "castrates" him by being more delinquent. Because of an unresolved Oedipus complex, Stanley's jealousy of his stepfather continues to cause school failure
4. Stanley's conflict with his stepfather would be expected to resolve in time, as he gains insight into why his stepfather is unable to work
5. Stanley's problems are due to his family's difficult financial situation
6. Stanley's problems can be explained by lack of an adequate masculine role model
7. Stanley's problems are due to his one mistake, stealing a bike, which no one will let him forget

    The symptoms of chronic lead poisoning would be incoordination, paralysis, abdominal or joint pains, wrist drop, etc. Also, there is no evidence that Stanley ate paint during his early years. The second answer, the best, incorporates significant problems affecting Stanley, including mother's immaturity at the time of his birth. The third answer is overinterpretive and incorrect. It is possible that Stanley's conflict with his stepfather would decrease as he gained insight, but this would more likely be insight into his own sadness and anger. The fifth and sixth answers are partially correct. The last answer is too simplistic and does not account for the history before the bike theft.

    Stanley's parents seemed unable to communicate. They lived from crisis to crisis. Although the father was unable to work, he "chauffeured" the rest of his family throughout the city daily for their many medical and agency appointments. Different interviewers obtained markedly different histories of growth, development, and family patterns. When the interviewers let her, Stanley's mother spent minute after minute haranguing Stanley for his misdeeds without any apparent empathy or understanding of how his feelings were being hurt. At such times he shrank into his chair and pulled his coat over his head with tears in his eyes.

QUESTION B:

A "WORKING FORMULATION" OF THE FAMILY WOULD INCLUDE:

1. The mother had never been able to accept the loss of her first husband through divorce. She has felt herself to be such a failure that she has not been able to make this marriage work. Her difficulties with her stepdaughters and stepson indicate her inadequate personality
2. The mother and father have had difficulties with finances, marriages, and communication. Becoming involved in the PTA and getting Stanley a "big brother" should solve the problems
3. Mother's obesity and the father's heart disease are indicative of defective genes. It would help if she had a tubal ligation to prevent future pregnancies
4. Stanley's parents have problems with communication, parenting and discipline. They need to be more consistent in their behavior
5. Stanley's problems are common when there are stepsisters and stepbrothers living together
6. Stanley's parents need to get a job if both of them weren't on "the dole," the family would be coping much better. Their laziness prevents all of the children from succeeding

CASE STUDY #3

7. Both Stanley's mother and stepfather have emotional difficulties. The mother's obesity, depression, and severe self deprecation indicate further evaluation and probable treatment. Stepfather's bombastic statements about how to handle his family may reflect a very poor self concept, possibly resulting from his status as an unemployed welfare recipient

The first part of answer one may be correct, but her difficulties with her stepchildren do not indicate an inadequate personality. In this chaotic family situation, answer two is naively overoptimistic. Neither obesity nor rheumatic heart disease are generally accepted as evidence of defective genes. Answer four is partially correct but the family's interaction was already too consistent in that it was always chaotic and punitive. Answer five may be true, but glosses over the problems. The sixth answer indicates common attitudes towards those most in need of our mental health services. The last answer is the most comprehensive.

QUESTION C:
STANLEY'S MOTHER WAS VERY CONCERNED ABOUT HIS HAVING TO RE-PEAT THE FIRST GRADE. SHE COMPLAINED OF HIS SCHOOL PERFORMANCE, HIS HITTING OTHER CHILDREN, AND HIS NEVER FINISHING HIS WORK. WITH THIS INFORMATION THE THERAPIST WOULD:
1. Contact the school and get all the information available
2. Talk with everyone concerned with Stanley
3. Reassure the parents that because of Stanley's ability to relate to people they need have no worry about his ability to get along in the world
4. Suggest to the parents that Stanley needs referral to a urologist
5. Recommend immediate hospitalization and three-year intensive psychotherapy in a behavior modification setting for Stanley's stealing, lying and enuresis
6. Establish an ongoing relationship with Stanley and his family. Efforts will need to be made to contact the school, the welfare agency, health care facilities and vocational rehabilitation concerning this family's problems
7. Hospitalize Stanley for intensive neurological work up

Obtaining school information may be done so routinely that the child's and the parents' feelings are not taken into consideration. Sometimes, involving the child and the parents in a conference at school would be advisable. The severe symptoms contraindicate reassurance to the parents. The fourth answer indicates an overly medical orientation to the boy's bedwetting and does not take into account his many other severe psychological problems. The fifth answer seems unrealistic. Answer six is best. The present trend towards brief therapy has value for some cases. However, families with a great deal of distrust need a long-term relationship. The last answer would be unproductive, poor medical economics, and possibly anti-therapeutic.

At certain times Stanley appeared slightly hyperactive. He always arrived thirty minutes early for his clinic visit, whether it was individual or group therapy. Sometimes he wandered up and down the halls and into doctors' offices, with many beguiling attempts to relate. He sold "PTA membership tickets," raffle tickets, candy for organizations, etc. On a few occasions he was chased out of the building by administrators for soliciting.

During both individual and group therapy, he often mentioned that he would never return again because he felt people were mean to him. He called his co-therapists obscene names, belittled other patients in group therapy, and lied repeatedly. He provoked all the other children in the latency-age group therapy to reject him.

CASE STUDY #3

QUESTION D:
WE CAN INTERPRET THIS BY SAYING THAT:
1. Stanley is getting some sort of payoff by getting others to reject him
2. Stanley has difficulties in trusting others
3. Stanley's mild neurotic problem of arriving too early is a symptom of obsessive-compulsive behavior which will help him in later life
4. Stanley has a huge "crush" on the therapist's secretary and comes early in order to get a chance to see her
5. Stanley's previous recurrent dreams, his early arrival at the clinic, and his ambivalence about wanting to be there indicate a psychosis of childhood secondary to damaged ego structure from the loss of his father during his mother's pregnancy
6. Stanley is ambivalent about people, especially his therapist. He wants very much to be dependent on the clinic and those he sees each week. His need to bring abuse upon himself reflects how severely distorted his self concept really is
7. Stanley has a seizure disorder which allows him to lose track of time, mutter obscene words, and fail at his schoolwork. He would respond to another anticonvulsant

The first answer was confirmed by a slight grin on Stanley's face whenever others rejected him. However, this and answer two are only partial and non-specific. There may be some truth in answer three, but Stanley's problems were not considered mild by the therapists who had to deal with him. The fifth answer is overly psychological. Answer six is the best. A seizure disorder is unlikely in view of the history, including a poor response to two anticonvulsants

After 50 sessions of group therapy once a week, Stanley was much less disruptive and aggressive than he had been previously. He frequently mentioned insights about his relationship with his mother and father and on one occasion was able to talk about his murderous rage. He bragged repeatedly about the promise of a farm to be bought with money which would come from his father's injury "settlement." One of the other boys in the group allowed Stanley to hit him at times and appeared to enjoy it. Stanley had temper tantrums, destroyed objects, and used obscenities when it seemed he could get his anger out in no other way. The co-therapists felt they must restrain him at those times, yet wondered about his response to the restraint. He cuddled up against the therapist and stopped struggling, while vehemently asking to be let go. When the restraint was loosened, he made no move to leave.

QUESTION E:
THE NON-RESTRAINING CO-THERAPIST COULD COMMENT ON THIS BEHAVIOR BY TELLING STANLEY:
1. Nothing. Often while a child is being restrained, any comment provokes increased struggling
2. That unless he immediately stops the obscenities his parents will be informed of his behavior
3. That "boys will be boys" and a certain amount of acting out is expected in a group. Then release him
4. That another brain wave test is needed to rule out the possibility that he is having seizures in the group
5. That his castration fear is unfounded. Remind him that the homosexual panic he feels when being cuddled by the male co-therapist is normal and that the co-therapist is not his father or his stepfather who abandoned him. Tell him the Oedipus myth and explain why he is "hung up"
6. That you are aware of his anger, the group's anger, and the anger that you feel as his therapist
7. That at times he smiles while being restrained, which might mean that he is enjoying it. Then ask him how he feels. It may be best if the restraining therapist not stimulate Stanley by talking with him

CASE STUDY #3

Though comments by the restraining co-therapist may indeed provoke more struggling, answer one does not consider the possibility of comments by the other co-therapist, who can often get away with a therapeutic comment. The second answer is a threat and is contraindicated because it violates confidentiality concerning his feelings. The third answer condones the inappropriate behavior. Even if Stanley appeared to be having seizures, an EEG outside the group could not rule out seizures in the group. That decision must be made on clinical grounds. The fifth answer would likely confuse and scare the patient. The sixth answer, being quite general, would be only slightly helpful. The seventh answer is the best.

Stanley continued to show gradual improvement in the group. He used fewer obscenities, was less provocative, needed less restraint, and was less hyperactive. However, his mother called to say that she felt his behavior was still intolerable. The co-therapists requested an interview with her. She came and immediately began a harangue against Stanley's misdeeds. When her direction was diverted to herself by asking about her other children, she was able to share both negative and positive information. She dwelt on her own inadequate parenting and gave many excuses for why the family was unable to cope. In a hopeless, helpless, depressed way she verbalized a desperate need of help. She mentioned that Stanley frequently lost his temper, hitting out at his brothers and sisters in a wild, disorganized manner. She recently again had complaints from the school that he was hitting other children there. In addition, he continued to sleep poorly.

QUESTION F:
ONE MIGHT SUGGEST THAT FOR THE FUTURE:
1. Stanley's progress has been good enough that the case should be terminated
2. His impulsiveness might be helped by the addition of a major tranquilizer
3. Additional chromosomal studies need to be undertaken
4. A therapist be made available for mother if she so desired. Stanley might benefit from a major tranquilizer for his impulsiveness
5. Since complex problems require complex solutions, we will not begin to understand fully Stanley's behavior for several years. It may take even longer to modify his behavior
6. Stanley's rebellion, hostile behavior, enuresis, school failure, and depression are related to the loss of his real father during mother's pregnancy. His fixation at the oral phase prevents growth of his superego. She should allow him to regress more fully during times of stress and not retaliate when he misbehaves
7. Stanley's problems are due to his race prejudice, which he has inherited from his mother and her husband. She should join a black-white sensitivity group

Stanley's symptoms are far from being markedly improved and termination at this point could only be seen as rejection. A major tranquilizer could be given on a trial basis, but answer two is incomplete. There is no reason to suspect a chromosomal abnormality. Even if there were, its discovery would have little therapeutic impact. The best answer is four. The fifth answer is too general and defeatist, the sixth too interpretive. The seventh answer would only antagonize the mother.

REFERENCES:
1. Alessi, S. L. and M. D. Kahn, 1972: Group psychotherapy with latency age boys: research training and practice in different settings. Paper presented at the Annual Meeting of the American Association of Psychiatric Services for Children, Washington, D. C., Nov. 5, 1972

CASE STUDY #3

2. Arnold, L. E., 1972: Levoamphetamine and dextroamphetamine: Comparative efficacy in the hyperkinetic syndrome. Archives of Gen Psychiatry 27: 816:822

3. Barcai, A. and E. H. Robinson, 1969: Conventional group therapy with adolescent children, Int J Group Psychotherapy 19:334-345

4. Berger, M. M., 1968: Nonverbal communications in group psychotherapy. Int J Group Psychotherapy 8:161-178

5. Berkowitz, I. H., 1972: Adolescents Grow in Groups, Brunner-Mazel, New York

6. Caudill, H. M., 1962: Night Comes to the Cumberlands, Little, Brown, and Co., Boston

7. Clement, P. W. and D. C. Milne, 1967: Group play therapy and tangible reinforcers used to modify the behavior of eight-year-old boys. Behavior Res and Therapy 5:301-312

8. Frank, M. G. and J. Zilbach, 1968: Current trends in group therapy with children, Int J Group Psychotherapy 18:447-460

9. Godenne, G. D., 1964: Outpatient adolescent group psychotherapy (Part I) Amer J Psychotherapy, 18:584-593

10. Godenne, G. D., 1965: Outpatient adolescent group psychotherapy (Part II) Amer J Psychotherapy 19:40-53

11. Grotjahn, M., 1971: Laughter in Group Psychotherapy, Int J of Group Psychotherapy 21:234-238

12. Kimsey, L. R., 1969: Outpatient group psychotherapy with juvenile delinquents. J Dis of the Nerv System 30:472-477

13. Kohl, H., 1967: 36 Children, Mentor and Plume Books, New York

14. Kozol, J., 1967: Death at an Early Age, Houghton-Mufflin Co., Boston, Mass.

15. Loof, D. H., 1971: Appalachia's Children, University Press of Kentucky, Lexington

16. McDonald, N. F. and P. L. Adams, 1967: The psychotherapeutic workability of the poor. J Amer Acad of Child Psychiatry 6:663-675

17. Minuchin, S., et al., 1967: Families of the Slums, Basic Books, New York

18. Vargas, F. and E. Gratz, (Unpublished) Group psychotherapy for parents in the child guidance clinic

19. Weller, J., 1972: Yesterday's People, University Press of Kentucky, Lexington

CASE STUDY #4

A 5-Year-Old with a Diagnostic Problem

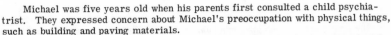

Michael was five years old when his parents first consulted a child psychiatrist. They expressed concern about Michael's preoccupation with physical things, such as building and paving materials.

While driving along in the car, he made many comments about such materials. He was also preoccupied with them when he played with toys or drew pictures; he almost always developed play that was in some way related to such things. As a matter of fact, on his way to the office he had picked up a half dozen stones from the parking lot, which he clutched in both hands throughout the initial review. During this interview he lay on the floor kicking his feet pleasantly in the air or resting them on a chair. His parents reported that he had no playmates and did not get along very well in kindergarten. He seemed more content to play alone than with others. Both parents also expressed concern about Michael's lack of affection.

Michael was the oldest of two children born to a prominent businessman and his sophisticated wife. Their marriage was superficially satisfactory but basically rather ungratifying to both parties. They both kept busy with social events, work, and frequent vacations to ski resorts. They were concerned about their children but were more interested in their active social lives than in their parenting roles. They consulted appropriate professionals and read avidly when they had questions about their children. Neither parent displayed any sign of mental illness.

After obtaining the initial history from the family, the therapist turned to Michael who was still lying comfortably on the floor. Generally, Michael confirmed in his own words what the parents had said, but he failed to give any explanation for his preoccupation. The therapist had no difficulty understanding Michael's words or in carrying on a meaningful conversation with him.

QUESTION A:
WHAT IS THE MOST LIKELY DIAGNOSIS?:
1. Obsessive-compulsive psychoneurosis
2. Early infantile autism
3. No mental illness
4. Personality disorder, passive-aggressive type
5. Mental retardation

The best answer is one. Autism can be ruled out in this case by the fact that the therapist was able to carry on a meaningful conversation with Michael. In early infantile autism language may be used, but not in a really meaningful interpersonal way by age 5. With this in mind, the therapist, who sensed the parents' anxiety, attempted to assure them that they need not be overly concerned about Michael's behavior. But the parents confessed that they already knew the diagnosis was early infantile autism. They said they had read many descriptions of this disorder in the lay literature. They had even consulted another psychiatrist, who had concurred in their diagnosis. Before beginning the long, complex, and expensive treatment program he had outlined, they wanted confirmation of the diagnosis; hence, their appointment with the author.

QUESTION B:
COMMUNICATION IN AUTISTIC CHILDREN IS CHARACTERIZED BY:
1. A repertoire of gestures used to convey meaning
2. The use of pantomime rather than verbal utterances
3. Persistently making sure the other person understands the gestures
4. Being monotonously repetitive and failing to convey meaning to others
5. Mutism

CASE STUDY #4

The lack of affective, human contact is the primary sign of early infantile autism. Children suffering from this disorder often avoid visual i. e., eye-to-eye contact with people and may be quietly absorbed in play with inanimate objects for hours. Though quiet for very long periods, they are not mute. The first three answers describe the communications of children with auditory impairment. Deaf children usually develop a repertoire of gestures as a means of communication, and are often very persistent about conveying their messages to others. The fourth answer is correct.

Michael's meaningful verbal communication ruled out the diagnosis of early infantile autism. He did act "autistic," the word being used as an adjective; but he was not autistic in the nosologic sense.

QUESTION C:
AT THIS POINT THE THERAPIST WOULD BE WISE TO:
1. Refer the family back to the first psychiatrist
2. Have further diagnostic or therapeutic sessions with Michael to confirm the impression
3. Start Michael on a minor tranquilizer
4. Start treatment with haloperidol, 2 mgm b. i. d.
5. Suggest a good nursery school

Referral back to a psychiatrist who made a serious diagnostic error is not in the best interest of the patient or his family. At this point there is not sufficient indication for medication. Nursery school would not be sufficient intervention in this case, although it would probably be helpful. The best answer is two.

Michael was taken into psychotherapy with a working diagnosis of psychoneurosis, which was confirmed in the next three months of weekly psychotherapy. It became apparent that some of his obsessive symptomatology was, in fact, a response to underlying anxiety and his parents' over-concern about his behavior. He was a lonely child, which probably was a result, at least in part, of the marital strife the parents were undergoing. The parents themselves were rather obsessive, tended to intellectualize constantly, and found it very difficult to relate to a five year-old on his level. Parenting was difficult for them.

In the very first individual play session Michael was attracted to a large, air-filled, plastic clown, which was weighted with sand so that it stood upright to just about his height. He grasped it, lay down upon it, and rolled back and forth rhythmically on the floor. When the therapist asked Michael if he and the clown were fighting, Michael responded: "No, I'm loving it." This little so-called autistic boy then explained that he was doing what he had seen his mother and father do in the dark in their bedroom without clothes on.

The parents later denied that this boy could possibly have witnessed the primal scene, but his description was quite vivid and was repeated on several other occasions. It seemed that his interpersonal relations had been colored by this experience. Further, it was clear that his anxiety over it was close enough to the surface to be brought out in psychotherapy. This could hardly be expected of an autistic child.

QUESTION D:
THE EARLIER DIAGNOSIS OF EARLY INFANTILE AUTISM HAD THE EFFECT OF:
1. Helping the parents by taking the problem out of their hands
2. Encouraging the parents to relax
3. Helping the parents get a proper school placement
4. Making the parents feel more adequate
5. Making the parents feel more inadequate

CASE STUDY #4

The diagnosis markedly increased the parents' anxiety; it made them feel much more inadequate. It confirmed their worst fears. It took the second psychiatrist six months to convince them that Michael was not autistic. Caution and conservatism are appropriate when dispensing diagnostic labels.

QUESTION E:
PRIMAL SCENE DATA IN AN INTERVIEW OR PLAY SESSION:
1. Usually indicate a psychotic process
2. Usually indicate the development of a sexual deviation or perversion
3. Is indicative of an incestuous relationship
4. Must be taken in context, for it can mean a lot of things
5. Must be de-emphasized because it is an attention-getting device

Only the fourth answer is correct. There are very few occurrences in therapeutic work with children which carry specific meanings and permit uniform interpretations. All behavior must be evaluated in terms of the context in which it occurs.

REFERENCES:
1. Arnold, L. E., 1973: Is this Label Necessary? J School Health, Oct. 1973, in Press

2. Bonaparte, M., 1945: Notes on the Analytic Discovery of a Primal Scene. Psa St of the Child 1:119-125

3. Chess, S., 1971: Autism in Children with Congenital Rubella. J of Autism and Child Schizo 1:33-47. Reprinted in Chess, S., Thomas, A., Annual Progr in Ch Psychiat and Ch Dev, Brunner & Mazel, 1972

4. Kanner, L., 1943: Autistic Disturbances of Affective Contact. Nerv Child 2:217-250

5. Kanner, L., 1946: Irrelevant and Metaphorical Language in Early Infantile Autism. Amer J Orthopsychiat 19:416-426

6. Kanner, L., 1949: Problems of Nosology and Psychodynamics of Early Infantile Autism. Amer J Orthopsychiat 19:416-426

7. Kysar, J. E., 1968: The Two Camps in Child Psychiatry: A Report from a Psychiatrist - Father of an Autistic and Retarded Child. Amer J Psychiatry 125:103-109

8. Niederland, W. G., 1958: Early Auditory Experiences, Beating Fantasies, and Primal Scene. Psa St of the Child 13:471-504

9. Treffert, D. A., 1970: Epidemiology of Infantile Autism. Arch Gen Psychiatry 22:431-438

CASE STUDY #5

A 16-Year-Old with a Hair-Trigger Temper

A 16 year-old black Catholic eighth-grade boy was accompanied to the clinic by his sister at his mother's insistence, with the chief complaint of "short attention span and quick temper." His mother had telephoned ahead to state that he was depressed, withdrawn, unhappy, easily triggered to violent temper outbursts, not able to get along with other kids, meddling, and possibly "schizophrenic."

His twenty year-old sister, who had been high school valedictorian, felt that their parents had always spoiled him so that even after he grew up he still thought he should have his own way.

The school reported that he "felt persecuted and acted hostile." He had flunked twice, putting him with younger children, whom he bullied. They tended to agitate him, resulting in rage outbursts. His fighting was very difficult to stop once it started. He did not finish work, and lost his temper if corrected or crossed. When expulsion was considered, he pleaded for another chance. His IQ was 91 (Otis), his reading level eighth grade, arithmetic level fifth grade.

The patient presented as a six-foot, well-built, handsome young man with a faint, somewhat inappropriate smile, which vanished when he talked. There was no other inappropriate affect or evidence of thought disorder. He seemed to make affective contact, but in a resistant, cunning, denial-ridden fashion. He was coherent, relevant, and logical. He felt that his father did not understand teenage problems. He resented his mother taking half his paycheck each time "for bills." Though his parents argued a lot, he felt that the family was basically stable, with everyone loving each other.

When asked whom he would like to take on a trip to the moon, he said, "Someone I don't know, so that I would not be responsible for the death or injury of someone I know." If marooned on a desert island, he would want one of his girlfriends, with whom he had already experienced intercourse. On such occasions, he used two condoms to be safe against pregnancy and disease. His only open show of hostility was around the topic of medication, which he agreed bothered him so much because it would mean there was a weakness in him. For the same reason, it would disappoint his father. He was also reluctant to have an appointment made for his parents because this would mean there was something serious. Though he frankly admitted a problem with his temper, he felt he could overcome this himself.

Even though continuing to resist the idea of anything being wrong, he returned the following week with his mother. She was a well-motivated registered nurse who remarked that parents were the last to realize there was anything wrong with their children. Now that she knew there was something wrong, she wanted to get help. She described his problem as "short attention span." By this she apparently meant short temper. She described his flying into rages at the least provocation. He interrupted to explain that he got angry because he was constantly on call by the older members of the family. He seemed unable to get his mother to understand anything he was trying to say and eventually broke into tears. She then explained that sometimes he didn't get angry, he just broke into tears, and what she was really talking about was emotional lability, sometimes tears and sometimes rage.

His birth and developmental milestones were unremarkable. However, information from a follow-up study of premature infants, in which he had been a normal control, mentioned lower-than-average IQ levels, impairment of visual-motor skills on Bender Gestalt reproductions, and "personality aberrations." A home visit when the patient was nine had found "a houseful of children, mostly offspring of a retarded uncle and aunt." The patient was noted to be very active, always on the go, and mischievous. When the mother was asked if there were any problems with running away from home, she said, "Not yet, but I hope he goes soon."

The patient's uncle had epilepsy and his father had been in the State Hospital after having "cracked" in the penitentiary. The mother feared that this boy would turn out like his father and hoped that some medication would help prevent it.

CASE STUDY #5

QUESTION A:
THE ETIOLOGIC AND DIAGNOSTIC POSSIBILITIES AT THIS POINT WOULD
INCLUDE:
1. Maternal rejection, overprotection, and oversubmissiveness, epilepsy
   (temporal lobe), paranoid schizophrenia, unsocialized aggressive reaction,
   and explosive personality
2. Psychotic organic brain syndrome and paranoid schizophrenia
3. Nonpsychotic organic behavior disorder and paranoid schizophrenia
4. Minimal brain dysfunction, paranoid schizophrenia, unsocialized aggressive
   reaction and explosive personality
5. Adjustment reaction of adolescence vs. neurosis with acting out
6. Adjustment reaction of adolescence, explosive personality, paranoid schizophrenia, and psychotic organic brain syndrome
7. Epilepsy, temporal lobe behavior disorder, minimal brain dysfunction, explosive personality, and maternal rejection, overprotection and oversubmission

Adolescent adjustment reaction is a much-abused diagnostic wastebasket and
should not be further abused by trying to cram this case into it. "Adjustment
reaction" is by definition a "transient situational disturbance, " and we have
documentation in this case dating the problems back 7 years. Despite the family
history of schizophrenia and the mother's labeling of the patient as schizophrenic,
the clinical picture does not warrant a diagnosis of any type of psychosis; the
patient made good contact and was coherent, logical and relevant. Unsocialized
aggressive reaction resulting from maternal rejection and consequent overprotection and oversubmission should be considered in view of his sister's report
that his parents always let him have his own way. However, his tears and his
admission of his temper being a problem call this diagnosis into question.
A fragile case might be made for depressive neurosis with acting out of his
mother's expectation that he would be violent and crazy like his father. However,
seven seems the best answer. The clinical picture presents an organic flavor
(impulsiveness, episodic extreme reactions, visual-motor dysfunction on Bender
Gestalt, juvenile hyperactivity, short attention span) with longstanding personality
problems, probably exacerbated by the family situation and the mother's handling
of the boy.

QUESTION B:
A REASONABLE DISPOSITION AT THIS POINT WOULD BE:
1. Anticonvulsant medication, EEG, and psychological testing
2. Hospitalization for further evaluation and treatment
3. Psychological testing and a major tranquilizer
4. Electroencephalogram and family therapy
5. Family therapy, group therapy and individual psychotherapy

Though the problem is serious, it does not present enough urgency to mandate
hospitalization before a trial of outpatient therapy. The clinical value of an electroencephalogram (EEG) may be debated, since it fails to detect some cases of
frank clinical epilepsy and some persons with no symptoms may show an EEG
"seizure pattern. " The patient, not the EEG, should be treated. However, in
this rather complex case, an abnormal EEG could help clarify the suspected
neurological aspect of the patient's problem and provide a more secure basis for
future management. Therefore, anticonvulsant medication should be postponed
until after an EEG. A major tranquilizer is contraindicated for a suspected un-
treated seizure disorder, though it can sometimes be successfully added to the
anticonvulsant regimen of a treated case. Psychological testing could be helpful,
but did not seem urgent at this point. Enough evidence was already available to

CASE STUDY #5

conclude that a good bit of the boy's problem involved his family. Therefore
family therapy seemed warranted. The best answer is four. Group or individual
psychotherapy would not have been the most efficient, direct approach to this
problem.

The patient refused to come for the electroencephalogram at the scheduled
appointment time, claiming that an EEG made his "uncle's skin wave." He and
his mother at first agreed to come for family therapy and felt the rest of the
family would also cooperate. However, they never succeeded in keeping a single
appointment.

Several months later, the patient's mother called in desperation, describing
a deteriorating, intolerable situation at home, school and work. She pleaded for
a prescription for him. She felt that she could get him to take medicine even
though he refused to come to the clinic for an electroencephalogram or anything
else.

QUESTION C:
THE BEST RESPONSE TO THE MOTHER'S PLEA WOULD BE TO:
1. Give in to it and prescribe a trial of medication
2. Insist that she and the boy keep an appointment for re-evaluation. Explain
   her responsibilities for getting the boy to come
3. Hospitalize the boy for further evaluation and necessary initiation of treatment
4. Avoid being manipulated into cooperating with the mother's overprotection and
   overcontrol
5. Arrange psychological testing and another EEG appointment
6. Interpret to her that she and the boy showed by their missed appointments
   that they were afraid to work on the family problems, and that the boy was not
   likely to improve until they faced this

The serious situation has deteriorated into a crisis which cannot wait for
further testing or evaluation and will not be resolved by mere avoidance of mis-
takes. Positive, even dramatic, intervention is required. Answer 6, while ap-
pealing, does not seem to answer the need and may be a bit unfair in light of the
patient's suspected neurological problem. Hospitalization at this point could
easily be justified. However, a slightly better plan would seem to be a 2-week
trial of medication with the understanding that hospitalization would be necessary
if medicine did not help. Therefore, one is the best answer. This, of course,
risks reinforcing the medical orientation of the R. N. mother, who has repeatedly
stated she sees medicine as the answer to the boy's problem. However, there
is always the possibility that "the customer is right."

A prescription for diphenylhydantoin (Dilantin) 300 mg a day was given. At
the end of one week, the patient was showing neither side effects nor benefits.
Since he was rather large, the dose was increased to 400 mg per day. Within
two weeks he improved dramatically in all areas of his life. He voluntarily took
the diphenylhydantoin from that point on.

About a year and a half after his first clinic visit, with school and job successes behind him, the patient requested a letter to help him get into the Army. He
now appeared frank, open, and happy. He reported that, in contrast to his previous tendency to lose jobs by getting angry with the boss, he had been able to
hold both temper and job for a long time. He was getting along well at home also.
He was generally pleased with himself for being able to control his temper and
stay out of trouble. He planned to continue taking the diphenylhydantoin for several
more years, feeling that it had helped him to gain this control over himself. A
telephone check with his mother confirmed his excellent temper control and stability.

A letter was sent to Selective Service stating that his emotional problem was
well controlled with medication and he would be able to tolerate the stress of
military life as long as he continued his daily dosage. He called back later to

CASE STUDY #5

state with delight that he had been accepted into the service and was planning to take special training which would help equip him for a good job after his discharge.

QUESTION D:
THIS ADOLESCENT'S EMOTIONAL LABILITY MOST LIKELY RESULTED FROM:
1. Maternal overprotection, oversubmission, overcontrol, and possibly rejection
2. Minimal brain dysfunction
3. Temporal lobe epilepsy or temporal lobe behavior disorder
4. Maternal expectation of trouble
5. Failure to intervene effectively early in the development of his problems
6. Poor role-modeling by his father

All of these undoubtedly contributed somewhat to the development of the boy's troubles. However, the episodic nature of his outbursts and his otherwise good ego functioning in planning for future consequences (even using double condoms!) suggest a seizure-like disorder, possibly psychomotor "fighting" seizures triggered by emotional stress. This was the rationale for choosing diphenylhydantoin (Dilantin) as the medication. The dramatic response to this anticonvulsant tends to confirm the primacy of an epileptic etiology. Three is the best answer. Of course, we must suspect placebo effect in view of mother's repeated pleas for medication as the answer to his problem. However, the patient himself resisted the idea of medication. Further, there was no benefit reported at the 300 mg dose, which the R.N. mother must have known to be a "therapeutic dose." Therefore, the effect of the 400 mg dose appears truly pharmacologic. This phenomenon is reminiscent of similar experience medicating frank epilepsy. All this does not negate the obvious contribution of family influences to the boy's problem, nor the obvious value of family intervention in this case.

QUESTION E:
IF THE FAMILY HAD KEPT THEIR APPOINTMENTS, THE FIRST SESSION SHOULD HAVE BEEN DIRECTED TO:
1. An elucidation of the difficulties getting along together, as each member of the family saw them
2. An explanation of how the patient could not help what he did
3. Getting the parents to realize how they angered the patient and precipitated his temper outbursts
4. Supporting the parents in being very firm with the patient
5. Assisting the family to delineate the respective rights of the family members

Two, three, and four may each be appropriate eventually, depending on the information forthcoming after rapport is established. However, too quick or too complete an emphasis on one of these might be an inaccurate intervention and risks losing rapport with one or more members of the family. Five would be the safer and possibly feasible to begin working on by the end of the first session. However, it should logically and strategically be preceded by one, the best answer.

For an example of diphenylhydantoin failing to control behavior problems, see case 44.

REFERENCES:
1. Anderson, C. M. and H. G. Plymate, 1962: Management of brain-damaged adolescents. Amer J Orthopsychiatry 32:492-500

2. Haggerty, R. J. and K. J. Roghmann, 1972: Noncompliance and self medication: Two neglected aspects of pediatric pharmacology. Pediat Clinics of N Amer 19:101-115

CASE STUDY #5

3. Hertzig, M. E. and H. G. Birch, 1968: Neurological organization in psychiatrically disturbed adolescents. Archives of Gen Psychiatry 19:526-536

4. Johnson, A., 1952: Genesis of antisocial acting out in children and adults. Psychoanalytic Quarterly 21:323-343

5. Meletzky, B. M., 1973: Treatable violence. Resident and Staff 19:40-48

6. Menkes, M. M., J. S. Rowe and J. H. Menkes, 1967: A 25-year follow-up study on the hyperkinetic child with minimal brain dysfunction. Pediatrics 39:398

7. Missildine, H., 1962: Preventive psychiatry in emotional development Feelings Vol. 4, No. 6, Nov.-Dec., 1962

CASE STUDY #6

A 14-Year-Old Who "Didn't Grow Up in a Normal Way"

The parents of a fourteen year-old Jewish boy brought him to the clinic because of their concern about his poor school work despite above average intelligence as confirmed by a school psychologist. They were also worried because Adam had no friends and no interests even though many attempts had been made to get him into such activities as the Boy Scouts, YMHA, and school clubs. Other boys bullied him. In particular, one boy waited for him at school in order to sting him with rubber bands. He refused to fight back. Lack of interest and non-participation seemed to be the boy's attitude towards life, and he sat around complaining of "boredom."

Adam was a short, obese, pale boy whose nails were badly bitten. He showed no physical signs of approaching adolescence and looked younger than fourteen. He exhibited no spontaneity during the interview and seemed disinterested.

The father, who had immigrated, was self-educated and owned a chain of stores. He found it difficult to accept his son's problems and was reaching the point of hopelessness about him. He was also worried about his son's sexuality. The mother, too, was very concerned. She had a more accepting relationship with Adam and acted as his confidant when he received poor report cards or was teased by other boys. She overprotected him in many ways. His nineteen year-old sister had finished high school, was working, and was living at home. The two fought constantly, while at the same time they were very close and defended each other against outsiders.

Adam was born three weeks late. He gained weight rapidly and was a happy, contented baby. His developmental milestones were normal and there were no early illnesses or separations. Things went well until he entered the first grade at five years. Here he was the only Jewish child in the class, and his teacher, who was irritated when he was absent on religious days, made fun of him in front of his classmates. In the second grade he was held up by his teacher as "the boy who wouldn't learn." In the third grade his teacher often called him "crybaby."

The Children's Apperception Test (CAT) was administered in an attempt to understand some of Adam's feelings about himself. He seemed to be describing himself when he told a story about a "boy who didn't grow up in a normal way," a failure, and possibly a sissy in his father's eyes. Adam seemed to feel that his inadequacies, together with his struggles with his sister, were a terrible burden on his father, aging him and possibly making him ill. In his phantasies, his father would give him affection if only he were adequate, but withheld it because he was inadequate. In contrast, mother was seen as the giving one.

Food was used in responses to five of the cards. It was given in love, withheld as punishment, tricked away from father, and aroused paranoid fears that it would be stolen.

His stories also suggested that denial, in the form of a reaction formation, was the boy's main defense against his murderous impulses.

An example of his fears about what could happen if he lost control over these impulses was one of his stories in which he lost his temper and killed all of the other characters. He was then powerless to bring them to life again and was left with his own feelings of worthlessness and inadequacy.

QUESTION A:
ADAM'S SHORT, FAT, PALE, IMMATURE APPEARANCE WAS LIKELY DUE TO:
1. Thyroid deficiency
2. Hyperadrenalism (Cushing's)
3. Pituitary malfunction
4. Hypogonadism
5. Constitutional delay in puberty

Hypothyroidism could cause obesity and short stature, but it is not consistent

CASE STUDY #6

with nailbiting or high intelligence. Cushing's syndrome includes a flushed appearance, not pallor. An immature appearance at age fourteen would more likely result from constitutional delayed development than from hypogonadism or hypopituitarism, though the latter possibilities deserve investigation. Five is the best answer.

QUESTION B:
FOOD WAS MENTIONED SO OFTEN IN THE C. A. T. PROTOCOL BECAUSE:
1. The boy was hungry
2. The boy was overweight and possibly on a diet
3. It was the boy's only interest
4. In many ways it was symbolic of the affection from his father he so badly needed and felt he had lost
5. Such preoccupation is normal for growing boys

The earliest relationship a baby has with its mother is a feeding one. While feeding, the mother is also giving the baby affection, containment.and support. With growth to childhood, food becomes symbolic for love and affection. We can guess that the numerous references to food reflected Adam's feelings about the rejection he felt from his father and the withdrawal of his father's love. The best answer is four. See Case 32 for food in therapy.

QUESTION C:
ADAM SEEMED TO BE TALKING ABOUT HIMSELF IN ONE OF HIS C. A. T. STORIES WHEN HE DESCRIBED A BOY WHO DIDN'T GROW UP IN A NORMAL WAY. PERHAPS BEHIND THIS STATEMENT WERE HIS FEELINGS ABOUT:
1. Not being a good athlete
2. His physical immaturity and obesity when compared to boys of his own age
3. Being Jewish
4. Being bored
5. Being rejected by his peers

There are feelings of helplessness and despair in the boy's description. He seemed to be talking about his self-image and his awareness that he was physically different from his peers and that there was nothing he could do to remedy the situation. The best answer is two. One and five seem to be at least partially the results of two.

QUESTION D:
WHEN WE SPEAK OF A "REACTION FORMATION" WE MEAN:
1. That out of the many different ways in which a patient could react to a specific situation, he chooses one and uses it every time the situation arises
2. A process by which the patient imagines that specific wishes, feelings or other aspects of himself are characteristics of others and not his own
3. A situation in which a patient habitually tells lies in order to enhance his status in the eyes of others
4. A process by which a patient gives reasons for his behavior which conceals from others and sometimes from himself, the real reasons
5. An established pattern of behavior that is directly opposed to strong unconscious impulses or trends

In this case we have a boy whose attitude towards life seemed to be disinterest and lack of participation. In his CAT stories he revealed his deeper murderous rage over; 1) his physical stature, which he could not change, 2) his feelings that he had lost his father's love, and 3) the rejection by his peers. Thus, unconsciously, in order to deny the rage over which he feared loss of control, he be-

CASE STUDY #6

came the disinterested, non-participating boy, by means of a reaction formation. This case also illustrates that a reaction formation often covers larger areas of the personality than the other defenses.   The best answer is five.

REFERENCES:
1. Bellak, L. , 1954: The Thematic Apperception Test and the Children's Apperception Test in Clinical Use. New York, Grune & Stratton

2. English, H. B. and A. C. English, 1958: A Comprehensive Dictionary of Psychological and Psychoanalytical Terms, New York, Longmans, Green

3. Freud, A. , 1965: Normality and Pathology in Childhood, New York, International Univ. Press

4. Green, R. and J. Money, 1961: Effeminacy in pre-pubertal boys.   Pediatrics 27:286-291

5. Haworth, M. A. , 1966: The CAT: Facts about Fantasy, New York, Grune & Stratton

6. Mazzaferri, E. L. and T. G. Skillman, 1971: Endocrinology Case Studies, Flushing, New York, Medical Examination Publishing, Co. , Inc.

7. Pitcher, E. G. and E. Prelinger, 1963: Children Tell Stories: An Analysis of Fantasy, New York, International Universities Press

8. Redl, F. , 1966: When We Deal with Children, New York: The Free Press

9. Rycroft, C. , 1968: A Critical Dictionary of Psychoanalysis, New York, Basic Books

CASE STUDY #7

No Limits for Laura

Laura was a 15-1/2 year-old white Episcopal girl, the youngest of six siblings, brought for admission to the psychiatric hospital. For three years she had been a severe management problem for her parents, had failed some of the ninth grade courses three times, was suspended from school over 68 times, and was placed on probation for a phone bomb threat (a misdemeanor) to a public school. She admitted to promiscuity. Her parents could not maintain limits about where she spent the night and what hours she kept. She had spent several days in detention homes. She had tried outpatient psychotherapy four times with a variety of therapists.

Her mother stated that Laura had always been a behavior problem. Even at age one she was "difficult to control," not wanting to take a nap. When she brought her first report card home from first grade, it did not meet the parents' expectations; her siblings were frightened about what father would say. Her school memories included many different settings, few of them happy. Her intelligence was at least average, but her behavior was characterized by poor impulse control, suicide attempts, repeated runaways, truancy, and fighting with her parents.

Mother was a small, depressed-looking older woman who had been trained as a physical therapist. For most of her marriage she had not worked, but recently she had briefly taken up her profession in an attempt to assuage her depression. She had sought training in teaching remedial reading "to help Laura," and perhaps to keep the focus of Laura's problems at school rather than at home.

When seen by the psychiatric social worker, she complained of a lack of social outlets; her husband's isolation caused too many problems with house guests. Recently she had submerged herself in projects. It seemed that she was easily manipulated by Laura. She attempted to manipulate school excuses from physicians for Laura. Frequently she would leave the family and their difficulties to stay awhile with her well-to-do mother in a large city several hundred miles away. She was very ineffective in supporting Laura during times of stress. At times, when confronted with behavior problems, she would have hysterical panic reactions in which she would scream and shout.

Father was a highly trained man of letters who spent a great deal of time on professional tours. He characterized himself as an ambitious, driving man; he proudly described his hand-to-hand combat in World War II. He begged out of his responsibility for Laura by acknowledging his love of violence and saying that a fear of his own violent temper excused him from effective firmness when dealing with her; he feared he "might go too far." He admitted he had some difficulty in setting limits for himself with food, drink, and work. He worried about "certain ideas" of student groups which might lead to the "overthrow of the establishment." He remembered his own family as rather Spartan and independence-worshiping. He was quite proud of his daughter's prize-winning horsemanship. At times he seemed rather tired and depressed about the possible embarrassment his daughter might bring upon him.

Neither parent was able psychologically to support Laura's stay in residential treatment. When she would run away, their indecisive ambivalence interfered with their ability to bring her back. On one such runaway episode she threatened to "use a knife" on anyone who came near her and then fled the house.

QUESTION A:
LAURA'S MANY DIFFICULTIES IN COPING WITH LIFE ARE RELATED TO THE FACT THAT:
1. She rebels against her intellectual father's wishes for her to be a scholar

CASE STUDY #7

2. Laura has an unresolved oedipal complex and has never been able to identify with her weak, passive mother, who reinforces Laura's somatization and sense of failure. Laura's identification with her strong, masculine father continues to create severe problems for her. The horseback riding confirms this psychopathology

3. She has problems learning right from wrong and communicating in the family

4. The parents' ambivalence about Laura's misbehavior has impaired her sense of self-worth. Their inappropriate use of the detention home following an emotional upset and their inability to support psychotherapy in or out of residential treatment does not help Laura to improve her behavior

5. Laura's behavior in the first year of life indicates that she has a "constitutionally difficult personality."

6. Laura's behavior is very common among teenagers who are rebelling against the establishment. Time and maturation will lead to a normal life and a sense of success in later life if she is only left to work out her problems by herself

7. Laura should be taught karate and self defense by her father to help her develop a sense of success

In this case it did seem that Laura was rebelling against her father's emphasis on the intellectual. Her siblings also had rebelled, to a lesser extent. However, this answer is incomplete. Answer two may be correct in its interpretations, but is probably overly psychological; the last sentence about horseback riding would be very difficult to prove. Answer three is correct as far as it goes, but it is too general. Four is a slightly better answer than two and is the best when compared to the rest of the answers. Answer five may be correct, but fails to consider the important environmental influences in this case. Answer six sounds too optimistic. The glib ideas in answer seven do not relate to the question asked. Even as an answer for a treatment question, it would seem extremely unlikely that Laura and her father could work out a therapeutic program together.

QUESTION B:

MOTHER AND FATHER WERE SEEN IN FAMILY THERAPY. HOWEVER, MOTHER STATED THAT THE SCHEDULE WAS TOO DIFFICULT FOR FATHER TO COME REGULARLY AND MADE EXCUSES ABOUT HIS ABSENCE. IN A HOPELESS, HELPLESS MANNER SHE ALTERNATELY BLAMED HERSELF AND HER HUSBAND. SHE DID NOT SEEM TO BE IN TOUCH WITH HER ANGER TOWARDS HER DAUGHTER. MOTHER CAN BE DESCRIBED AS A PERSON WHO:

1. Will act out her frustration through Laura and by overprotection will foster helplessness and infantilization. Her hysterical panics illustrate why her daughter finds her so irrelevant and hopeless

2. Creates dependency and by not sharing feelings provokes paranoia and mistrust around her. Her inability to deal with her daughter at age one is a sign of her inadequate personality

3. Has many communication problems with her daughter and cannot be supportive during times of stress

4. Is correct in her continuing attempt to find what is wrong with her daughter by taking her for repeated physical checkups

5. Is reacting to an adolescent going through a phase of parental rejection. She is no more depressed than most mothers of teenage daughters

6. Wants the best for her daughter but has difficulty in carrying out correct decisions

7. Could help her daughter if only she would continue to overcome her phobia about horseback riding and join in the girl's sport

The first answer was confirmed during treatment. Answer two is partially correct but sounds overstated. The third and sixth answers are correct as far as

CASE STUDY #7

they go. Answer four incorrectly indicates that mother's diagnostic "merry-go-round" should continue. Not all mothers of teenage daughters are depressed. Answer seven is unrealistic.

QUESTION C:
LAURA PRESENTED AS A DEPRESSED GIRL WHO RECENTLY HAD HER LONG BLOND HAIR CUT SHORT. IN RESPONSE TO VERBAL APPROACHES, SHE EITHER RETORTED ANGRILY WITH A HOSTILE PUT-DOWN OR READILY AGREED WITHOUT THINKING AS IF SHE FELT SHE MUST. SINCE SHE HAD RUN AWAY SO MANY TIMES IT SEEMED LIKELY SHE WOULD SOON RUN AGAIN. THE BEST COURSE OF ACTION WOULD BE:

1. An intense regressive, dependency-producing, infantilizing technique which would allow her to begin all over again constructing an adequate ego
2. A behavior modification routine, rewarding her with additional riding time for every week that she does not run away from the hospital
3. A therapeutic relationship. Unless this is established soon, she will destroy herself
4. For her to return to her local junior high school with her normal peers. In this way she would be able to bring her behavior in line
5. To set limits on her behavior and give her a trial of a major tranquilizer, which might decrease her impulsivity and allow her to count to ten. The staff will have to work together in order to help this difficult patient
6. To establish a trust relationship
7. For her to enter into a Doman-Delacato program to improve her learning ability

An intense regressive technique would seem contraindicated in this girl. Her mother had already given her too much of that kind of "therapy." The second answer might have worked if the parents cooperated and if Laura continued her great interest in horseback riding. However, her depression had become so great that this reward no longer interested her. The third answer is correct but not as good as five, which is more comprehensive. Answer four is unrealistic. Answer six is correct but not specific enough. Answer seven implies that Laura's problems were all neurological rather than mostly behavioral and emotional.

QUESTION D:
LAURA HAD CONSISTENTLY PICKED BOYFRIENDS WHO HAD DIFFICULTIES WITH THE LAW, ABUSED DRUGS, AND WERE SEVERAL YEARS OLDER THAN SHE. THIS CREATED A SITUATION IN WHICH THE PARENTS OFTEN FORBADE HER FROM SEEING THEM. THE BEST WAY OF UNDERSTANDING THIS WOULD BE TO SAY THAT LAURA:

1. Is not attractive to boys her own age
2. Has difficulty relating to male figures
3. Is following the norm for our society: girls usually go with boys older than themselves
4. Is sexually precocious and because of her early maturation has selected older boys
5. Selects boys who have been in difficulty with the law because she is getting mixed messages from her parents
6. Is selecting this type of boy in order to prove to her father that there are others who are able to break the law and get away with it. Her rebellion against parental authority is a search for a male figure who will dominate her
7. Repetitively selects "loser" boyfriends because of unconscious desires to hurt herself and her family

Laura was attractive to boys her own age. The second answer is too general. The third and fourth answers do not explain why Laura had always to pick losers.

CASE STUDY #7

No evidence was given that Laura was sexually precocious. Answer five may be correct, but is not specific or comprehensive. The sixth answer is overinterpretive. Answer seven's explanation was frequently confirmed by the patient later in therapy.

QUESTION E:
DURING THERAPY LAURA WAS VERY ERRATIC IN HER STATEMENTS. THOUGH ON ONE OCCASION SHE STATED THAT SHE WANTED TO FINISH HIGH SCHOOL AND GO TO COLLEGE, AT OTHER TIMES SHE STATED THAT SCHOOL WAS NOT WORTH MUCH TO HER. EARLY ON SHE TALKED ABOUT HER HORSEMANSHIP IN A SELF-DEPRECATING WAY. THE THERAPIST COULD HELP THE THERAPEUTIC RELATIONSHIP BY:
1. Suggesting that when Laura fell off a horse, she damaged her brain, causing her learning disabilities
2. Suggesting that she make a commitment and stick to it. Laura is too ambivalent about many things
3. Suggesting she have a slumber party. Laura is a typical teenager who shifts from time to time, varying her interests
4. Showing an interest in horses
5. Arranging for Laura to ride her horse to school to increase her self esteem
6. Ordering further psychological testing. Laura's ambivalence about school demonstrates that she is schizophrenic. Her interest in horses is an effort to gain control of her weak ego
7. Developing the real meaning of her interest in horses and strengthening her self-esteem by reinforcing the successes that she had in this area

The confusion that Laura shows in the interviews is not normal. She is trying desperately to sort out her feelings about school and her life. Laura did not fall off a horse. The second answer is not specific enough. A slumber party would have put the parents into a situation which they had never been able to control. Showing an interest in horses might help build rapport, but this is not a very comprehensive therapeutic strategy. Answer five, of course, is unrealistic. Ambivalence about school is not enough to demonstrate schizophrenia, and Laura would have rejected further psychologic testing at this point. The best answer is seven, which actually proved helpful.

QUESTION F:
WHEN LAURA'S PARENTS WERE NOT ABLE TO BRING HER BACK TO THE RESIDENTIAL TREATMENT SETTING AFTER AN AWOL, OUTPATIENT THERAPY WAS GIVEN A TRIAL. WITH GREAT EFFORT THE PARENTS WERE ENTICED TO A FEW FAMILY TREATMENT SESSIONS. LAURA GOT A JOB AT A HAMBURGER STAND, WHICH INCREASED HER SELF-ESTEEM. SHE BEGAN USING THE PSYCHOTHERAPIST TO HELP HER SORT OUT HER LIFE. AT THIS POINT THE PARENTS STOPPED COMING TO THERAPY. LAURA NEEDS:
1. Electroshock treatments and an antidepressant to keep her from suicide
2. For her parents to stop sabotaging her treatment
3. To be allowed to return to junior high to finish her credits. The parents should be encouraged to hire a tutor to help pull up her scholastic work. On returning to the normal peer group, Laura will straighten herself out
4. A friend
5. Psychoanalysis. A strong dependency relationship will be necessary for her to get a hold on herself and begin to restructure her psychic apparatus
6. To know that one therapist in the clinic will be available to her no matter what kind of difficulty she creates. The therapist may need to prevent the parents from interfering with treatment by maintaining some distance from them
7. Laura needs to have complete freedom to come and go as she pleases. Her parents' restrictions are unrealistic in this day and age

CASE STUDY #7

Laura responded to continued therapy only when she found that she could miss appointments and call her therapist erratically without resulting retaliation. The parents briefly continued to interfere with treatment. Answer six seems the best. Electroshock is rather uncommon in treating adolescents and would not be recommended here. Answer two is correct but incomplete. Answer three seems highly unrealistic. Four is true as far as it goes. Analytic treatment for this adolescent seemed unfeasible because of her highly erratic behavior and inconsistent, ambivalent motivation. The last answer had already been tried by the parents and did not seem to work.

REFERENCES:
1. Beiser, H.R., 1971: Pretesting as a teaching tool in a child psychiatry clerkship. J of Amer Acad of Child Psychiatry 10:444-463

2. Johnson, A.M., 1952: Genesis of antisocial acting out in children and adults. Psychoanalytic Quarterly 21:323-343

3. Johnson, A.M., 1949: Sanctions for superego lacunae of adolescents. In K.R. Eissler (Ed.), Searchlights on Delinquency, New York, International Universities Press

4. Kaufman, I., Makkay, E.S. and J. Zilbach, 1959: The impact of adolescence on girls with delinquent character formation. Amer J Orthopsychiatry 29: 130-143

5. Keith, C., 1968: The therapeutic alliance in child psychotherapy. J Amer Acad of Child Psychiatry 7:31-43

6. Meeks, J.E., 1971: The Fragile Alliance. Williams and Wilkins Co., Baltimore

7. St. John, R., 1968: Developing a therapeutic working alliance with the adolescent girl. J Amer Acad of Child Psychiatry 7:68-78

8. Thomas, A., Chess, S. and H.G. Birch, 1968: Temperament and Behavior Disorders in Children. New York University Press, New York

CASE STUDY #8

The Adolescent Barker

Chuck, a 15 year-old white high school boy of strong Catholic upbringing, was brought to a psychiatrist by his parents with the chief complaint of "making noises and having twitching movements."

Chuck seemed well until about age six when his father began noting a rather unusual movement of his head, a slight twist to the right. This occurred especially in church. His family physician assured the parents that he would grow out of this habit, and the movement did disappear. However, at age 13, he developed other "habits": blepharospasm (repeated, forceful, momentary eye closing) and grunting tics. The blepharospasm also disappeared but was replaced by a facial contortion. About six months prior to the psychiatric consultation the grunts changed to explosive sounds which Chuck described as "barks."

His father stated that the barks increased in frequency when Chuck was under stress and usually disappeared during sleep. He thought that Chuck felt pressure both in school and at church, where he played the organ three times a week for various services. The father further stated that he had been advised to be more accepting of Chuck and to relax some of his very high expectations.

Chuck's developmental milestones were normal, with no early illnesses nor separations. However, when Chuck was four, the father acquired a gas station which kept him occupied 80 hours a week away from home for the next ten years. It was when the father sold the station in order to devote more time to Chuck that Chuck's grunts changed to barks.

QUESTION A:
THE BEST WORKING DIAGNOSIS AT THIS POINT IS:
1. Kleinfelter's syndrome
2. Obsessive-compulsive psychoneurosis
3. Gilles de la Tourette syndrome
4. Rowe's syndrome
5. Anxiety psychoneurosis

The combination of tics and coprolalia (obscene language) was described in 1885 by Gilles de la Tourette as a specific nervous disorder which he felt was due to central nervous system disease. Since other tics have been found to be caused psychogenically, and since children with Gilles de la Tourette's syndrome often have neurotic features, a controversy has developed regarding the etiology of these symptoms. Answer three is correct.

Chuck's relationship with his mother was unusually close. She explained this on the basis of the father's absence. She rarely, if ever, said "no," and she sometimes became so distraught when Chuck became upset with her that she would weep for several days. This relationship became mutually "clinging." Chuck also developed a close attachment to his maternal grandmother, who encouraged his interest in music, especially the church organ.

There was always considerable tension between Chuck and his father. The latter said he felt inadequate and dominated at home. Therefore, he withdrew to his gas station, where he felt more competent and effective. Every time he had tried to relate to his wife and son, he felt rebuffed and left out, as Chuck grew closer to his mother and grandmother. He felt that Chuck as a small boy had never responded to him. He never looked forward to seeing Chuck when he came home because seeing him made him feel less adequate as a father.

Father also had a number of tics (blinking, mouth movements, and foot movements) and a peculiar articulation similar to Chuck's explosive speech.

In pre-school years Chuck characteristically sat on the back porch watching other children play. When he entered school he failed to make friends, and the children teased and rejected him.

CASE STUDY #8

QUESTION B:
AT THIS POINT THE MOST APPROPRIATE TREATMENT FOR THIS BOY
WOULD BE:
1. Group therapy to help him relate to his peers
2. Family therapy to deal with the disturbed relationships
3. Individual psychotherapy
4. Use of a major tranquilizer
5. Use of an anti-depressant medication

Each answer is logical, but at this point the fourth is best. Group therapy or individual therapy alone is not likely to be as effective. Very intensive in-patient treatment might succeed in reducing his anxiety and relieve the intensity of the tic. Family therapy seems very reasonable in light of the history, and would be an important adjunct therapy in this case, but is not as specific as four. Anti-depressants are not the treatment of choice although exceptional cases of Gilles de la Tourette's have been known to respond to imipramine. The anti-dopaminergic haloperidol (Haldol) is currently the pharmacologic treatment of choice for this syndrome, believed to be related to an excess of dopamine or other catecholamine.

Chuck was admitted to a psychiatric hospital. He had many obsessive fears about his parents dying. Psychological testing suggested obsessive and phobic qualities in a passive, feminine personality. Haloperidol treatment had limited success. The focus was shifted to intensive family therapy, but this too was disappointing. He was then transferred to an adolescent unit, where he remained for 14 months.

Because of anxiety about being separated from his mother, he found it very difficult to accept hospitalization. Within a short time his vocal tics began to include cuss words. However, when he became verbally aggressive towards his psychotherapist, his barking decreased. Such angry, verbally aggressive outbursts usually led to guilt feelings and apologies. He was never able to relate to peers and was never accepted by them. Instead, he hung around the nursing station, pestering the staff and constantly seeking physical contact with them. When his privileges were restricted for pestering the nurses, his bark took on a "fuck you" quality. In another instance his visiting mother became very upset when his barking resembled the word "make." This seemed to represent to him "make her live," or "make her die," related to his fear of his mother's dying and his belief that the barking would ward off this disaster. Chuck later discussed with his psychotherapist how fearful he was that his parents might be killed in an automobile accident after he had been angry with them for leaving him in the hospital. The nursing staff's most vivid memory of Chuck was his outburst of barking each Sunday morning as he read the obituaries.

Chuck unquestionably improved during his hospital stay. His fears about his destructiveness abated considerably, although he continued to have difficulty handling his angry feelings. His sexual identity also continued to be a problem.

He visited the hospital about two years and a half following his discharge. Although his speech was hesitant and jerky, he was not barking. He had worked full time for one of the political parties in a presidential campaign and was planning to enter a technical school upon graduation from high school.

QUESTION C:
THE PROGNOSIS FOR THIS DISORDER IS:
1. Good if treated adequately with haloperidol
2. Good if the combined individual, family, and group psychotherapies are intensive enough
3. Guarded despite treatment
4. Poor
5. None of the above

CASE STUDY #8

Haloperidol is usually the treatment of choice in this disorder and represents a rational biochemical approach. Unfortunately, as this case illustrates, it is not always successful. Also, some patients become reversibly tolerant to the drug after a period of time (DiGiacoma, 1971). The various forms of psychotherapy can be helpful, as in this case, but are rarely curative. In this case, the third answer is correct; at best, the prognosis is guarded.

REFERENCES:
1. DiGiacomo, J. N., et al., 1971: A Case with Gilles de la Tourette's Syndrome: Recurrent Refractoriness to Haloperidol and Unsuccessful Treatment with L-Dopa. J Nerv and Ment Dis 152:115-117

2. Kanner, L., 1972: Child Psychiatry, 4th ed., Charles C Thomas, Springfield, Ill., p. 409

3. Knopp, W., Arnold, L. E. and F. Messiha, 1972: Tourette's Disease: Implications for Research in Huntington's Disease. Huntington's Disease Symposium, in Press, Edited by Barbeau, A., Raven Press

4. Lucas, A. R., Kauffman, P. E. and Morris, E. M., 1967: Gilles de la Tourette's Disease: A Clinical Study of Fifteen Cases. J Am Acad Ch Psychiatry 6:700-722

5. Meyerhoff, J. L. and S. H. Snyder, 1972: Catecholamines in Gilles de la Tourette's Disease. Huntington's Disease Symposium, in Press. Edited by Barbeau, A., Raven Press

6. Mohler, M. S. and L. Rangel, 1943: A Psychosomatic Study of Maladie des Tics (Gilles de la Tourette's Disease). Psychiat Quart 17:579-603

CASE STUDY #9

A Substitute Child

Polly, a pretty, lively, six year-old girl, was brought to the clinic by her rather tired-appearing, middle-aged adoptive parents. They complained that this child completely dominated their family. Things were fine as long as she was humored and given attention, but she was unable to play by herself for any length of time. When she was reprimanded, she became violently aggressive and attacked with any available object. They had a natural daughter in her teens with whom they had never had any trouble.

The parents had always wanted a second child, but the mother had difficulty conceiving. A few months before the adoption, the mother had given birth to a severely malformed baby. She was told of this tragedy about eighteen hours after its birth. The parents were advised that the infant would not survive and that it should be placed in a home. Father made the decision for his wife and himself, and it was placed without mother seeing it. The parents kept their sorrow a secret, and several weeks later they went to the home to see it. The nurse picked the baby up and offered it to the mother, but she refused to hold it. The infant died two months later.

Mother became severely depressed following the birth and often reproached herself, saying that if she had just taken her infant and mothered it, it might have lived. Father refused to talk about it, saying, "You make your decisions and then forget about them." Hence, mother was left with no support in her feelings of guilt and despair.

About that time the obstetrician suggested that they adopt the baby of one of his unwed patients. They agreed to consider this, but insisted on seeing the pregnant woman before the adoption was initiated. So, it was arranged for the mother to observe the mother-to-be without her knowing it by taking a tour of the home for unwed mothers.

Polly was adopted and the parents left her with a live-in baby sitter while they took a six weeks' vacation in Florida. Things went well and developmental milestones were normal until Polly was about eighteen months old. She then became wakeful, screamed, and seemed to panic if forced to remain in her crib. She also started sleepwalking. In desperation the parents moved her into their bedroom, but this didn't reassure her. She continued a difficult sleeper and started having temper tantrums if she didn't get her own way. These gradually developed into more aggressive outbursts.

Mother felt frightened and helpless in the face of these tantrums because she was unable to soothe her. She found herself unable to say "no"; the child dominated her. In contrast, the father wasn't disturbed by her aggressive behavior and was usually able to calm her. He also was able to set limits for her. The fact that mother was often irritable and moody seemed to play into the child's explosiveness.

A school report described the patient as a gay, happy little girl who got along well with everyone. Only rarely did she exhibit slight stubbornness. She participated fully in all activities and was well liked by the first-graders.

During projective testing with the Children's Apperception Test (CAT) and Rorschach, the patient's controlling behavior immediately became apparent. She refused to give any stories to the CAT cards. Instead, she said she would tell a story of her own. It was a story full of despair and sadness about a fat little hoptoad. The little toad suddenly hopped onto its mother's lap in what was apparently an appeal for bodily contact and warmth. Mother threw the little one off, calling him "naughty and ill-mannered." This was followed by aggressive, messy, and destructive behavior on the part of the little toad. Mother reacted to this by threatening to call a policeman and to make the little hoptoad pay for the damage he had done.

The patient then sang a series of nonsense songs which she made up as she went along, and which she accompanied with dancing. Finally, she seemed to project all of her angry feelings onto the psychologist and demanded that the psy-

CASE STUDY #9

chologist obey her, as if attempting to control the aggressive impulses and feelings within herself.

The Rorschach, which she seemed to enjoy, closely corroborated the dynamics of the story she told. In general, her world wasn't a very happy place and all her efforts to change it failed. Her despair over lack of containment and warmth was evident, and these depressive feelings were most often followed by a kind of aggressive and manic acting out. The Rorschach also contained suggestions of her confusion and anxiety about sex, more specifically about babies and who has them.

QUESTION A:
POLLY WAS:
1. Suffering from a childhood psychosis
2. Reacting normally to her parents' problems
3. Mildly emotionally disturbed
4. A hyperkinetic child who probably would have responded to medication
5. A severely disturbed child

QUESTION B:
IN THIS FAMILY THE "PATIENT" WAS:
1. The family and each of its members
2. The child
3. The mother and child
4. The mother and father
5. The father and child

Although the "identified patient" was the child, it would seem that both the parents and the child could have used psychiatric help. The little girl was severely disturbed in that her gay, happy behavior bordered on a manic defense against her despairing feelings of lack of acceptance, warmth, and containment. She had difficulty in controlling her aggressive impulses and projected these and her feelings of badness into others, and then controlled the other person in order to control what she felt were the bad parts of herself.

The mother, who was often moody and irritable, suffered severe bouts of depression. She also needed help to work through her angry and guilty feelings in order that she might find her inner world a more comfortable place, which would allow her to give more of herself to the child. The father, who was the decision maker, seemed to use repression and denial as defenses. Hence, he possibly "bottled up" feelings and was not in touch with them. Thus, it must have been very difficult, if not impossible, for him to feel for the child.

The best answer to Question A is five. The best answer to Question B is one.

QUESTION C:
IN ADDITION TO THE PARENTS' EMOTIONAL PROBLEMS, WHICH THEY HAD PRIOR TO THE ADOPTION, ONE OF THE CORE PROBLEMS OF THIS FAMILY WAS:
1. That they had not taken the time to mourn the tragedy and loss of their natural infant
2. That they had attempted to replace the lost infant
3. That they feared that their friends would find out that mother had given birth to an abnormal child
4. That they waited too long before seeking help
5. That they should have known more about the infant before adopting her

The parents had resigned themselves to not having another child due to mother's inability to conceive. When the mother became pregnant, their hopes and plans came alive again, only to be dashed by the birth of a malformed infant

CASE STUDY #9

incapable of surviving.

The ordinary mourning process which enables the individual to work through his loss usually consists of three stages, although their demarcation lines are somewhat blurred. The earliest is a combination of protest and denial in which the mourner in his anger casts about, attempting to place the blame on the physician or the hospital, and attempts to deny that the loss has occurred. The second stage usually consists of acceptance of the reality of the loss, and is accompanied by intense sorrow and feelings of emptiness, as though part of oneself has been lost with the love object. The third stage gradually leads to detachment: the mourner slowly develops other interests and adapts to living without the lost object. Only when this stage has been worked through is the individual emotionally ready for and capable of new attachments.

In this case the parents did not work through, via the mourning process, the loss of their infant for whom they had so many hopes and plans. Rather, they seemed to stop at the first stage when they attempted to deny the loss of their infant by adopting a replacement for her. The adopted infant undoubtedly increased the family pathology as well as suffered intense emotional pain due to the fact that the parents were neither emotionally ready nor capable of accepting and attaching themselves to her, which they possibly further denied.

QUESTION D:
THE MOTHER WAS UNABLE TO BE FIRM OR TO SET LIMITS FOR HER ADOPTED DAUGHTER BECAUSE:
1. She was afraid of her own anger
2. She thought that Polly wouldn't like her if she said "no" to her
3. She thought that discipline was father's job
4. She felt the child would feel rejected if she said "no" to her
5. She had ambivalent feelings towards the child

This mother certainly did have ambivalent feelings about Polly. Often an ordinary, menopausal mother would like to have one more child, while at the same time another part of herself feels that another baby would be a burden. These ambivalent feelings were demonstrated when immediately following the adoption of this very young infant, the parents left her with a baby sitter while they went off on vacation.

This mother must have had some feelings of resentment and anger towards Polly because she was replacing her own infant. She also felt tied down and controlled by her. She possibly found it difficult to keep these feelings suppressed and may have been afraid of what she might do if she expressed them. So, one way to protect Polly from her anger was not to set limits. However, in Polly's hoptoad story, we can see how aware Polly was of her mother's feelings toward her. The best answers are one and five.

REFERENCES:
1. Bellak, L., 1954: The Thematic Apperception Test and the Children's Apperception Test in Clinical Use. New York, Grune & Stratton

2. Bixler, R.H., 1965: Limits are therapy. In: Child Psychotherapy Practice and Theory. Edited by Haworth, M.R., New York, Basic Books

3. Bowlby, J., 1951: Maternal Care and Mental Health. Geneva: World Health Organization Monograph #2

4. Feinstein, S.C. and E.A. Wolpert, 1973: Juvenile manic-depressive illness: Clinical and therapeutic considerations, Am J Child Psychiat 12:123-136

5. Frank, G., 1965: The role of the family in the development of psychopathology. Psychol Bull 64:191-205

CASE STUDY #9

6. Freud, S., 1917: Mourning and melancholia. Standard Edition, 14:243-258. London: Hogarth Press, 1957

7. Gardner, Richard, A., 1971: Therapeutic Communication with Children, The Mutual Story Telling Technique. New York, Science House, Inc.

8. Halpern, F., 1953: A Clinical Approach to Children's Rorschachs. New York, Gruen & Stratton

9. Haworth, M.A., 1966: The CAT: Facts about Fantasy. New York, Grune & Stratton

10. Klein, M., 1948: Mourning and its relation to manic-depressive states. In: Contributions to Psychoanalysis. London: Hogarth Press, pp. 311-338

11. Pitcher, E. and E. Prelinger, 1963: Children Tell Stories: An Analysis of Fantasy. New York: International Univ. Press

12. Solnit, A.J. and M.H. Stark, 1961: Mourning and the birth of a defective child. Psycho-anal Study Child, 16:523-537

13. Winnicott, D.W., 1958: The Manic Defense. In: Collected Papers Paediatrics to Psycho-analysis. London, Tavistock Publications, Ltd

CASE STUDY #10

A Pseudosophisticated, Suicidal Second-Grader

Linda was an attractive 7-1/2 year-old white second grader referred to the Child Psychiatry Clinic by her pediatrician. She had ingested a large amount of oil of wintergreen in an apparent suicide attempt foiled when her father made her vomit. When Linda was interviewed by her pediatrician, she admitted that she had wanted to kill herself because she had "no friends" and was having "school problems."

Linda was the third of four children with a brother age 12, a sister age 11, and a sister age 6. The father was an inspector in the space industry. A few weeks prior to the child's suicide attempt, the mother had taken an evening job at a local grocery store in order to help with the family finances. One of their greatest financial problems was a large medical debt incurred because of the mother's severe headaches.

The parents had a history of recurring tense, angry arguments, the mother claiming that the father was "callous and indifferent" to her problems. These quarrels took place in the presence of the children and were followed by the parents separating. However, during the interview they stated that they were a "child-centered family," and their wish was to work together.

QUESTION A:
THE MOST LIKELY CAUSE OF THE CHILD'S SUICIDE ATTEMPT WAS:
1. Since her mother had gone to work, Linda was lonely for her. She thought that by trying to attract attention to herself the parents' arguments might subside
2. Linda was furious at her mother for abandoning her. She thought that by attempting suicide she would be making it obvious to her father not to argue with her mother
3. Linda's suicide attempt was a message about how she felt about herself.
4. Linda had an upper respiratory infection and thought that the oil of wintergreen would help it
5. Linda was acting like any other second grader whose parents often fight
6. Linda was responding to stress
7. Linda probably has an early brain tumor

It is unusual for children to tell their parents directly about their rage or other feelings of abandonment, as is implied in answer two. (This, however, may be an example of egocentric thinking.) Answers three and six are correct but need to be more specific. From the history given, there is no evidence for answers four or seven. Answer five is "too normal"; it is unusual for a child at this age even to make an hysterical gesture of suicidal nature. One, the best answer, is a common finding in juvenile suicide.

Linda's mother spoke in a hesitant manner and seemed preoccupied. She had difficulty bringing Linda regularly for individual therapy. She cancelled many appointments with the excuse that the children had the mumps or other illnesses or the car had broken down. She presented a recurring theme of "difficulty with doctors": she stated that she had been advised not to have any more children because of Rh incompatibility, Linda received the wrong medication once when ill, she herself had delivered before the doctor was able to get there, and she had received inappropriate advice about surgery.

QUESTION B:
THE MOTHER'S RELATIONSHIP WITH LINDA COULD BE BEST EXPLAINED BY WHICH OF THE FOLLOWING STATEMENTS?:
1. The mother is cancelling appointments because she wants the girl to commit suicide

CASE STUDY #10

2. The mother's narcissistic preoccupation has impaired the patient's sense of self-worth. Should the mother continue to be unable to hear Linda, she will attempt suicide again soon
3. Linda's mother is too wrapped up in herself
4. Linda's mother is preoccupied with herself but her concern for Linda is strong enough so that she will be able to understand her daughter without outside help
5. Linda's mother is wrapped up in herself. She is a "martyr type" who frequently says, "Woe is me." Perhaps Linda must go to drastic means in order to gain her mother's attention
6. Mother's frequent illnesses have depleted her stores of energy, and therefore she is unable to help with her daughter's problems
7. The mother has difficulty in communication with both her husband and Linda

Number one is incorrect because it is very unlikely that the mother would have brought Linda in the first place if she really wanted her to kill herself. The next answer, although partially true, implies a more severe pathology than seems to be evident. Answer three would be more correct if followed by the phrase "to notice Linda's needs." Answer four is incorrect; since Linda's mother was unable to cope with her own marital difficulties, it is doubtful that she would be able to support Linda with adequate insight to prevent recurrence of her problems. Answer five, the best answer, is most specific about the psychopathology. Parents rarely are consciously aware of their resistance in treatment. Answer seven is only a partial answer.

QUESTION C:
ONE OF THE FACTORS THAT GOOD CASE MANAGEMENT MUST CONSIDER IS THE DISTANCE THE FAMILY LIVES FROM THE CLINIC. IN THIS CASE THE FAMILY HAD TO DRIVE SEVERAL MILES. THEREFORE:
1. The mother should be told that she is angry; 1) at her daughter because of Linda's dependency and 2) at herself for her own dependency upon her husband, who, she feels, may abandon her
2. Linda should be seen by her pediatrician to rule out a respiratory illness; there is no need for further exploration
3. Linda should be seen at a guidance clinic which is closer to home
4. All of the children should be seen in family therapy to prevent a suicide attempt by one of them
5. Linda's problem, although apparently mild at this time, needs further exploration. Weekly visits for short-term crisis intervention might be helpful. An honest explanation of the parents' financial situation and the need for mother to return to work could prove helpful to Linda
6. Linda could benefit from play therapy
7. Linda should be hospitalized at a referral hospital for a neurological work-up

The interpretations in answer one are accurate but it is rarely helpful to confront this directly or use jargon such as "dependency" early in psychotherapy. The case does not seem to warrant long-term therapy. Answers two and seven are irrelevant, too organically oriented; Linda's problems are emotional. Answer three is incorrect for two reasons: 1) there was no closer clinic and 2) the case did not seem to warrant long-term therapy and therefore the family would not be faced with the prospect of driving the distance over a long time period. Answer four is incorrect since, although hysteria in families may be somewhat contagious for children, it is much more common that one child is designated the scapegoat or "clown." Such a child sometimes repeats a parental pattern. Answer five is best. An honest, logical explanation of financial matters is often forgotten by parents when they are under stress. Answer six is only partially correct; help is also needed for the parents.

CASE STUDY #10

When the child psychiatrist and psychiatric social worker initially interviewed the mother and child, Linda immediately began tearing. Linda appeared to be an attractive, slightly seductive, pseudosophisticated girl, who was inhibited in play and afraid to share her feelings directly. She shared many facts about home, school and peers, but related them in a detached tone. She shared a dream readily and had a sense of humor. She did not like her mother's work taking her "away from the family almost every night." Her earliest memory was of a "new baby in the neighborhood who came home from the hospital" and how she and her mother had "talked about it the next day." This was one of the few times she spoke with enthusiasm. She then said, "The kids never wanted to play with me," but didn't know the reason why. She had frequent fights with her sister and brother. Sometimes she said to herself "in her mind" that her "mother shouldn't work." She had nightmares and talked of how scary they were. She related positive feelings about the father taking the family bike riding, sometimes visiting the mother at work. She revealed her three wishes: 1) "to be real rich," 2) to "have school be all math and reading," and 3) that her "mother wouldn't have to work." She also wanted "a large house with a swimming pool and a large farm with many horses."

QUESTION D:
WE CAN INTERPRET THIS CHILD'S COMMENTS TO SUGGEST THAT:
1. Linda is reacting to feelings of sibling rivalry, murderous rage about mother's abandonment, and penis envy about father's autonomy
2. Linda is dependent on her mother and is acting out some of her anger
3. Linda's genetically determined temperament is such that she will always have inhibitions characterized by an inability to be playful
4. Linda is a latency child whose daily life is within normal limits
5. Linda is upset over family matters
6. Linda likes to ride her bicycle and has temper tantrums whenever she cannot have her way
7. Linda is able to talk about her life rather well. However, she is inhibited in the playroom, which makes one wonder if too much is expected of her at home and whether she is not allowed to express anger in normal ways

Even though the strong statement in answer one may be true, it is not based on adequate evidence. Answer two does not give a full explanation of the problem. Rather than being permanently unable to be playful, Linda seemed to be pseudosophisticated and needed permission to be able to let herself play (as implied in number seven, the best answer). Answer four gives a "too normal" impression, and answer five, although true, is an understatement. Answer six is irrelevant as well as incorrect.

QUESTION E:
THE BEST TECHNIQUE TO CONTINUE THE INTERVIEW WITH LINDA WOULD BE:
1. Encourage her to use the toys whenever she feels able. Fingerpaints and drawing might allow her to play and discuss her deeper angry feelings. The mutual storytelling technique might help her see other ways of handling anger
2. Confront her with her inability to show angry feelings toward her punitive parents
3. Encourage her to be more specific about the indirectly expressed anger whenever possible. A variety of forms of activity therapy might help
4. Take her on a brisk walk or vigorous bike riding session
5. Silence; Linda will talk about her angry feelings without encouragement, since she has done so well relating to her other feelings
6. Tell her that she seems angry at the world and is acting it out in many ways
7. Tell her to write a story about her life during the therapy hour

CASE STUDY #10

Answer one is the best answer since it gives specific techniques as well as telling why they are used. A confrontation at this time as suggested in answer two, will probably not be helpful. Answer three tells what should be done, but not how. Linda may not like to walk and may prefer to play. Answer five is superficial; a correct answer would indicate that what Linda talks about is more important than whether she talks. Answer six is wrong; Linda may not be angry at the world, only her parents. It is likely that answer seven will provoke anger rather than allow anger to be understood.

QUESTION F:
IN REGARD TO LONG-TERM MANAGEMENT OF LINDA'S CASE:
1. It is likely that Linda will be able to share angry feelings with her family after role modeling in therapy. The psychiatric social worker will help the parents to accept some of the child's anger
2. Linda will need to be in play therapy for many years to change her personality from an inhibited, depressed pattern
3. Linda needs play therapy for two or three sessions during the crisis, with some gentle suggestions
4. Linda needs continued neurological examinations with skull X-rays, since suicide attempters often have brain tumors
5. It is highly unlikely that Linda will ever again have emotional problems because she is only going through a phase
6. Linda's suicidal tendencies will spread to her siblings and all of the family will need treatment
7. Linda needs residential treatment for three years to keep her from destroying herself

Children Linda's age often are able to transfer quickly into the family setting the role-modeling from puppet play, mutual story-telling, or direct counseling. This makes answer one the best answer. Answer two seems too pessimistic and answers three and five too optimistic. There is little evidence to suggest that suicide attempters have brain tumors. Suicide attempts in children are not a phase of normal behavior. Suicide attempts are not usually epidemic. Answer seven is incorrect; Linda's problem, if treated properly, would not likely require such prolonged therapy.

REFERENCES:
1. Baruch, D. W., 1952: One Little Boy, Dell Publishing Co., New York

2. Gardner, R., 1969: Mutual story-telling as a technique in child psychotherapy. Science and Psychoanalysis 14:123-136

3. Mack, J., 1970: Nightmares and Human Conflict, Little, Brown & Co., Boston

4. Piaget, J., 1965: The Moral Judgment of the Child, Free Press, Glencoe, Ill.

5. Sabbath, J., 1969: The expendable child. J Amer Acad Child Psychiatry 18:272-289

6. Thomas, A., Chess, S. and H. G. Birch, 1968: Temperament and Behavior Disorders in Children, New York University Press, New York

7. Winnicott, D. W., 1971: Playing and Reality, Basic Books, New York

CASE STUDY #11

"We Didn't Want this Baby"

Bonnie was the last of five children in an upper-middle-class white Protestant family. She was born nine years after the fourth child. The pregnancy proceeded without complications, and the baby appeared quite healthy when the pediatrician examined her in the newborn nursery.

When the pediatrician entered the hospital room to visit the mother, she immediately confronted him with the statement: "Doctor, you know we didn't want this baby." Her dissatisfaction with the pregnancy was clear, but she did seem resigned to the fact that she needed to love this baby just as much as she had loved the others.

At a regular "well baby" visit, when Bonnie was two months of age, the pediatrician realized that her development was not progressing optimally. For the next three months the developmental quotient was approximately 50%, but the parents still denied the existence of a problem. Therefore, the pediatrician felt compelled to refer the baby to a children's hospital for evaluation of possible causes of mental retardation. After a two-week hospitalization, no specific cause had been discovered. The child was discharged with a diagnosis of "mental retardation, severe, idiopathic."

QUESTION A:
WHEN THIS THOROUGH EVALUATION FAILED TO ALTER THE PARENTAL ATTITUDE, THE PEDIATRICIAN SHOULD HAVE:
1. Continued to care for the child and ignore the parents' denial
2. Requested a psychiatric consultation in the hopes that the psychiatrist could help the parents accept the reality of the situation
3. Referred the family to the child welfare services
4. Suggested referral to an institution for retarded children where the child would receive better all around care
5. Begun a therapeutic trial of thyroid in the hope that this was a sub-clinical case of cretinism

Severe to moderate mental retardation is not sub-clinical, and cretinism should have been ruled out by the pediatrician even prior to referral to the children's hospital. Referral to a state institution or to the welfare services would have been inappropriate, since the family was able to provide for the infant's material needs. The four other children in the family played a good deal with Bonnie, a benefit she might not receive elsewhere. Removal from the home was contraindicated. A psychiatrist might have been able to help penetrate the parents' denial; hence the authors feel that two is the best answer. Whether or not a pediatrician continues to follow such a child without psychiatric help would depend upon his skills in providing supportive psychotherapy.

As it turned out, this pediatrician was psychologically oriented and attempted to follow Bonnie without a psychiatric consultation, but he failed to alter the parents' attitude.

When Bonnie was eighteen months old, she fell against a coffee table and sustained a laceration 1/4 of an inch long extending laterally from the juncture of the eyelids. Whereas most parents are extremely anxious about injuries in or about children's eyes, this family did not seek medical help. The injury was only discovered by the pediatrician 10 days later during a routine office visit. The laceration, although superficial, had severed the elevator muscle of the lower lid, which caused the lid to droop and the cornea to dry out. As a result, the cornea had become infected, and it was already cloudy by the time the pediatrician saw it. The laceration itself was also infected, so that several attempts at surgical repair were unsuccessful. As a result the child became blind in this eye, developed a complication of sympathetic opthalmia and finally became bilaterally blind. At three years of age it was necessary to institutionalize this blind, retarded child.

CASE STUDY #11

QUESTION B:
THE TERM APPLIED TO DESCRIBE THE RELATIONSHIP CHARACTERIZED BY
SUCH REJECTING PARENTAL NEGLIGENCE IN THE PRESENCE OF APPARENT
ACCEPTANCE IS:
1. Ambivalence
2. Maternal deprivation
3. Undoing
4. Sublimation
5. Introjection

   Many pregnancies are unplanned and unwanted, yet most couples adjust during
pregnancy to the idea of having a baby. But for some couples, nine months are
insufficient. Infants can also become unwanted when they fail to measure up to
parental expectations. When parents make a modicum of adjustment to the child's
presence but still resent it, they are said to be ambivalent; the first answer is
correct.
   Maternal deprivation is also a correct answer and can be used to refer to any
degree of deprivation from complete absence of the mother (Spitz, 1945) to a
lesser degree of neglect, as exemplified in this case. When the negative aspect
of ambivalence outweighs the positive, the infant is in danger of rejection, injury
(battered children), and even death. Pediatricians must be alert to such possibilities and be prepared to deal with parental feelings and to seek psychiatric consultation when necessary.

QUESTION C:
THE ESTIMATE OF MENTAL SUBNORMALITY IN THE GENERAL POPULATION
OF THE U.S. IS REPORTED TO BE:
1. 12-15%
2. 8-12%
3. 5-8%
4. 2-5%
5. Less than 2%

   Only approximate estimates can be reported since precise data are very
difficult to obtain, and authors report different figures. Friedman and Kaplan
(1967) put the figure at three percent. On this basis, the fourth answer is the
best.
   The World Health Organization's term of "mental subnormality" is divided
into two separate and distinct categories: mental retardation and mental deficiency. Mental retardation is reserved for subnormal functioning due to environmental causes alone while mental deficiency indicates central nervous system pathology. Mental deficiency is often used also as a legal term, applied to
people with an IQ below 70.

QUESTION D:
A PSYCHIATRIST MIGHT DEAL WITH THE DENIAL OF BONNIE'S PARENTS BY:
1. Threatening legal action
2. Adopting an understanding attitude while concentrating on the relationship of
   the parents to the older children
3. Recommending treatment for the marital problem that may be the cause of the
   ambivalence
4. Adopting an understanding attitude while confronting the parents with their
   rejection of the unwanted and retarded child, interpreting their ambivalence
   to them
5. Getting an IQ test to prove she is retarded

CASE STUDY #11

The therapist who threatens legal action will in all likelihood alienate his patients and thereby become most ineffective. The second answer is also wrong, because it permits the parents to continue their defensive denial. There is no evidence that marital discord is the basic problem. The fourth answer is the best one; the therapist must deal with the issue but be understanding and supportive. He must support the positive aspects of the family relationships while helping the parents work through their disappointment in the unwanted pregnancy as well as in the child's limitations. If answer five had worked, psychiatric referral would not have been necessary in the first place.

REFERENCES:
1. Friedman, A. M. and H. I. Kaplan, 1967: Comprehensive Textbook of Psychiatry. Williams & Wilkins, Baltimore

2. Menaloscino, F. J., 1970: Psychiatric Approaches to Mental Retardation. Basic Books, New York

3. Spitz, R. A., 1945: Hospitalism: An Inquiry into the Genesis of Psychiatric Conditions in Early Childhood. Psa St of the Child 1:53-72

4. Spitz, R. A., 1946: Hospitalism: A Follow-Up Report on Investigation Described in Volume I. Psa St of the Child 2:113-117

5. Spitz, R. A. and K. M. Wolf, 1946: Anaclitic Depression: An Inquiry into the Genesis of Psychiatric Conditions in Early Childhood II. Psa St of the Child 2:313-339

6. Solnit, A. J. and M. H. Stark, 1961: Mourning and the Birth of a Defective Child. Psa St of the Child 16:523-537

CASE STUDY #12

A 16 Year-Old Gang Leader Sees a Shrink

A 16-1/2 year-old white Protestant working-class eleventh-grade boy came to the clinic on his own volition because of "anxiety feelings" at unexpected times. These consisted of palpitation, shakiness, and stomach cramps. They had occurred at least several times a week for the previous 5 months.

The first such anxiety attack occurred when he was approaching his father's cabin with some friends. Because of these feelings he stopped doing many things he previously enjoyed, like fishing, riding motorbikes, and going places with friends. In fact, he began withdrawing from friends, girls, and family. He ate and slept irregularly. He had suicidal ideas of driving his car into a bridge abutment. He often wished himself dead.

Past history showed that he was suspended as early as the first grade for aggression against teachers. By age 12 he had become so aggressive, with both sexual acting out and verbal and physical abuse towards parents, neighbors, teachers, and classmates, that he was put in the state hospital for 9 months. There he was at first assaultive, but eventually seemed to make a satisfactory adjustment.

Unfortunately, he had to be discharged to an unfavorable home situation. His parents often fought, each accusing the other of inadequate functioning. The father's usual way of settling an argument was either to leave or to punch the mother in the mouth. The patient, who was the second of six children, was given many overt and covert messages of rejection. He and his brother, one year younger, both had many scrapes with the law, and his brother eventually also spent some time in a psychiatric hospital. This younger brother seemed to have been favored by the mother and was consequently hated by the patient.

The patient presented as a thin "greaser" of moderate height who dressed and acted tough, with slicked-down hair and leather clothes. Though he avoided looking people in the eye, he seemed basically friendly and cooperative. He easily verbalized feelings of wishing himself dead, of being willing to kill someone else to help out a "true friend," and of planning revenge on the police for an incident of alleged brutality. He hated his parents and avoided the family by staying in his room when they were around.

In contrast, he had feelings of great loyalty to his friends. He was the leader of a 17-member delinquent gang which had an intricate system of keeping in touch. Even during the initial interview, he checked his two watches repeatedly and said that he had to make telephone calls at certain times to check on the safety of his members. One of his foremost wishes was to be reunited with a close friend who had moved away two years before.

Though he and this friend had joined in girl-hating, he had experienced sexual relations with five girls and felt some guilt over this. He mentioned other feelings of guilt and worry. He disclaimed any use of drugs or alcohol, feeling it would be bad for his health. He did not even like prescription medicines, because he once told off a friend after taking a sedative.

Though he was the gang leader, he reported being referred to as "Loser." The apparent basis for this title was that he had been run over; 1) by a truck, resulting in a three-day coma with "blood clot in the skull" (he insists someone he knew intentionally ran over him); and 2) by a large lawnmower that accidentally stuck in gear. He punched the doctor in the mouth over this latter incident when he fantasied that the "sawbones" might amputate his leg without warning him. He was also frightened of any needle since having a "Baker's cyst" removed.

He wrote poems about loneliness and war which he fantasied were valuable enough to be in danger of being stolen. Nevertheless, he would not publish them because that would be mercenary and spoil the poems' purity.

A Minnesota Multiphasic Personality Inventory showed mixed disturbance, primarily neurotic, with hysterical concerns over physical ills, as well as denial and rationalization. He appeared egocentric, hyperactive, and passive-aggressive, with insecurity and guardedness. His intelligence tested in the average range.

CASE STUDY #12

QUESTION A:
AT THIS POINT THE MOST LIKELY DIAGNOSTIC IMPRESSION IS:
1. Unsocialized aggressive reaction
2. Prepsychotic paranoid schizophrenia
3. Psychophysiologic reaction
4. Depressive neurosis
5. Hysterical neurosis, conversion type
6. Anxiety neurosis
7. Antisocial personality
8. Group delinquent reaction and brain damage from the truck accident
9. Panneurosis (pseudoneurotic schizophrenia)

This boy shows such a complex tangle of psychopathology that most of the answers might be defended as at least partially correct. However, the diagnosis should reflect the chief complaint as well as the auxiliary information from the history and mental examination, and should parsimoniously explain as many manifestations of the patient's problem as possible. Unsocialized aggressive reaction would have been worth considering during his violent early school years, but does not seem appropriate in view of the presently manifesting neurotic symptoms. The latter also make group delinquent reaction and brain damage inadequate diagnoses. The chief complaint of anxiety is incompatible with antisocial personality. Though there are some paranoid elements in this boy's expectation of harm from other people, the latter are not a prominent enough part of his symptomology to warrant a diagnosis of paranoid schizophrenia.

The diagnosis which seems to account best for most of the patient's symptoms, including the chief complaint, is pseudoneurotic schizophrenia, also known as panneurosis. The patient shows elements of depressive, anxiety, obsessive-compulsive, phobic, and hysterical neuroses, a long history suggestive of severe disturbance, and a history of probable deprivation, all compatible with such a diagnosis. Nine is the best answer. The individual neurotic diagnoses do not do justice to the severity and complexity of his problem.

QUESTION B:
THE BEST THERAPEUTIC INTERVENTION AT THIS POINT WOULD BE:
1. A tranquilizer and psychotherapy
2. Group or individual psychotherapy
3. Family therapy
4. Hospitalization
5. Behavior modification

Though tranquilization may eventually become necessary, it would not seem immediately appropriate in view of this voluntary patient's reservations about drugs. Family therapy would not appear feasible from what we know about the family and from the fact that the patient apparently did not wish to involve the family, coming alone. Straightforward behavior modification would be rather hard to manage with no parent or school contact, and does not seem appropriate here. [However, see Clements, 1973. Also, the somewhat related desensitization by reciprocal inhibition (Wolpe, 1969) might be feasible for the neurotic symptoms]. Hospitalization could await a trial of outpatient therapy. The best answer appears to be number two. Since there was no immediate opening available in a group at the time this patient presented, individual psychotherapy was initiated as the best available treatment.

The patient quickly developed a dependent relationship with the student therapist and came on time regularly, even if it meant driving 120 miles per hour after a late start. He worked regularly, got a girlfriend (which he had been afraid to do before) and made good enough grades to pass to the senior year. When the first therapist rotated off the service after six weeks, the patient reported that he had

CASE STUDY #12

lost his girlfriend and his job and cited these as reasons for wanting to continue with another therapist.

QUESTION C:
AT THIS POINT THE PATIENT IS STRUGGLING WITH:
1. Dependency feelings and separation anxiety
2. Feelings of rejection and neglect
3. An inferiority complex
4. Ambivalence about whether to continue in therapy
5. Excessive dependence

Though the patient may be ambivalent about many things, he does not appear ambivalent about his wish and need to remain in therapy. One appears to be the best answer, but a case might also be made for two insofar as he has formed a dependent relationship with the therapist who he may have hoped would provide the gratifications of which he had been deprived by his rejecting, neglectful parents, and who now likewise appears to be abandoning him. He was undoubtedly suffering an increase of anxiety because of his separation feelings regarding the therapist. The loss of girlfriend and job seems a thinly disguised manipulation to insure a replacement for the therapist he was losing, and perhaps an unconscious attempt to keep the same therapist.

QUESTION D:
THE BEST INTERVENTION AT THIS POINT WOULD BE TO:
1. Interpret his dependency and separation anxiety and show confidence in his ability to handle his problem by refusing to assign another therapist
2. Hospitalize him
3. Tell him he can have another therapist if he gets his girlfriend and job back
4. Arrange for the original therapist to continue carrying the case even after rotating off the service
5. Tranquilize him
6. Arrange for another therapist, perhaps prescribe a tranquilizer to tide him over the difficult transition, and alert the new therapist to the psychodynamics

The situation does not seem urgent enough to warrant hospitalization at this point unless the patient requests it. On the other hand, the patient is burdened with a serious enough problem that it would be destructive to cut him adrift without a therapist. To pressure the original student therapist into continuing the case, even if he wanted to, might set up another unhealthy "rejecting parent" situation, as obligations of the next rotation impinge on his time. To make assignment of a new therapist contingent on his behavior would not respect the unquestionable motivation for therapy he has already demonstrated. Further, regaining the same job and girlfriend might be impossible, reinforcing his role of "Loser." Six is the best answer.

He was assigned another student therapist and was given a prescription for thioridazine (Mellaril) 50 mg. q. i. d. He found another girlfriend and another job. Several times bodyguards accompanied him to therapy in order to protect him from ambush from a rival gang. His gang members apparently saw nothing wrong with their leader consulting a "shrink" for his anxiety. The latter became so intense whenever he would ride in a car that he had to refrain for awhile from going anywhere out of the city. This cramped his style somewhat as leader of the gang, and he began relinquishing that role. After one month with the new therapist, he revealed that he had not been taking the medicine, but then did start taking it, with some reduction in anxiety attacks. He claimed that the thioridazine did not faze him, and reported no side effects. However, he continued to have great reservations about taking any drug and continued to worry about losing control.

CASE STUDY #12

As the end of the second therapist's two-month rotation drew near, the patient reported that he had lost his new girlfriend and thought he was going to lose his new job. When he was confronted with the similarity of these complaints to those he had at the time of termination with the first therapist, he insisted that though he had obtained no help from therapy he wanted to continue with another therapist because it was his last hope. He refused to consider the possibility of hospitalization.

QUESTION E:
A MAJOR TRANQUILIZER RATHER THAN A MINOR TRANQUILIZER WAS THE APPROPRIATE MEDICATION IN THIS CASE BECAUSE:
1. The patient had a major problem, not a minor one
2. He was suspected to be basically schizophrenic
3. A major tranquilizer is safer
4. Minor tranquilizers are not useful for adolescents
5. None of the above

All psychotropic medications found useful in adults have also been found useful in adolescents, though not always to the same degree. Except for addiction with minor tranquilizers, major tranquilizers carry more risk. The choice between a minor and a major tranquilizer for anxiety is best predicated on whether or not schizophrenia is suspected. The best answer is two. Some people would accept the patient's tolerance to the drowsy side effect in the dose used as confirmation of the suspicion that he was basically schizophrenic.

QUESTION F:
THIS CASE ILLUSTRATES THAT GROUP DELINQUENTS:
1. Are often neurotic
2. Are often schizophrenic
3. Can suffer from other psychiatric problems which can be treated independently of the delinquency problem
4. Usually cooperate with psychiatric treatment
5. Usually dislike drugs

The diagnosis of group delinquency implies no other psychiatric disturbance. As in this case, individual gang members may have other psychiatric problems. For these they may be willing to cooperate with treatment if the symptoms are distressing. The group delinquency itself, they usually do not see as a problem. Though drugs tend to lead to gang disintegration, some gangs nevertheless experiment with them. Three is the best answer. See case 2 for an isolated delinquent.

QUESTION G:
LONG-TERM PATIENTS TREATED PSYCHOTHERAPEUTICALLY BY STUDENTS ON TWO-MONTH ROTATIONS MUST CHANGE THERAPISTS ONE OR MORE TIMES, AS IN THIS CASE. SUCH THERAPIST CHANGES:
1. Are destructive to the therapeutic process
2. Promote the process of therapy
3. Mobilize feelings of separation anxiety, deprivation, fear, or anger, and may bring out the patient's psychodynamics more clearly
4. Should be avoided
5. Must be taken in stride as a fact of life

Such rotating therapist changes are sometimes destructive, sometimes helpful. They usually mobilize feelings which need to receive careful attention. The best answer is three. See case 52 for an example of therapist changes promoting the progress of therapy, and case 32 for a 7 year-old with intense feelings about therapist change.

CASE STUDY #12

REFERENCES:
1. Bowlby, J., 1944: 44 Juvenile Thieves. Int J Psychoanalysis 25:107-128

2. Clements, P., 1973: Teaching children to be their own behavior therapists. J School Health, In Press

3. Coleman, J.S., 1961: The Adolescent Society, Free Press, Collier Mac-Millan Ltd, London

4. Haggerty, R.J. and K.J. Roghmann, 1972: Noncompliance and self medication: two neglected aspects of pediatric pharmacology. Ped Cl N Amer 19:101-115

5. Healy, W., 1915: The Individual Delinquent, Little-Brown, New York

6. Hoch, P. and J.P. Cattell, 1959: The diagnosis of pseudoneurotic schizophrenia. Psychiatric Quarterly 33:17-43

7. Johnson, A., 1952: Genesis of antisocial acting out in children and adults. Psychoanalytic Quarterly 21:323-343

8. Redl, F., 1966: When We Deal With Children, Free Press, New York

9. Redl, F., 1951: Children Who Hate, Free Press, Glencoe, Ill.

10. Wilkerson, D., 1963: The Cross and the Switchblade, Geis Associates, New York

11. Wolpe, J., 1969: The Practice of Behavior therapy, Pergamon Press, New York

CASE STUDY #13

"Twiggy"

Rosalind was 14 years old when referred to the medical center by her pediatrician, who was concerned about her sudden weight loss. In a four-month period she had lost 49 pounds (from 125 to 76 pounds). Previous to this weight loss, she had always enjoyed good health. When she weighed 125 pounds, a few boys in the neighborhood had allegedly called her "fatso"; therefore, she went on a diet and reduced to 115 pounds. In retrospect, she said that she was satisfied with that weight, but for some reason kept right on losing until the time of admission.

QUESTION A:
AT THIS POINT THE MOST LIKELY WORKING DIAGNOSIS IS:
1. Primary hepatoma
2. Lymphosarcoma
3. Dextroamphetamine overdosage
4. Rowe's syndrome
5. Anorexia nervosa

Rosalind was admitted to a pediatric unit, where no endogenous cause of weight loss was discovered, and the diagnosis of anorexia nervosa was correctly made. She was discharged after gaining a few pounds, but at home she promptly lost weight again. Therefore, she was readmitted to the pediatric service, and a psychiatric consultation was requested. Except for the obvious weight loss, there were no significant physical or laboratory findings.

A careful psychiatric evaluation failed to discover any really remarkable findings. Rosalind was shy and somewhat resistant to revealing her feelings and personal thoughts. She felt that she had no emotional disturbance, tearfully asked to be discharged, and promised to eat and gain weight at home. During the interview she expressed the usual amount of interest in boys, careers, etc., but constantly used her intelligence to give the socially acceptable reply rather than her own opinion. An hour's interview left one with the feeling that he knew no more about Rosalind than at the outset. She maintained that she had plenty of friends, enjoyed school, and had a healthy family life.

When the parents were interviewed, they generally confirmed Rosalind's statement that she was psychologically healthy. Her birth history and early development were unremarkable. According to the parents, she was characteristically shy and usually confined herself to a few close friends. Rosalind was bright and had enjoyed school all through the elementary grades. In junior high school she seemed to become somewhat less outgoing, but could not be described as schizoid. She had menstruated once, a year prior to admission, but since then she had experienced only a little "spotting." Rosalind did not enjoy dancing. Both she and her parents felt she was too young to date boys.

QUESTION B:
THE UNDERLYING PSYCHIATRIC DIAGNOSIS USUALLY SEEN IN CASES OF ANOREXIA NERVOSA IS:
1. Schizophrenia
2. Psychoneurosis, obsessive-compulsive type
3. Psychoneurosis, anxiety type
4. All of the above
5. None of the above

The fourth answer is probably the best. Obsessive-compulsive features are often present to some degree in anorexic children, but such symptoms can also be seen in schizophrenic children and to a mild extent in otherwise healthy children. The obsessions reach delusional intensity at times, and the patient's behavior becomes dominated by obsessive rituals. The delusions often involve the

CASE STUDY #13

patient's self-image. Such youngsters have been known to stand naked with legs together before a mirror in order to examine in detail the spaces between various portions of their legs. Such behavior is much more reminiscent of schizophrenia than any of the neuroses. Thus, some children with this disorder are very seriously disturbed, while others, such as Rosalind, seem only mildly disturbed.

QUESTION C:
THE TREATMENT OF CHOICE SHOULD BE:
1. Group psychotherapy
2. Behavioral modification therapy
3. Individual psychotherapy
4. Careful medical management
5. Family therapy

One can find some rationale for all of these forms of therapy, but in the author's experience a behavior modification program, as described below, is by far the most effective. Rosalind's case is typical in terms of her resistance to psychotherapy in any form. Most authors agree, though, that hospitalization on a psychiatric ward is indicated. (An outstanding exception to this is presented by John Reinhart 1972.) In general, treatment of anorexics is difficult in most pediatric settings, because these girls are so manipulative. They often "cheat" and are difficult to watch on pediatric floors. They may hide weights in their clothes before weighing in, make themselves vomit after eating, throw their food away, or give it to other children. Psychiatric nurses are better able to cope with this type of behavior.

At Ohio State University we have developed a program based on the ideas of Hilde Bruch (1965). We focus our attention first on the symptom, namely the eating disorder, and place the psychological exploration in a secondary position. The therapist begins by calculating the patient's ideal weight, based on age, height, and sex; and then draws a chart (Fig. 13.1) which illustrates very clearly how long it will take to attain the desired weight if the patient gains half a pound daily.

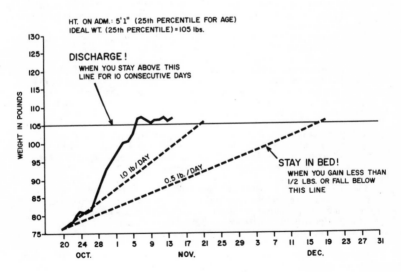

FIGURE 13. 1

CASE STUDY #13

This plan is discussed with the patient in detail, and she is told that she will be discharged when she stays above the desired level for ten consecutive days. These statements are also written down on the chart, and the patient is given a copy as a contract.

Another tool to motivate anorexics to gain weight is their tremendous drive to be moving or exercising at all times. These patients seem to be bent on expending every possible calorie - quite in contrast to obese persons who seem to want to conserve every ounce of energy - and often show compulsive foot-tapping or other rituals. Consequently, we tell the patients that we are worried about their weight and that if they have not gained their half pound at the morning weigh-in, they will be confined to bed all day "in order to conserve every calorie." They must lie still and not read or play cards, etc., for all these activities use up calories.

It is surprising how effective this regimen is in helping such youngsters gain weight. In fact, it is rather disconcerting, almost frightening, how they can control their weight. It forces the therapist to consider the question of their underlying psychological problem. (For other uses of behavior modification, see cases 13, 37, 41, 48 and 52).

QUESTION D:
THE MOST COMMON PSYCHODYNAMIC ISSUE IN ANOREXIA NERVOSA IS:
1. Fear of oral impregnation
2. Fear of sexuality
3. Fear of development into adolescence
4. Suicidal ideation
5. Manipulation of parental behavior

Although most authors feel that these girls suffer from a fear of oral impregnation, which is translated into a fear of eating, it is often hard to get confirmation from the patient. Anorexics are concerned about sexuality, and they are very manipulative. Their capacity to control their weight drives one to the conclusion that they may be truly suicidal. But none of these possibilities can be easily established in the course of psychotherapy. The onset of anorexia nervosa often occurs just prior to or just after pubescence. Sometimes the decision to start on a diet is made while anxiously overhearing girl friends discuss boys, dating, etc. It may be that the girl then decides not to grow up but to remain forever in the safety of pre-adolescence. The best answer is three.

As an interesting illustration of the oral impregnation fantasy, we offer this supplementary vignette:

Susan was a sweet 10 year-old girl who had lost 12-13 pounds in three months. She was interviewed along with her mother. During the interview, she spontaneously described her strong wish to have a baby sister with whom she could play, and said that her mother was unable to have any more babies, due to a hysterectomy. She also knew that babies occur after one is married, but had read about a girl in India who had a baby at age nine. About a year ago, she continued, she had been told of a 5 year-old who had "wished for a sister so much that she had a baby of her own." She also said that she felt that babies begin to grow in mothers' stomachs when they "eat enough for two."

The fantasy of oral impregnation was interpreted to this girl as the cause of her fear of eating, but no change occurred until a month later, when this interpretation was given to her again. She subsequently gained 10 pounds in two weeks and continued to do well over the following two years.

The reader is cautioned not to make an interpretation of oral impregnation to older girls in the early stages of treatment because they are unable to accept such a psychoanalytic concept. Too early interpretation may do them more harm than good, possibly prompting them to drop out of treatment.

CASE STUDY #13

Rosalind did well for two years and seemed at that time to be making a very fine adjustment to adolescence. She began menstruating at age 15-1/2. Her weight fluctuated between 120 and 130 pounds, depending mostly on her activity, which varied a lot, since she was a member of the high school track team. She was also active in other school activities, the marching band, the French Club, and the yearbook staff.

In looking back, Rosalind feels she needed the hospitalization, even though she didn't like it. At the two year follow-up she told of dating and of enjoying contact with boys. She thinks they are sometimes too serious; one boy wants to marry her. At 16 she feels she is too young to think of such things and is more interested in a career as a physical education teacher.

The prognosis in this disorder is guarded. Rosalind has done very well and was one of our best patients. Although never interested in psychotherapy, she benefited from our hospital milieu and behavioral modification approach. She was psychiatrically healthier than our other patients. Some other girls remain very thin at age 17-18 and seem to have very poor interpersonal relationships. One was clearly schizophrenic and required a prolonged psychiatric hospitalization.

REFERENCES:
1. Blinder, B. J., et al., 1970: Behavior Therapy of Anorexia Nervosa: Effectiveness of Activity as a Reinforcer of Weight Gain. Am J of Psychiatry 126:1093-1098

2. Browning, C. H. and S. I. Miller, 1968: Anorexia Nervosa: A Study in Prognosis and Management. Am J Psychiat 124:1128-1132

3. Bruch, H., 1965: Anorexia Nervosa and its Differential Diagnosis. J of Nervous and Mental Diseases 150:51-67

4. Bruch, H., 1970: Psychotherapy in Primary Anorexia Nervosa. J of Nervous and Mental Diseases 150:51-67

5. Crisp, A. and D. Toms, 1971: Weight Phobia in the Adolescent Male. Presented at the Soc. for Psychosomatic Research, London, October 1, 1971

6. Reinhart, J. B., et al., 1972: Anorexia Nervosa in Children: Outpatient Management. J Am Acad Child Psychiatry 11:114-131

CASE STUDY #14

A 12-Year-Old Who Lost Everything

Charles, the 12 year-old son of white working class parents, was brought to the clinic because he was always losing things. His parents recited a long list of objects: coats, shoes, sportswear, keys, school books and money. When queried, the boy would say that he couldn't find them or that they had been taken. Both mother and father referred to their son as "odd," and said that he lied a great deal.

When asked what they meant by "odd," they described the boy as being afraid to be in a room by himself and refusing to go from one room to another if the next room were empty. They thought this amusing, not a problem, but rather one of their son's eccentricities. He was also afraid of the dark and that burglars would enter the house. The parents dealt with this fear by pointing out that the windows and doors were locked.

Throughout the interview both parents seemed cheerful and unconcerned. They joked and laughed about everything, especially Charles' protruding ears and his oddities. Mother, who seemed hypomanic, suffered Addison's disease and was taking steroids and thyroxine. Father had occasional periods of depression but was not on medication. There was also a five year-old daughter in the family.

The boy enjoyed anything violent and spent several hours each evening watching television. He was particularly fascinated by a monster on one program and talked about it at every opportunity. He loved knives; he would take his mother's from the kitchen and practice throwing them. He had tried to borrow five hundred dollars from father "to buy a one-man tank."

Developmental milestones were normal with the exception of age 2-1/2 when he went into trance-like states which lasted several minutes. Although these states occurred for seven or eight months, medical advice was not sought. When he started school at age five, he refused to eat and became very thin. However, this too passed, and parents weren't very concerned. One teacher described the boy as being "shy and not very honest" while another spanked him for "laziness."

When pressed for real concerns, father felt that Charles "wasn't very bright," perhaps like himself. He had tried to get him to share in building models, but after failure to arouse his interest, he built them himself. Mother's concern was that the boy wasn't conforming and that he would appear "peculiar" to others.

He enjoyed playing with younger children and his companions ranged in age from two to four years old.

Charles was given a Stanford-Binet (L-M), the Children's Apperception Test (CAT) and the Bender-Gestalt. He was found to be of average intelligence and there were no indications of cerebral dysfunction in either the test data or in a follow-up EEG. However, the CAT protocol suggested rather severe emotional problems. The quality and structure of his stories deteriorated progressively, and in several instances perceptual distortions and confusion about the identity of the figures occurred. An unusual feature was that he included himself in some of the stories, which is an indication of rather weak ego boundaries.

In general, Charles seemed to feel that his younger sister got all of mother's good things, while he seemed to get all the bad. He had angry, aggressive feelings toward mother because of this grievance, but for the most part was able to conceal them by a kind of manic denial similar to his parent's.

Charles saw father as unpredictable, which must have added to the boy's confusion. At times he was punitive, but more often irresponsible, giving little support to the family.

Much of the boy's disturbance seemed concerned with sexual areas. His stories became more confused. He began to rhyme his response to Card V, which is a picture of a darkened room with two little rabbits in a cot next to a shadowy bed in which the outlines of two adult figures under the covers can be seen. Masturbation was also probably an area of conflict.

Finally, his stories contained disguised aggressive and possibly destructive feelings in relation to younger children, which was rather alarming in a boy who was accustomed to playing with children much younger than himself.

CASE STUDY #14

Following the testing, Charles was able to discuss how uncomfortable and frightened he often felt. He seemed quite introspective and eager for help. The fact that he was able to relate and that he was aware that he had problems which made him uncomfortable, suggested that he might have been able to make good use of psychotherapy.

QUESTION A:
THE FATHER SEEMED UNPREDICTABLE AND UNDEPENDABLE TO THE PATIENT BECAUSE:
1. He wouldn't give the boy money to buy a tank
2. He occasionally went into depressions and the patient never knew what his mood would be
3. He had rather given up on the boy
4. He laughed at his son's fears
5. He became angry when his son lost things
6. He teased his son about his ears

Father certainly didn't seem to be a very dependable figure on whom the boy could rely nor did he seem to be a sympathetic person. His manic defenses against his own feelings of despair probably did not allow him to know about his son's pain lest these feelings should be aroused in himself. Hence, he laughed at the boy and made fun of him in order to ward off his own feelings of depression, which may have been quite frightening to him. Two, three, and four are correct.

QUESTION B:
THIS PATIENT MAY HAVE CONSTANTLY LOST HIS POSSESSIONS BECAUSE:
1. He was trying to manipulate his parents by claiming he lost things
2. He was so preoccupied with his own inner world of fantasies that he forgot them
3. His possessions had no value to him
4. He was unconsciously aware that this caused consternation in his parents, whereas his "odd" behavior, as his fear of empty rooms, was only joked about by them
5. He didn't realize that his parents had paid for these things and thought they could easily provide new replacements

Manic parents can seem very undependable: little that happens to the child arouses their concern. We see in this boy's history their lack of concern over his trance-like states at two years, or over his loss of weight at five years. Perhaps he quickly discovered after the first few objects were lost that this was a way to arouse his parents' attention to his needs. The best answer is four. Two is also a possibility.

QUESTION C:
THERAPEUTIC INTERVENTION IN THIS CASE SHOULD HAVE BEEN:
1. Hospitalization for the boy in a residential treatment facility
2. A major tranquilizer for the boy
3. Individual psychotherapy for the boy and parental guidance
4. To have taken all of the boy's possessions away from him until he learned to take care of them
5. None of the above

This family had problems in communication, possibly due in part to the parents' illnesses. It would have been important to mother to have consulted with a physician in order to determine if part of her behavior was due to side effects of her medication. It is possible that psychotherapy for the parents might have

CASE STUDY #14

helped them to get in touch with their own feelings, which would have given them a better understanding of their son.

Individual psychotherapy for the boy might have helped to sustain him during the period of his parents' therapy in that he would have felt supported and that someone was "listening" to him.

Eventually, a series of family therapy sessions which included the younger sister might also have been helpful in that they could have learned to communicate. Unless changes could have been brought about in this family, she too could easily have developed emotional problems. The best answer is three.

QUESTION D:
CHARLES' RHYMING TO CAT CARD V INDICATES:
1. Literary ability
2. Precociousness
3. Defensiveness
4. Denial
5. Echolalia

Sometimes it is difficult to understand exactly what is going on when a child suddenly starts to rhyme his stories. In this instance, Charles' stories were becoming progressively disintegrated and loss of mental control was apparent. It would seem that two dynamics were simultaneously occurring. The first was that Charles was rhyming as a defense against his anxiety and further loss of control. The second seemed to be denial or a device he was using to appear adequate, in collusion with the psychologist. He was giving the psychologist something (rhymes), and the psychologist was accepting that which he gave. The best answers are three and four.

REFERENCES:
1. Armstrong, M. A., 1954: Children's responses to animal and human figures in thematic pictures. J Consult Psychol 18:67-70

2. Bellak, L., 1954: The Thematic Apperception Test and the Children's Apperception Test in Clinical Use. New York, Grune & Stratton

3. Bender, L., 1938: A visual-motor gestalt test and its clinical use. Amer Orthopsychiat Assn. Monogr. Series No. 3

4. English, O. S. and G. H. J. Pearson, 1972: Irrational fears and phobias in Childhood Psychopathology, edited by S. Harrison and J. F. McDermott, New York, International Universities Press pp. 375-381

5. Frank, G., 1965: The role of the family in the development of psychopathology. Psychol Bull., 64:191-205

6. Freud, A., 1967: About losing and being lost. Psychoanal Study Child 22:9-19, New York, International Universities Press

7. Haworth, M. A., 1966: The CAT: Facts about Fantasy. New York, Grune and Stratton

8. Klein, M., 1948: Mourning and its relation to manic-depressive states in: Contributions to Psychoanalysis. London, Hogarth Press, pp. 311-338

9. Plotsky, H. and M. Shereshefsky, 1960: An isolation pattern in fathers of emotionally disturbed children. Am J Orthopsychiat 30:780-787

CASE STUDY #14

10. Terman, L. M. and M. A. Merrill, 1960: <u>Stanford-Binet Intelligence Scale, Manual for the Third Revision Form L-M.</u> Boston, Houghton, Mifflin

11. Winnicott, D. W. , 1972: Basis for self in body. <u>Int J Child Psychother</u> 1:7-16

12. Winnicott, D. W. , 1958: The Manic Defense. In: <u>Collected Papers Paediatrics to Psycho-analysis.</u> London, Tavistock Publication

CASE STUDY #15

14 Year-Old Bart's "Affair" with his Pastor

Bart Q., a nearly 14 year-old white rural middle-class ninth-grade boy, was brought by his father and his father's 19 year-old fiancee, Helen, because of the discovery one week before that he had submitted to homosexual relations with his 54 year-old pastor.

He was the middle of three children of a 38 year-old widower. His 17 year-old sister was closest to their father. His 9 year-old brother had been closest to their mother, who died of cancer three years previously. Bart's recollections of the death were rather confused because he thought she had died when she lapsed into coma the day preceding her actual death. Prior to the coma, he had not expected her to die.

After Mrs. Q.'s death, Bart's sister was put in charge of the younger children. Bart would often be punished for not obeying her and also for failing to add "sir" or Ma'am" to his yes's and no's. He described his father as very strict. Mr. Q. did not even want Bart to spend his own money on what he wanted, and occasionally searched his room to make sure that he hadn't bought things without permission.

Mr. Q., seen separately, broke into tears at several points, verbalizing feelings of having been an inadequate father, not giving Bart enough love, and always being too quick to anger with him. His anger had been more explosive since his wife's death, particularly when Bart seemed to interfere with his getting close to his daughter, on whom he wanted to lean. He was hurt by all the children's attitudes about their mother's death. Though they cried at the funeral, they did not since then ask to visit the grave.

Mr. Q. felt that he had been inconsistent with Bart, sometimes too strict and other times not strict enough. He cancelled the children's allowances because chores weren't getting done. Since then the children had to ask for money for each thing. Though he seldom refused his daughter "because she gets her chores done," he often refused Bart.

Ten months previously, Helen, Mr. Q.'s niece, came to live in the house. She had left home because her parents (Mr. Q.'s sister and brother-in-law) objected to her planned marriage to Mr. Q. The wedding was scheduled for approximately one month after the initial clinic appointment. Bart had always got along well with cousin Helen both before and after she lived at the house. His only concern about the marriage was whether he would still be allowed to use the kitchen. In addition to helping clean the kitchen and liking to cook, he also had masculine chores such as cutting grass and cleaning the basement.

The pastor starting taking an interest in Bart about a year previously, treating him to bowling, swimming, etc. They had to sneak to do this because Mr. Q. did not want Bart going places so much. Bart used to tell the minister how his father treated him. The minister would sympathize, saying that Mr. Q. was wrong and that he would treat Bart differently if he were his son.

Soon the minister persuaded Bart to undress and let him put his penis between Bart's legs. Bart felt he should let him do this because he owed it to him after the minister had been so kind. Bart recalled being rather scared and curious about the situation at first. He never had an erection except when the minister would play with him. However, on other occasions, away from the minister, he would sometimes masturbate while thinking about girls, never while thinking about the minister or any other male. He denied any oral-genital contact, and did not know any other homosexuals.

When the minister's wife found out, about a month before the clinic appointment, they quit having physical contact but corresponded with each other even when the minister and his wife went on vacation. He left a whole pack of these letters in an open drawer, and his sister found them when she was cleaning his room a week prior to the first clinic visit. He thought his father found them while snooping in his room. After his father had talked with him about them, he allowed another letter to be seen in his pocket and taken away from him before he opened it. Therefore, his father and Helen felt that he deliberately allowed these things to be

CASE STUDY #15

discovered, wanting help. Mr. Q. brought one of the letters, which contained a reference to wanting to eat something which Bart made, but it was not clear whether this referred to fellatio or some of Bart's famous cooking.

Bart presented as a tall, lanky, almost "pretty," early adolescent of quietly tense appearance. Neither his handshake nor his voice suggested effeminacy. Despite apparent anxiety, he slouched along the hall in a rather passive manner. Once seated, he nondefensively and frankly discussed the details of the relationship with the minister and other problems he felt he had, particularly with his father and sister. He picked at his fingertips while talking. He seemed rather disturbed about having to sneak to do so many things and indicated he had gone along with the homosexual activity because of a feeling of obligation to the minister. He showed no evidence of thought disorder, disorientation, or loss of contact with reality. He had previously been afraid to tell his father about the problem, expecting him to get angry. He was gratefully surprised to see his father weep and be more concerned about what Bart was doing to ruin himself than what he was doing to the father. Bart wished that his father were marrying someone older, because it was hard to think of a 19 year-old as his mother.

QUESTION A:
THE FIRST THERAPEUTIC INTERVENTION WAS WEEKLY INDIVIDUAL PSY-
CHOTHERAPY FOR BART AND OCCASIONAL CONFERENCES WITH HIS FATHER
AND COUSIN-STEPMOTHER. MATERIAL COMING OUT IN SUCH THERAPY
CONFIRMED THAT BART HAD ALL BUT WHICH ONE OF THE FOLLOWING
PROBLEMS?:
1. Homosexual urges
2. Feminine identification
3. Passivity
4. Submissiveness
5. Dependency
6. Feelings of deprivation
7. Having to compete with his sister and Helen for his father's love

Interestingly, the only item above for which no evidence appeared in therapy was number one, the one we might have expected most, judging from the chief complaint. However, his heterosexual masturbation fantasies should have tipped us off that homosexual urges would not be prominent.

Bart's feelings of envy towards his sister and eventually towards his step-mother became more and more prominent. He spent most of his therapy time complaining about his unfair treatment from his father, at times appearing much like a petulant, whining little girl. Since the homosexual affair did not appear to be an important part of his problem, since his complaints about his father appeared to be a good entree to group therapy, and since some peer feedback would appear therapeutic for his querulousness and passivity, he was entered in group therapy in addition to the individual therapy.

He soon opted to stop individual therapy and rely completely on group therapy after it was pointed out that he was using individual therapy to discuss things which he should be discussing in group therapy, thereby avoiding participating in the group. In group therapy he made rapid progress. At first silent and passive, he began participating, and eventually verbalized that he thought his problem was being too submissive and passive. Unfortunately, at this time his father, who was resistant to the expense and bother of getting Bart to the clinic, pressured him into withdrawing from treatment.

QUESTION B:
THIS CASE ILLUSTRATES:
1. A negative oedipal situation
2. How allowing boys to do feminine things like cooking leads to homosexuality

CASE STUDY #15

3. How the loss of the opposite-sex parent in early adolescence can interfere with the usual formation of sexual identity
4. The early stages of homosexuality
5. The middle child syndrome

   Homosexuality is not this boy's main problem, so 2 and 4 are not good answers. Five is partially right. Though this case is not typical of the middle child, the patient's ordinal position probably helped set the stage for the feeling of deprivation he suffered at his mother's death. The negative oedipal situation is one where the child develops an attachment for the parent of the same sex (in this case, probably because of the untimely loss of his mother) and tries to win that parent's affection by reversing his own sex roles. This is shown by Bart's assumption of many housewifely duties and his envy of his older sister and cousin-stepmother, to whom his father showed more affection. It is well known that loss of the same-sex parent in early adolescence can interfere with sexual identity formation. It is less well known that loss of the opposite-sex parent can do the same through a different mechanism. Answers one and three are both correct, and overlap.

QUESTION C:
THE 38 YEAR-OLD MR. Q.'S MARRIAGE TO HIS SISTER'S 19 YEAR-OLD DAUGHTER ILLUSTRATES:
1. A subcultural norm deviating from the larger culture
2. The natural interest of any man in a beautiful young woman
3. Magical thinking, because his age was exactly twice hers
4. Breach of the incest taboo
5. Preservation of the incest taboo

   Helen's parents' objection seems enough evidence that such a marriage was not a subcultural norm for the Q. family. Two seems too "normal" and shallow an explanation. Three's "logic" doesn't hold up, because the ages were 37 and 18 at the time of engagement. Mr. Q.'s marriage to his niece, though incestuous, was not as incestuous as the one initially wanted. It is rather obvious, from his initial remarks and from information gained in therapy, that Mr. Q. had a strong attachment to his daughter, Bart's sister, expecially after Mrs. Q.'s death. Marrying his sister's daughter instead of his own provided a more acceptable displacement of these feelings to a very similar love object of the same age. Thus, this marriage appears to be more a preservation of the incest taboo than a breach of it.

QUESTION D:
WHEN AN ADOLESCENT LEAVES PERSONAL THINGS LIKE LETTERS OR DIARIES WHERE ANOTHER MEMBER OF THE FAMILY FINDS THEM:
1. They should be opened and read for his own good
2. They should be left untouched
3. It should be interpreted as a subtle plea for help
4. His carelessness should be called to his attention
5. The finder need not worry about confidentiality, because the adolescent obviously wants them read

   Such an adolescent may want the finder to read the material, as Bart seems to have wanted, but this cannot be assumed. He may merely have been careless and trusting. On the other hand, it may be an unconscious attempt to get help, so it should not just be ignored. The most prudent course would be to apprise him of his carelessness in a manner that lets him know the finder did not read the material, e.g., "If you don't want anyone to read these, better not leave

CASE STUDY #15

them lying around. Suppose someone had found them who would read them?" If
he has a problem for which he is looking for help, his response to such an apprisal
(guilt, anxiety, etc.) will provide an opportunity for inquiry. Four is the best
answer, with three also correct.

QUESTION E:
THIS CASE SHOWS THAT ADOLESCENT HOMOSEXUAL SYMPTOMS:
1. Can usually be treated in group therapy
2. Have a good prognosis
3. Come from a dominating, punitive father
4. Are elicited by contact with ministers
5. Often cover up deeper problems of submissiveness, passivity, dependency,
   or love deprivation, which can sometimes be treated in group therapy after
   the presenting symptom has been dealt with individually

Though this case was suitable for group therapy, many homosexual problems
would not be as suitable for a diagnostically heterogeneous group. (See case 22
for further discussion of this.) Prognosis, of course, varies from case to case.
A passive, ineffectual or absent father seems more common in homosexuality
than a dominating, punitive one. Five is the best answer.

REFERENCES:
1. Berkowitz, I. H., 1972: Adolescents Grow in Groups. Brunner-Mazel, New York

2. Obesey, L., 1969: Homosexuality and Pseudohomosexuality. Science House,
   New York

3. Ollendorf, R., 1966: The Juvenile Homosexual Experience and Its Effect on
   Adult Sexuality. The Julian Press, Inc., New York

CASE STUDY #16

An 8-Year-Old Who Couldn't Get Anybody To Listen

Peter's mother brought him to the clinic at the school's insistence. A third-grader, he was small for eight years. Dressed in a soiled shirt and tattered dark trousers, he looked grubby and dejected. His fingernails were badly bitten.

The school doctor had called the clinic in advance to say he felt a crisis was rapidly approaching for the boy and that help was urgently needed. Peter had been soiling and wetting himself for the past few weeks, and most recently completely soaked his trousers while in the health office. A short time previously he had run out of school and spent his lunch money on candy. When the principal asked Peter to come to talk with him about the incident, he ran home, saying he thought school was out. His teacher felt sorry for him; she regarded him as mentally retarded. He didn't participate in classroom activities, seemed unable to do his work, was "backward in reading," and for the most part sat quietly in his seat daydreaming.

Peter was the youngest of three children, with a 12 year-old brother and a 13 year-old sister. The parents lived together, but each had extra-marital sexual partners.

Mother, a rather pleasant, plump lady in her late thirties, talked constantly and seemed to hear little of what was said to her. She had taken over father's job as a taxi driver about two years previously, and worked from 9:00 a. m. to 9:00 p. m. each day. She seemed quite unconcerned, and said she wasn't worried about her son; he would grow out of it.

Father, a rather short, muscular man, had taken over mother's role and re-mained at home keeping house. They had made the change because father had been ill and needed free time for doctor's appointments. He blamed the boy's problems on mother's pampering, and boasted that he stopped Peter's encopresis by giving him a "good wallop" each time he soiled and then forcing him to wash his pants. He had strong views about raising children. They shouldn't be pam-pered and should be brought up as tough as possible. There was nothing wrong with Peter that he couldn't correct with a little discipline. His only problem was that he was lazy.

Peter had been a normal, full-term baby with an easy birth. Developmental milestones were normal. Mother had first potted him at five months when he was introduced to solids. Unfortunately, at a year he became severely anemic, which necessitated frequent trips to a clinic for a two-year period. His anemia was eventually cured by femoral vein injections of iron. Although mother did not resume training, he was controlling himself fairly well by the time he entered nursery school, with only occasional nighttime wetting. He had been a fussy eater and mother had always given in to his food wishes. This included a bottle until he was five, when father suddenly announced that he had had enough and took it away from him.

The boy's encopresis and enuresis had started about two years prior to the referral and had become progressively worse during the past year. He wet him-self while playing and was more often wet than dry at school. He had also started telling lies.

Peter needed constant support and encouragement from the psychologist throughout the psychological evaluation. Otherwise, he immediately gave up when confronted with any task. He often muttered to himself. He obtained an I. Q. of 117 on the Stanford-Binet, L-M.

His Bender-Gestalt contained no signs of cerebral dysfunction, but did sug-gest severe anxiety, as did his figure drawings. The female figure was dominant and phallic, while the male figure suggested dependency and immaturity. Both figures were drawn with robot-like stances. The body outlines were broken and worked over in many places.

The Children's Apperception Test (CAT) indicated that Peter was a seriously disturbed little boy who was finding withdrawal into himself the only way of coping in a world which he found cold, frightening and unsupportive. There was evidence

CASE STUDY #16

of denial of reality and rather strong indications that he was self-punitive and had many fantasies about self-damage and death. His stories raised many questions about his relationship with his father. He was apparently terrified of him and felt completely defenseless and helpless when confronted with his anger. He was also caught in his ambivalence between wishes for his father's demise and terror lest something should happen to him. In general, father was seen as distant and violent-tempered, and there was no escape. However, in one story there was a good male figure who saved the boy.

Peter was also muddled about his parents' sexual identities. He described a picture of a mother and father bear lying close together with a baby bear nearby as a "father, brother and a baby bear."

The Rorschach also raised concern about Peter because six out of ten cards were seen as the "insides" of people who were not only sinister, but were run by wires inside them to make them move. The Father Card (Card IV) was seen as "the inside of a monster who overheats and has pinchers." Allusions were made to mother or an adult female on two cards, and in each she was seen as having stone-like qualities. The Rorschach strongly supported the findings of the CAT that Peter's reality ties were very weak.

The hopeful signs were that the boy had been able to use the psychologist and to work very hard with her support; he saw one good male figure who saved him in one of his CAT stories, and he had good intelligence.

QUESTION A:
THE MOST LIKELY REASON PETER'S TEACHER MISTAKENLY CONSIDERED HIM MENTALLY RETARDED RATHER THAN EMOTIONALLY DISTURBED WAS THAT HE:
1. Often wet his pants and soiled himself in school
2. Didn't pay attention, seemed disinterested and didn't do his work
3. Was dirty and unkempt in appearance
4. Ran out of school and said he thought school was out
5. Muttered to himself

His teacher may have misjudged the boy's withdrawal symptoms for lack of intellectual capacity. She may also have linked his soiling and wetting to the behavior of a much younger child. This is understandable when she compared Peter to the other children in the class who were able to cope. The signs of emotional disturbance which he manifested and which may have been overlooked by the school were: lying, running away from the principal, muttering to himself, daydreaming, biting his fingernails, isolation and his dejected appearance. The best answers are two and one.

QUESTION B:
ALTHOUGH FATHER ACCUSED MOTHER OF PAMPERING THE BOY, SHE SEEMED COLD AND UNGIVING TO PETER BECAUSE:
1. She disagreed with father on how to raise children
2. She was away all day
3. Rather than trying to help Peter, she denied he was having difficulties
4. She talked all the time, made pleasantries and didn't listen
5. She drove a cab

There are several suggestions in the history that mother, as well as being accepting and lenient, may have been avoiding the role of ordinary mothering for her own convenience. It can be postulated that allowing her son to have a bottle until five may have been easier and less demanding then teaching him to drink from a cup, which would have involved relating to him. She also appeared unconcerned that Peter was not coming for his meals. She never did resume his toilet training following his anemia, which would have necessitated a mothering relation-

CASE STUDY #16

ship with him. Finally, during the intake, she expressed little interest and said, "Peter will grow out of it." Her willing reversal of roles with her husband also hints of a reluctance to mother. The best answers are three and four.

QUESTION C:
THE BEST EXPLANATION OF THIS BOY'S SOILING AND WETTING WAS:
1. He suffered a neurological impairment of sphincter control secondary to malnutrition
2. He was never trained
3. He was trying to keep people at a distance
4. It was a way of letting the world know that he felt he was in a mess
5. He was scared of the school restroom
6. He was trying to get out of school

It is not possible to provide an exact answer because some of the facetious choices may have partially contributed to Peter's soiling and wetting. E. J. Anthony (1957), in comparing "discontinuous" with "continuous" soilers, found that the latter group had experienced very low toilet training pressures and that continuous soiling was due to defective socialization rather than a neurotic symptom. However, this boy had been able to control himself fairly well by the time he entered nursery school. This, together with his intense anxiety revealed in the projective tests, suggests his wetting and soiling may have been more a loss of control due to anxiety. He was also such a fearful boy that it is not unreasonable to suspect that he may have been afraid of going to the school restroom. Finally, as Dare (1969) suggests, this was certainly a way of letting the world know he felt he was in a mess although it was probably an unconcious signal. There is no best answer.

QUESTION D:
THE DIAGNOSIS WOULD BE:
1. Overanxious reaction of childhood
2. Unsocialized aggressive reaction of childhood
3. Social maladjustment
4. Withdrawing reaction of childhood
5. Childhood schizophrenia

Overanxious reaction of childhood could be ruled out. Although Peter was anxious and fearful, he didn't have enough ego strength to be conforming or approval seeking. Rather, he paid little attention to what was going on in the classroom, soiled himself and seemed, for the most part, to respond to the anxieties of his inner world rather than to the demands of his environment.

He was neither quarrelsome nor hostile; nor was he aggressive or destructive. Although he was starting to tell lies at the time of the referral, he had no relationships with peers which would allow for hostile teasing, verbal aggressiveness or destructiveness. Thus, unsocialized aggressive reaction of childhood can be ruled out, as can social maladjustment.

In some ways Peter's symptoms fit the diagnostic category of withdrawing reaction of childhood in that he was unable to form close personal relationships. However, this category does not provide for his autistic behavior, his loosening of ties with reality and his feelings that he was being controlled by wires. The latter symptoms suggest that this boy was suffering childhood schizophrenia. The best answer is five.

REFERENCES:
1. Adams, P. L., Schwab, J. J. and J. F. Aponte, 1965: Authoritarian parents and disturbed children. Am J Psychiat 121:1162-1167

CASE STUDY #16

2. Ames, L. B., et al., 1952: Child Rorschach Responses: Developmental Trends from Two to Ten Years. New York: Hoeber

3. Bellak, L., 1954: The Thematic Apperception Test and the Children's Apperception Test in Clinical Use. New York: Grune & Stratton

4. Bender, L., 1938: A visual motor gestalt test and its clinical use. Am Orthopsychiat, Assn. Monogr. Series No. 3

5. Bender, L., 1947: Childhood Schizophrenia. Am J Orthopsychiat 17:40-56

6. Burns, R. C. and S. H. Kauffman, 1970: Kinetic Family Drawings (K-F-D) and Introduction to Understanding Children Through Kinetic Drawings. New York, Brunner/Mazel

7. Dare, C., 1969: Your 6 Year Old. London, Corgi

8. DiLeo, J. H., 1970: Young Children and Their Drawings. New York: Brunner/Mazel

9. Frank, G., 1965: The role of the family in the development of psychopathology. Psychol Bull 64:191-205

10. Gordon, E. M. and A. Thomas, 1967: Children's behavior style and the teachers appraisal of their intelligence. J Sch Psychol 5:292-300

11. Halpern, F., 1953: A Clinical Approach to Children's Rorschachs. New York, Grune & Stratton

12. Haworth, M. A., 1966: The CAT: Facts about Fantasy. New York: Grune & Stratton

13. Kanner, L., 1952: Emotional interference with intellectual functioning. Am J Ment Def 56:701-707

14. Meyers, D., 1962: Psychiatric appraisal of parents and siblings of schizophrenia children. Am J Psychiat 118:902-915

15. Piaget, J., 1954: The Construction of Reality in the Child. New York: Basic Books

16. Tapia, F., Jekel, J. and H. R. Domke, 1960: Enuresis: An emotional symptom? J Nerv Ment Dis 130:61-66

17. Warson, S. R., et al., 1954: The Dynamics of Encopresis (Workshop), Am J Orthopsychiat 24:402-415

18. Wolff, S., 1969: Children Under Stress. London: Penguin Press

CASE STUDY #17

The Ugly Duckling

Vera, a 16 year-old, white, Protestant girl, from a middle class family, was psychologically well adjusted when discharged from an adolescent psychiatric unit after one year of treatment. She was the oldest of three children but had always been viewed as the one who required the most nurturing. In a figurative sense, she was the ugly duckling who became a beautiful swan.

Ever since infancy, Vera had suffered from a convulsive disorder. This was characterized first by a few grand mal seizures but eventually by petit mal attacks consisting of staring spells and apparent lapses of thought processes for several seconds. The electroencephalogram was abnormal, and she was success-fully treated by a neurologist with anti-convulsants. The neurologist reported that by age 11 the seizures had been completely controlled, and he added, "It looked as if a lot of the recent episodes were largely functional."

At age 14 Vera had begged the neurologist to stop the medication, and the primidone (mysoline) was discontinued, but phenobarbital was continued at a dosage of 30 mg T. I. D. Vera refused to take some of her pills at age 16, and the neurologist agreed to discontinue all medication over a five-month period. Vera's mother felt ambivalent about this and became quite anxious, since she had come to view Vera as a vulnerable child.

At age 7, Vera began having episodes of abdominal pain, and a peptic ulcer was diagnosed. Medical treatment was periodic, ". . . when the ulcers came back." She was still bothered by intermittent abdominal pain in her early adolescence. It was this symptom which eventually brought her to the attention of a psychiatrist.

In the meantime, Vera's sister, who had a heart murmur, had been scheduled for cardiac catheterization. This procedure was performed at a distant hospital on Vera's 15th birthday and caused the cancellation of her birthday party. When Vera's sister returned home, Vera chided her, "Wait and see, I'll be in the hospi-tal when it's your birthday." During the ensuing four months, Vera had two or three attacks of abdominal pain. First, a diagnosis of colitis was made by the family physician. On another occasion he concurred with the mother that it might be acute appendicitis and referred Vera to a surgeon, and as Vera had predicted, she was in the hospital on her sister's birthday. An appendectomy was performed but the abdominal pain continued unabated for six months. She was admitted to a hospital for evaluation on two more occasions, and on the second occasion she was transferred to a university setting with a diagnosis of a possible peptic ulcer, which was not demonstrable by radiologic techniques.

During the latter hospitalization, her mother, while making Vera's bed, dis-covered a suicide note which was hidden between the mattresses. When the note was shown to Vera, she recognized her own handwriting, but disclaimed any mem-ory of writing it. This discovery and the absence of a definitive diagnosis to ex-plain the abdominal pain resulted in a psychiatric consultation.

During the psychiatric evaluation Vera was very quiet and passively coopera-tive, but did not contribute spontaneously. There was no explanation for the ap-parent "cry for help" symbolized by the suicide note. She was transferred to the psychiatric service. Vera's psychiatric hospitalization was marked by a para-dox: Despite her apparent willingness to accept the rules and regulations of both her therapist and the adolescent unit, she gave a general impression which prompt-ed many of the staff to remark that Vera was being "her usual hostile self." On innumerable occasions Vera could have obtained more privileges if she had merely asked for them. In almost every instance she refused to assert herself, thereby undoubtedly prolonging her therapy and hospital stay. She liked her therapist and several members of the nursing staff, but usually said she had nothing to talk about because "there is nothing on my mind." She behaved as though she had made some secret vow to herself that she would not truly cooperate in any form of psychotherapy.

It was this appearance of stubbornness that prompted staff to perceive her as hostile; they felt she was consciously refusing to cooperate in therapy. Though

CASE STUDY #17

Vera witnessed many adolescents express hostility openly, she herself was never able to. She occasionally joined in AWOL's and group delinquency towards the hospital staff when such were instigated by other patients but never spontaneously expressed negative feelings towards authority figures.

She made fifteen to twenty suicide gestures during her hospitalization, usually when angry, but she was never able to discuss these incidents in any great detail. On one occasion she left a suicide note unsigned on her therapist's desk.

Vera became mildly obese while she was in the hospital, but was unconcerned about this until her discharge drew near. When she began to make preparations to leave, she asked her therapist to prescribe a low calorie diet. After some discussion, they agreed on a 900 calorie diet, which was to begin the following Monday. Vera told her parents about this over the weekend, and in Monday's family therapy session, her mother expressed her disagreement with such a strict diet. She asserted that Vera should have 1200 calories. She backed this up by offering Vera a piece of cake she had brought along for her.

Vera's parents believed her to be the shy, quiet child she pretended to be, and her various medical problems had reinforced their contention that her needs were greater than the other children's. Furthermore, the parents seemed to like her that way, as the constant patient who needed their care. They had resisted the discontinuation of the anticonvulsants, and they resisted the 900 calorie diet. As Vera improved in the hospital and expressed herself more openly and directly, they failed to listen. It seemed as if maintenance of the status quo within the family, including Vera's role of "ugly duckling," was more important to them than the satisfaction of seeing her mature. They were threatened by the development of this eldest child into womanhood.

QUESTION A:
THE BEST EXPLANATION FOR VERA'S APPENDECTOMY ON HER SISTER'S BIRTHDAY, AS PREDICTED BY VERA, IS:
1. This case of appendicitis was psychogenic
2. The diagnosis was wrong, and her appendix was normal
3. Vera wanted to be a martyr in order to spoil her sister's birthday celebration
4. The appendicitis resulted from a psychological stress to the pituitary-gonadal axis with subsequent inflammation into the adjacent appendix
5. None of the above

A psychogenic explanation as the cause of acute appendicitis is currently not accepted. One exception to this general attitude is the finding that children who suffer from appendicitis have often undergone an unusual number of significant life events prior to the development of appendicitis. (Heisel, et al., 1973). But this is only a correlation and one should not conclude that appendicitis is a psychosomatic disorder. Vera apparently did consciously wish to spoil her sister's birthday, as evidenced by her prediction, but hospitalization is a very unusual way for most children to act out hostility towards siblings. The concept in answer four is not supported by present medical knowledge. Surprisingly, answer two is correct. The pathology report showed that the appendix was normal, with no sign of acute or chronic inflammation.

QUESTION B:
THE BEST EXPLANATION FOR THE ABDOMINAL PAIN FOLLOWING THE APPENDECTOMY IS:
1. It was psychogenic
2. It was a smoldering but non-demonstrable ulcer crater in the duodenum
3. It was an attention-getting device, a feigned symptom
4. It was probably due to a food allergy
5. None of the above

CASE STUDY #17

The question of the abdominal pain following the appendectomy is most interesting. Vague abdominal pain is a common complaint in childhood. After an unrewarding investigation, the physician too often suggests that the pain is "faked," "put on" or "imaginary," a practice which is unfair to the patient. The normal pathway of pain of any kind is as follows: A nerve ending is stimulated; the impulse travels along afferent fibers into the brain; there connections are made with associative neurons and with efferent motor fibers which may result in withdrawal from the noxious stimulus. Very rarely, if ever, does pain sensation originate in the brain itself. Many kinds of internal stimuli representing normal physiologic variations, such as gastric contractions, distention of organs by gas or fluid, and increased abdominal pressure, stimulate afferent fibers to the brain. Such afferent messages, while being "processed" in the brain, may be misinterpreted or distorted, and perceived as pathological. Therefore, pain thresholds vary considerably amongst different individuals and within a single individual at different times, depending upon other external and internal conditions. It is the physician's responsibility to evaluate what factors are influencing the patient's perception of whatever afferent impulses are arriving at the brain. Vague or ill-defined abdominal pain is often psychogenic, but not imaginary. In this case, the first answer is correct.

QUESTION C:
VERA'S INABILITY TO RECALL WRITING A SUICIDE NOTE WAS MOST LIKELY DUE TO:
1. Fear of punishment
2. Confusion secondary to the organic lesion which also caused her convulsive disorder
3. Confusion due to the anticonvulsant medication
4. True amnesia, i.e., dissociative episodes
5. None of the above

At the time that Vera wrote the suicide note, she was taking only phenobarbital t.i.d. and had not had a seizure for four years. Hence, confusion on an organic basis is unlikely. Fear of punishment may initially have prevented Vera from remembering, but after considerable psychotherapy it is unlikely that she would have continued to have amnesia on this basis. The most likely explanation is that for this rather shy girl the very idea of writing a suicide note which correctly expressed her feelings was so shocking that it became necessary for her to bury it, first beneath the mattress and secondly in her unconscious (repression), thereby forgetting it. It was a dissociative episode; answer four is correct.

QUESTION D:
THE SUICIDE NOTE PROBABLY REPRESENTS:
1. Depression
2. Hostility
3. Another attempt to manipulate the parents
4. A common adolescent act
5. An attention-getting mechanism

The suicide note most likely represents depression in this child. As a general rule, any suicide gesture or attempt by an adolescent should at first be taken seriously. It should not be considered merely a common adolescent act. Suicide gestures by adolescents are sometimes attempts to get across the message that they want professional help. Only after every other possibility has been ruled out can we safely dispose of a suicide threat by an adolescent as merely a manipulative gesture or an attention-getting mechanism. An adolescent who makes suicidal attempts often harbors considerable hostility towards one or both parents

CASE STUDY #17

or towards other authority figures. If he is the kind of person who finds it difficult to express this hostility directly, he will sometimes turn it inward on himself, more or less as punishment for his hostile thoughts, and might attempt to kill himself. In other words, suicidal attempts might be hostile acts, expressions of depression, or both.

QUESTION E:
VERA'S FINAL DIAGNOSIS IS:
1. Hysterical neurosis
2. Chronic brain syndrome
3. Passive-aggressive personality disorder
4. Depressive neurosis
5. Schizoid personality

Despite her epilepsy, there is no real evidence that Vera's current problem resulted from a chronic brain syndrome. Her last two EEG's, taken during the previous year, were normal, and she did not have a seizure for four years. The amnesia regarding the suicide note does point towards a diagnosis of hysterical psychoneurosis, dissociative type, but there is little other evidence of this. Similarly, Vera has seemed depressed and might be diagnosed as depressive psychoneurosis, but this is probably not the best diagnosis. It is true that she is somewhat detached and distant from others, particularly authority figures, so that the diagnosis of a schizoid personality can logically be entertained. However, she is able to make friends with some peers, a fact that argues against this diagnosis. By far the bulk of her behavior can be explained on the basis of a passive-aggressive personality disorder as evidenced during her psychiatric hospital stay. She obeyed all rules and never asserted herself to ask for additional privileges, but at the same time impressed the staff as hostile. Both of her parents were also rather passive. We can see her hiding of the suicide note as a passive way of sending an aggressive message, an act so threatening to her that she was forced to repress it. Her concurrent abdominal pain might have resulted from her inability to express aggression appropriately.

During her hospital stay, treatment was focused on helping her to express all her feelings more openly, including negative ones, such as hostility. As she succeeded in learning new ways of coping with angry feelings, her abdominal pain disappeared, and she made no more suicidal gestures. Eventually she was discharged from the hospital with a good prognosis.

REFERENCES:
1. Carter, V. E. and S. Chess, 1951: Factors Influencing Adaptation of Organically Handicapped Children. J Orthopsychiatry 21:827-837

2. Drye, R. C., Goulding, R. L. and M. E. Goulding, 1973: No-suicide Decisions: Patient Monitoring of Suicidal Risk. Am J Psychiatry 130:171-174

3. Freud, A., 1952: The Role of Bodily Illness in the Mental Life of Children. Psa St of the Child 7:69-81. Reprinted in: Harrison, S. I. and J. F. McDermott, (eds.) Childhood Psychopathology, An Anthology of Basic Readings, International Univ. Press, New York, N. Y.

4. Heisel, J. S., et al., 1973: The Significance of Life Events as Contributing Factors in the Diseases of Children, III. A Study of Pediatric Patients. J Pediatrics, in Press

5. Jessner, L., 1959: Some Observations on Children Hospitalized During Latency. In: Dynamic Psychopathology in Childhood, pp. 257-268. Jessner, L. & E. Pavenstedt (Eds.), Grune & Stratton, New York, N. Y.

CASE STUDY #17

6. Lambert, J. P., 1941: Psychiatric Observations in Children with Abdominal Pain. Am J Psychiatry 98:451-454

7. Pavenstedt, E., 1956: The Effects of Extreme Passivity Imposed on a Boy in Early Childhood. Psa Study of the Child 11:386-409

8. Pleso, I. B. and K. J. Roghmann, 1971: Chronic Illness and Its Consequences: Observations Based on Three Epidemiologic Surveys. J of Pediatrics 79:351-359

9. N. B. For references on suicide, the reader is referred to the bibliography for case 44

CASE STUDY #18

A 6-Year-Old Babbles and Behaves Bizarrely

A 6 year-old white, Protestant, Appalachian boy was referred by his local speech and hearing clinic because of bizarre behavior, stereotyped mannerisms, and encopresis. Five months earlier he had been rejected for kindergarten and referred to the speech clinic because his vocalization consisted entirely of babbling, which was unintelligible even to his family.

He was the oldest of three siblings. His sisters appeared normal despite their undesirable sleeping arrangements: one shared his bed and the other slept with the parents. The patient had been hospitalized several times in infancy for malnutrition. This was apparently associated with the mother's depression regarding her difficulty separating from her own family after her marriage at age 17. After the family moved to another state, the mother apparently recovered from her depression and became the dominant parent. She admitted to doing things for the patient in ways which suggested that she was overindulgent and oversubmissive to him.

QUESTION A:
FROM THIS LIMITED INFORMATION, THE BEST EXPLANATION OF THIS MOTHER'S RECOVERY FROM HER OWN DEPRESSION IS:
1. Depressions are self-limited
2. She finally grew up
3. She identified with the child and by overindulgent care of him vicariously enjoyed the care she craved herself
4. She resolved her "oedipal depression" on leaving the state where her father lived
5. Her husband threatened to leave her if she didn't snap out of it, and this acted as a psychological "shock treatment."

There is no evidence for answers four or five in the material presented. Though depressions are indeed self-limited, answer one does not make use of the available information. Maturation (answer two) undoubtedly contributed to the recovery. At age 17, the mother had probably not matured emotionally (perhaps not physically or intellectually) and was not ready for the stress of maternal responsibility; this is one of many reasons for the failure of most teenage marriages. However, a better explanation for the mother's recovery in this case is answer three. The mother's depression was related to her dependence on her family and she later overindulged her son. Identification with the child and vicariously caring for oneself by caring for him is a common psychodynamic of mothering. It may be normal in moderation, but in excess, as in this case, it can be one cause of overindulgence and oversubmission. (For discussion of other causes, see cases 28, 37, and 55.) We have not considered here the possibility that the mother's recovery was related to the birth of a daughter. Some mothers find it stressful to care for a baby of one sex, but can mother the other sex with ease and gratification.

Though neither parent showed striking pathology, both appeared rather passive and accepting of events as they occurred. Neither had been particularly concerned about the patient's development until the school refused to accept him in kindergarten. The mother was bothered by his daytime enuresis and encopresis, which she attributed to laziness, but both parents considered his failure to talk intelligibly at age 6 a variation of normal. In the extended family there were other examples of children who did not talk until this age, including one of the father's brothers.

The patient presented as an affectively withdrawn, noncommunicative, but overactive boy who failed to relate to the interviewer as a person. He seemed more interested in objects, to which he "talked" in unintelligible gibberish.

CASE STUDY #18

There was some question of retardation, but his intelligence was difficult to assess because of his inability or unwillingness to communicate. Recent school psychological testing placed him at the mental age of 3 years, 5 months.

He was seen in individual therapy and his mother was counseled regarding his home management. He started taking thioridazine (Mellaril), eventually reaching a dose of 300 mg a day. There was steady improvement. Improved rapport was noted at the fourth visit and good interpersonal interaction by the end of two months (with speech still mostly unintelligible). The parents not only cooperated with clinic suggestions, such as getting his sisters their own bed, but also responded to constructive pressure from relatives, who had become more forthright in their criticisms of maternal overindulgence and oversubmission.

After four months of treatment, the patient related well, but remained over-active and was still speaking in only one or two-word utterances. Therefore, dextroamphetamine, 15 mg per day, was added to the Mellaril. With this, the hyperactivity lessened. He was enrolled in a Head Start program, in which he did well. In an effort to keep his drugs to a minimum, the thioridazine was gradually decreased, with a continuation of the improvement. When it had been decreased to 200 mg per day, he entered the hospital for a physical ailment, at which time all psychiatric medication was stopped.

QUESTION B:
SUCH ABRUPT DISCONTINUANCE OF PHYSICALLY "UNNECESSARY" MEDI-CINES IS COMMON PRACTICE ON ADMISSION TO A MEDICAL OR SURGICAL SERVICE. IN THE CASE OF A MAJOR TRANQUILIZER LIKE THIORIDAZINE, WE WOULD EXPECT THIS TO RESULT IN:
1. Immediate mental deterioration
2. Possible mental deterioration in days, weeks, or months
3. Gradual mental deterioration over 18 hours' time
4. No change
5. Withdrawal symptoms

In contrast to minor tranquilizers, major tranquilizers are not addictive and have no withdrawal symptoms. Furthermore, they can usually be abruptly stop-ped without immediate consequences. Even for schizophrenics who need a major tranquilizer to maintain psychological compensation, serious deterioration may not show for weeks, occasionally even months. Because of this time lapse, such patients often do not see the connection between their deterioration and cessation of drug therapy. Sometimes deterioration never comes, as will be seen in this case. In contrast, we would expect day-to-day behavioral reflection of changes in this boy's dextroamphetamine. Of course, the best way of electively discon-tinuing any psychotropic drug is by gradual tapering down. Two is the best answer.

On discharge, the patient returned to the Head Start Program without medi-cation. Though the thioridazine was not restarted, he appeared to maintain his improvement, except for reappearance of the hyperactivity. The latter was successfully treated by restarting the dextroamphetamine.

Eight months after his first clinic visit, he began to speak in complete, intelligible sentences and draw in an age-appropriate manner. The school agreed to accept him into a regular kindergarten at mid-year after further work in the speech and hearing clinic, thus allowing him to enter first grade only one year later than his age-mates.

QUESTION C:
THIS PATIENT'S INABILITY TO TALK WAS PROBABLY A MANIFESTATION OF:
1. Elective mutism
2. Conversion hysteria
3. Catatonic stupor

CASE STUDY #18

4. Mental retardation
5. Childhood psychosis or childhood schizophrenia

There may be some mental retardation, but it does not appear that this diagnosis alone would account for the symptoms seen. Elective mutism implies speaking only to selected intimates (see case 52), but this boy spoke intelligibly to no one. Though catatonia is a common cause of adult mutism, it is rare in children, and this boy was not really mute -- just unintelligible. Conversion hysteria can result in speech disruption, but not in the psychotic picture presented by this boy. He showed some autistic features, not only in his failure to communicate verbally, but also in his attempts to relate to objects more than to the interviewer. Though he did not appear to be a classical case of early infantile autism, some workers might thus diagnose him. At least, the more general term of childhood psychosis appears appropriate. Some authors consider autism a subtype of childhood schizophrenia while others consider autism and schizophrenia mutually exclusive subcategories under the generic heading of childhood psychosis. The possibility of brain damage, or at least brain dysfunction, should also be considered here, possibly related to severe infantile malnutrition and deprivation.

QUESTION D:
IN THE TREATMENT OF CHILDHOOD PSYCHOSIS, MAJOR TRANQUILIZERS AND OTHER MEDICATIONS:
1. Are not usually as effective as with adult psychotics
2. Are usually dramatic in their benefit
3. Are incompatible with a psychotherapeutic approach,
4. Can be profitably substituted for a psychotherapeutic approach
5. Are safe

Major tranquilizers carry risks, but their risks are warranted when the benefits are sufficient, as in this case. Animal research has supported the clinical impression that drug treatment can facilitate psychosocial therapy and that the combination of drugs and psychosocial therapy can effectively result in improvement which is often maintained after gradual withdrawal of the drugs (Corson, 1972; McKinney, 1972). One is the best answer. Unfortunately, drugs are not as helpful with some psychotic children as they appear to be in this case.

QUESTION E:
MATERNAL DEPRESSION DURING THE FIRST TWO YEARS OF THE CHILD'S LIFE:
1. Can, if it is severe enough, result in severe psychopathology in the child through maternal deprivation
2. Usually results in severe psychopathology in the child
3. Usually has no effect on the child
4. May have little noticeable effect on the child if another mothering figure is available
5. Results in irreversible psychological damage to the child

A depressed mother may be too preoccupied with her own depression to offer adequate mothering. At our present state of knowledge, "maternal deprivation" proper can occur only from the age of six months, after the infant is able to distinguish his mother from strangers. Prior to six months, however, maternal depression can result in stimulus deprivation, also disastrous. The latter type of deprivation is more easily prevented. Effective stimulation can be provided by any combination of affectionate people, not necessarily requiring one constant mothering figure. Even appropriate toys can help provide stimula-

CASE STUDY #18

tion. However, from the age of six months the infant requires a consistent "mother." If the natural mother is "unavailable," either physically or emotionally, someone else must supply the consistent, round-the-clock mothering necessary between the sixth and eighteenth month to prevent damage from maternal deprivation. Such deprivation usually leaves some permanent residual, but much of the apparent damage can often be reversed by appropriate treatment, both psychosocial and pharmacological, if it is supplied early enough. One and four are correct.

REFERENCES:
1. Aug, R. G. and B. S. Ables, 1971: A Clinician's Guide to Childhood Psychosis. Pediatrics 47:327-338

2. Bowlby, J., 1944: 44 Juvenile Thieves. Int J Psychoanalysis 25:107-128

3. Brown, R., 1965: Social Psychology, Free Press, New York

4. Clarke, A. D. B., 1961: Some Recent Advances in the Study of Early Deprivation. Child Psych & Psych 1:26-36

5. Corson, S., Corson, E. O'L., Kirilcuk, V., Arnold, L. E. and W. Knopp, 1972: Psychopharmacologic Facilitation of Psychosocial Therapy of Violent Behavior. Proceedings of Crime Prevention Through Environmental Design Workshop. June 19-23, 1972, Columbus, Ohio. Available from: Program for Study of Crime & Delinquency, 1314 Kinnear Road, Suite 214, Columbus, Ohio 43212

6. Crumley, F. E. and R. S. Blumenthal, 1972: Children's reaction to temporary loss of father. Paper 212, 1972 APA Convention Abstracts

7. Giovannoni, J. M. and A. Billingsley, 1970: Child Neglect Among the Poor: A Study of Parents' Adequacy in Families of Three Ethnic Groups, Child Welfare 49:196-204

8. Kanner, L., 1949: Primary Infantile Autism. Am J Orthopsychiatry 19:416-426

9. McKinney, W. T., Young, L. D., Suomi, S. J. and J. Davis, 1972: Reversing the irreversible, Paper NR-14, 1972 APA Convention

10. Reiser, D. C., 1963: Psychosis of Infancy and Early Childhood as Manifested by Children with Atypical Development. NEJM 269:790-798

11. Spitz, R., 1945: Hospitalism. Psa Study of the Child 1:43-74

CASE STUDY #19

A 15-Year-Old from the Gastroenterology Service

Gail was a 15 year-old, Jewish, female patient on the gastroenterology service, who became known to a psychiatric consultant through his friendship with the internist. A formal psychiatric consultation was not requested, but when the psychiatrist showed an interest in the case, the internist asked him if he would see the patient. Gail had suffered from ulcerative colitis for two years and was currently diagnosed as having granulomatous disease of the bowel, which was slowly progressing. The internist predicted that if she did not improve very rapidly, she would have to undergo a major bowel excision. The internist also felt that this patient and her family had some psychiatric problems.

QUESTION A:
IF THIS INTERNIST HAD NOT BEEN THE FRIEND OF A PSYCHIATRIST, HIS BEST TECHNIQUE IN MAKING A REFERRAL WOULD HAVE BEEN:
1. To tell the family and the patient that he wanted the opinion of a psychiatrist before proceeding with further treatment
2. To say nothing to the family and let the psychiatrist introduce himself, since a psychiatrist is more skillful at such things
3. To ask the patient and/or her family whether or not she/they would consent to a psychiatric consultation
4. To give a therapeutic trial on a major tranquilizer, and if it works, send for the psychiatrist
5. To send for the psychiatrist and introduce him as a neurologist
6. To tell the family that he wants a psychiatrist to help prepare the patient for the psychological adjustment to possible surgery

The primary physician, be he internist, pediatrician, or family practitioner, must, in the case of all psychiatric referrals, consider how much of his reluctance to call in a psychiatrist is due to his own feelings, and how much is due to the patient's and the family's. Although adolescents often willingly accept a psychiatric consultation and attach no stigma to it, parents may feel that if their child has an emotional disturbance, they have not behaved properly as parents. Physicians, too, may feel that calling in a psychiatrist implies they are not able to handle all aspects of the patient's care, and may therefore hesitate to make the referral. In other words, physicians can feel the same as the parents of an emotionally disturbed child; both may feel that if they had done their jobs well, the referral would not be necessary. Whether or not the physician uses the impending surgery and the psychological adjustment necessitated by a colostomy or colectomy as the justification for his psychiatric referral is immaterial. His own desire for a psychiatric opinion is quite sufficient as a reason for such consultation, and he really does not need to justify his opinion on some sort of scientific basis. If he really wants to do what is best for the patient, and if he thinks a psychiatric referral may be indicated, then he only needs to express his feelings, and in most cases his suggestion will be accepted without further ado. In the author's opinion, children over the age of 10 and certainly over the age of 12, should be included in such conversations, but the conversation should be couched in language which they can understand. The first answer is the best one.

The initial psychiatric evaluation, which took place in a general hospital, revealed that Gail had been well throughout the first twelve years of her life. As a matter of fact, when she was twelve years old, she had been involved in many rather active pursuits in conjunction with the program of a Jewish day camp. Included in these activities were her first two trips away from home, during which she suffered from minor diarrhea. At her 13th birthday, Gail was still in good health and looking forward to her 8th grade. At the beginning of the school year, she again developed diarrhea, which was diagnosed as ulcerative colitis in October.

CASE STUDY #19

The only life event which was chronologically related to the onset of her disease was the death of her paternal grandfather - actually the father of her step-father - who died in November after a long terminal illness. Her stepfather, with whom she was very close, spent considerable time with his own father at the time the patient developed diarrhea.

The patient's early development had been normal with no sign of psychiatric illness. She had developed at an accelerated pace from a psychological stand-point and appeared pseudomature by the age of 15. At the interview, she was able to give a very accurate medical history. She seemed so mature that she probably would have very little fun during her adolescent years. Apparently she had always been quite the little lady, very sophisticated and reluctant to "let her hair down" and enjoy life. She really lived a rather restricted life, although she forced her-self to participate as much as she could in various local and church-organized activities. Her illness, of course, prevented her from taking part in very active programs. She was, as a matter of fact, a semi-invalid.

QUESTION B:
THE BEST PSYCHIATRIC DIAGNOSIS IS:
1. Schizophrenia with granulomatous disease
2. Obsessive-compulsive personality disorder with psychophysiologic manifesta-tions
3. Passive-aggressive personality disorder with psychophysiologic manifestations
4. Psychophysiologic disorder in an otherwise healthy girl
5. Psychoneurosis, hypochondriacal type

The diagnosis is two-fold; she is suffering from a psychophysiologic disorder, gastro-intestinal type (ulcerative colitis or granulomatous disease), and she has a personality disorder, compulsive type, of many years standing. Answer two is the best. Passivity and hypochondriasis are clinically apparent in Gail, but they are not well enough established and prominent enough to warrant the diagnoses in answers three and five. Nothing in the history indicates schizophrenia.

QUESTION C:
THE QUESTION OF WHETHER OR NOT PSYCHOTHERAPY IN ONE FORM OR OTHER IS INDICATED COMES UP IN MOST CONSULTATIONS. WHAT WOULD BE THE BEST THERAPEUTIC APPROACH IN THIS CASE?:
1. Treatment of the personality disorder through psychoanalytically oriented therapy
2. Preparation of the child and her family for the predicted bowel surgery
3. A cautious psychotherapeutic effort aimed solely at helping the child to be less inhibited and more expressive of her feelings in conjunction with some family therapy
4. Group psychotherapy with the goal of helping the child relate to her peers
5. No psychotherapy, because the stress of uncovering psychological problems might endanger the bowel still further

Psychoanalytic therapy would very likely be effective but might require such a long period of time that it would be impractical in view of the patient's physical disease, which might necessitate the removal of her bowel shortly. Psycho-therapy with an understanding therapist would probably not be so stressful that it would aggravate her physical condition. Group psychotherapy with the limited goal of helping her relate to her peers as well as individual therapy aimed at helping her express her feelings better, might be quite appropriate. The authors would not accept the very limited goal of preparing her for surgery unless it had already definitely been decided for her. If the decision to remove her bowel in the next two or three weeks had been made, the therapist would not have enough time to bring about any psychological change and could only work toward the goal

CASE STUDY #19

of preparing her for surgery. Three is the best answer, and four is a close second. The caution suggested in answer three is meant to remind the reader that patients who have suffered from a chronic physical disease for a period of time and have undergone considerable treatment must make an important adjustment when their treatment is shifted towards psychiatric care. They may become depressed if they feel that their doctor has given up on them, or they may be strongly resistant to the notion that some of their suffering is psychogenic and might have been avoidable. These feelings may cause the patient to reject treatment. Hence the therapist must use a cautious approach.

In this case weekly individual therapy was begun, and at the same time the mother was seen regularly by a social worker who worked on supporting the notion that the patient must be given an opportunity to gain a certain amount of independence. If she was ever to become independent, she would have to learn to express herself more openly to family members and friends. This would be true whether or not the patient ever lost a large portion of her bowel.

While her medical status was being re-evaluated, the treatment goals had to remain tentative. Working closely with the internist, the therapist felt compelled to work as rapidly as possible in order to avert the surgical intervention. As the crisis lessened, the therapist and the patient could turn their attention to more basic psychological issues. After 10 months, Gail's individual psychotherapy was discontinued in favor of group psychotherapy with adolescents, which continued for 4 additional months. Gail did fairly well in group psychotherapy, and during her senior year in high school she became involved in a theatre group, a hobby which required that one express feelings quite openly. She graduated from high school. Eighteen months after the cessation of treatment she enrolled in a university away from home, where she was again involved in the theatre program and thinking seriously of acting as a career. Her bowel function had improved steadily since the beginning of therapy. Currently she has neither diarrhea nor bleeding, but she does experience occasional abdominal pain. The internist sees her three times per year and is somewhat concerned about an area of bowel that may be developing a stricture. She still takes a variety of medications.

QUESTION D:
IN GAIL'S CASE ONE WOULD EXPECT THE PROGNOSIS TO BE:
1. Poor with development of carcinoma within 2 years
2. Poor with relapse of the colitis within 2 years
3. Guarded with a tendency to relapse frequently but mildly
4. Good since she seems almost well now
5. Good as long as medications are continued

Carcinoma of the colon does occur in a certain number of these children, so their survival rate is somewhat diminished. This neoplastic change occurs on the average nine years after onset of the ulcerative colitis (Michener, et al., 1961). One would not expect such changes in two years. The prognosis must be guarded, because relapses do occur, but there is no need to be so pessimistic as the second answer. Number three is correct.

REFERENCES:
1. Blom, G. E., 1955: Ulcerative Colitis in a Five Year Old Boy. Emotional Problems of Early Childhood, Edited by Gerald Caplan, London, Chapt. 8, pp. 169-198

2. Broberger, O. and P. Perlman, 1962: Demonstration of an Epithelial Antigen in Colon by Means of Fluorescent Antibodies from Children with Ulcerative Colitis. J Exp Med 115:13-25

CASE STUDY #19

3. Davidson, M., Bloom, A. A. and M. Kugler, 1965: Chronic Ulcerative Colitis of Childhood; An Evaluation Review. Jr of Pediatrics 67:471-490

4. Engel, G. L., 1954: Studies of Ulcerative Colitis, I: Clinical Data Bearing on the Nature of the Somatic Process. Psychosom Med 16:496-501

5. Engel, G. L., 1954: Studies of Ulcerative Colitis, II: The Nature of the Somatic Processes and the Adequacy of Psychosomatic Hypotheses. Amer J of Medicine 16:416-433

6. Engel, G. L., 1955: Studies of Ulcerative Colitis, III: The Nature of the Psychological Processes. A Review and Formulation. Amer J of Med 19:231-256

7. Engel, G. L., 1956: Studies of Ulcerative Colitis, IV: The Significance of Headaches. Psychosomatic Medicine 18:334-346

8. Michener, W. M., et al., 1961: The Prognosis of Chronic Ulcerative Colitis in Children. The New England J of Med 265:1075-1079

9. Prugh, D. G., 1951: The Influence of Emotional Factors on a Clinical Course of Ulcerative Colitis in Childhood. Gastroenterology 18:339-354

10. Sperling, M., 1946: The Psychoanalytic Study of Ulcerative Colitis in Children. Psychoanalytic Quarterly 15:302-329

11. Sperling, M., 1969: Ulcerative Colitis in Children. J Am Acad Child Psychiatry 8:336-352

CASE STUDY #20

Rejection is Hard to Swallow

Roberta, a 5-1/3 year-old white girl, was brought to the clinic by her parents because of cyclic vomiting, which often resulted in dehydration and many hospitalizations.

The problem dated from the age of 18 months. The first episode had occurred during a viral illness, thought to be roseola. Roberta's typical pattern was to vomit at least once a month for several hours, sometimes days. When she was hospitalized, the parents worried that she might die. They were very frightened of her periods of dehydration. Though the parents had been told that the problem was psychological, they had sought help only through medical channels. Roberta's most recent pediatrician referred her to the child psychiatry clinic after finding no organic explanation for the recurrent vomiting.

Mother was a short, wiry, grey-haired 48 year-old ex-Catholic former Wave of Sicilian descent. She was a high school graduate, and had been a swimming instructor. She had met her husband while they were both in the military. Her own mother, who could not speak English, had to support herself after Roberta's grandfather abandoned the grandmother for a young "god-daughter" who had been brought into the home. Roberta's mother remembers her early childhood as being very deprived, with not enough to eat, not enough clothes, and harsh, punitive interchanges with her own overworked, rigid mother.

Roberta's mother as a child had recurrent nausea and difficulty gaining weight. A retrospective diagnosis of anorexia nervosa could be postulated. She was the only child to move away from the family setting. After her mother died, she was able to accept her father (Roberta's grandfather) and attended his funeral even though she "still carried a grudge." She conceived Roberta when she was premenopausal at age 42. She said she had expected her husband to "take care of" contraception. During psychotherapy, mother was often angry, and began to share her previous reluctance to have a baby at that age: she was "too old."

Father was a 50 year-old Presbyterian graduate of business college. He worked in a print shop. His psoriasis caused frequent hospitalizations and interfered with sunning or swimming. The skin shedding was of constant concern to his wife and was a symbol of underlying conflicts. He was a passive, quiet, red-haired, freckled man who laughed after teasing his wife. He described himself as a second son of a railroading alcoholic father and a domineering mother. Frequently he spoke of his rivalry with his older brother, who was "more successful" than he.

Roberta's oldest sibling, age 24, was married and had a child almost Roberta's age. The parents remembered being especially strict with him. He had experienced difficulty in school.

The middle sibling, age 20, had been a rebel and resented Roberta. The parents felt somewhat guilty about sending him to a military prep school where he improved academically and behaviorally. His relationships with both his sister and his parents were strained.

Roberta was a small girl who showed no physical abnormalities. She seemed passively controlled, somewhat mechanical, with stilted speech. She was blaming in her play with dolls. Gradually she was able to share that she did not like to have her mother and father yell. There were morbid and melancholy themes in individual psychotherapy.

QUESTION A:
THE CAUSE OF ROBERTA'S CYCLIC VOMITING COULD BE:
1. An undiscovered pyloric stenosis which needed operation
2. The parents' rigid behavior
3. Overexaggeration by her pediatrician and her parents. Her vomiting was not to be expected from a child who vomits for a few hours
4. Feelings that she was pregnant. She thought that by vomiting she could get rid of the baby

CASE STUDY #20

5. Her overconcerned parents
6. Her anxiety and anger toward her older parents, who were ambivalent about wanting her. She obtained a "payoff" when she frightened them about her death
7. A very prominent gag reflex which was easily triggered whenever she coughed

A previously undiscovered pyloric stenosis at this age would be worth publishing. Answer two may be correct, but is not very specific or complete. The third answer would be very unlikely. Pediatricians rarely refer children with such symptoms without clear documentation of the child's difficulties. The fourth answer, although possible, would be very difficult to document. Pregnancy fantasies are common in childhood, but until the child confirms this, we cannot be sure of her feelings. Since this child's symptoms began before her second birthday, this rather complex fantasy seems unlikely. Roberta's parents were overconcerned and most likely this feeling was present even before the onset of the symptoms. However, answer five is not as specific as the best answer, number six. Although children often vomit when they gag with a cough, this child did not do so every time. Rather, the vomiting seemed directly related to some psychologically significant event.

Throughout more than 50 psychotherapy sessions the parents had great difficulty in looking at their marital relationship. They frequently teased each other, and father demonstrated "gallows humor" (Berne, 1972). Mother frequently took a martyred, helpless-hopeless, "woe is me" attitude, stating that she "would die soon anyway;" that "people would not be able to do without" her when she left. She was somewhat hysterical. During an important phase of therapy, she contracted pneumonia in combination with a "nervous breakdown" as described by her general practitioner. She was treated with amytryptiline (Elavil) and in a few weeks regained her vigor.

Mother repeatedly blamed herself for many of the family's troubles. Frequently she demonstrated difficulty in abstraction. Father's passive behavior changed markedly when the male child psychiatrist joined the female psychiatric social worker. He became more assertive. He stated that following the sessions he changed at work and was able to get along with his employees much better. His psoriasis improved more than anytime since the onset of the condition.

QUESTION B:
THE BEST COMBINATION OF DIAGNOSTIC LABELS FOR BOTH MOTHER AND FATHER WOULD BE:
1. A passive-dependent oral character disorder in the father and a narcissistic, paranoid personality in the mother
2. A father with low energy levels and inability to play and a mother with hereditary anorexia
3. A passive-dependent father and a borderline schizophrenic mother, both with obsessive-compulsive characteristics
4. Passive father with psoriasis and an inadequate older mother
5. A pair of older parents with a difficult child
6. An emotionally disturbed mother and father
7. A schizophrenic father and an unliberated mother

Although father seemed to exhibit passive-dependent personality characteristics, use of the word "oral" to describe the father and "paranoid" to describe the mother would be inaccurate for the amount of data given in this case. The father apparently did have low energy levels and in the beginning didn't play very much with his daughter, but at present anorexia is not considered hereditary. The best answer, three, is supported by the father's life history and the mother's persistent thought disorder. The fourth answer is accurate but not as good as three. Not all older parents have difficulty with their children. Answers five and six are too general. There was no evidence to indicate the father was schizophrenic.

CASE STUDY #20

QUESTION C:
DURING THE INITIAL SESSIONS, MOTHER RELATED THAT SHE ALWAYS HAD
ROBERTA CLEAN UP AFTER HERSELF AND WOULD FREQUENTLY ABANDON
HER WHEN SHE BEGAN VOMITING. SHE FELT SHE WOULD FALL APART IF
SHE STAYED IN THE ROOM. MOTHER SHOULD BE ADVISED TO:
1. Hire a homemaker and allow all the parenting to be taken over by someone
   else
2. Try to communicate with the child
3. Ignore the child's vomiting
4. Ask the pediatrician to give Roberta another physical checkup
5. Begin to sort out the feelings that occur in her while the child is vomiting
6. Tell Roberta that she is vomiting because she is angry at her mother and
   because of sibling rivalry with the middle brother
7. Try to allow herself to become aware of the feelings she has during the child's
   vomiting episodes. Try to be warm and supportive to the child without giving
   the child too much "payoff" for the vomiting
8. Leave the situation and have father care for the child

In a sense, the mother was allowed to back off from the angry episodes with
her daughter and the father did assert himself some as a result of the parent
guidance. However, the first and eighth answers would have only enhanced the
mother's feelings of inadequacy. The mother was trying very much to communicate with Roberta, but in her harsh way was not succeeding. She had tried,
without success, to ignore the child's vomiting. The pediatrician's repeated
physical checkups had yielded neither diagnosis nor improvement. The fifth
answer is correct, but not as complete as seven, the best answer. The sixth
answer is over-interpretive. The mother was not psychologically oriented. Even
if she were, such an interpretation through the mother, even if accurate, would
not likely be effective. Answer seven enabled Roberta's mother to lessen her
own panic. She became somewhat aware of her anger and frustration with Roberta.

QUESTION D:
AFTER ABOUT 40 SESSIONS OF INDIVIDUAL PSYCHOTHERAPY, ROBERTA,
IN A LOUD, ANGRY VOICE, TOLD HER MOTHER THAT SHE DID NOT WANT
TO COME HOME DURING A GAME WITH ONE OF THE NEIGHBORHOOD CHIL-
DREN. THIS WAS THE FIRST TIME THIS HAD HAPPENED, AND THE MOTHER
WAS SURPRISED. IN THE PSYCHOTHERAPY SESSION SHE ASKED THE MEAN-
ING OF THIS BEHAVIOR. ANSWERS MIGHT INCLUDE THAT ROBERTA IS:
1. Acting out anger due to role-modeling in individual therapy. This may be a
   necessary phase through which Roberta must pass
2. Acting out the anger for her neighborhood friends
3. Upset about having to come home from play
4. Having her playtime cut too short
5. Needing more excercise and knows her own limitations
6. Showing assertiveness that is a sign of progress
7. Expressing the murderous rage that she feels about her mother's controlling
   behavior

It is possible that Roberta was acting out for angry neighborhood friends,
but the second answer misses the point. The first answer is the most complete.
The mechanical interpretations made in answers three, four and five do not take
into account changes in Roberta. Answer six is correct but incomplete. Answer
seven is overinterpretive.

QUESTION E:
ROBERTA USED A PENCIL TO DRAW HER FEELINGS ON THE WALL OF THE
THERAPY ROOM. WHEN SHE STARTED THERAPY, SHE MADE HERSELF A

CASE STUDY #20

TINY SPECK IN CONTRAST TO HER LARGE PARENTS. AFTER A FEW MONTHS OF THERAPY SHE MADE A LARGER STICK FIGURE, STILL SMALL IN RELATION TO THE PARENTS. ONE COULD INTERPRET THIS TO ROBERTA, THUS:
1. Roberta likes to draw on the therapy room wall
2. Roberta's small size in relationship to her parents is a continuation of the pregnancy fantasy
3. Roberta's self-concept is damaged
4. Roberta has a perceptual difficulty
5. Roberta sees herself small compared to her parents, like any other 5-1/2 year-old
6. Roberta feels better about herself now and sees herself as more equal to parents
7. Roberta should have waited until a blackboard was put up on the therapy room wall

The first answer may be true and it may also be true that Roberta's therapist liked for her to draw on the wall. However, answers one and seven miss the question of why she drew herself so differently on the two separate occasions. The third answer would seem correct, but not very complete. No evidence was given for a perceptual deficit. The fifth answer is partially true. Answer six, the best, is the interpretation made by the therapist at the time.

QUESTION F:
THE PARENTS' MARITAL RELATIONSHIP GRADUALLY IMPROVED. REPORTS FROM THE SCHOOL INDICATED THAT ROBERTA BECAME MORE ASSERTIVE AND LESS OBSESSIVE IN HER PLAY. MOTHER ALLOWED HERSELF TO BE LESS OVERPROTECTIVE. ROBERTA STOPPED COMING HOME FOR LUNCH EVERY DAY AND WALKED HOME FROM SCHOOL BY HERSELF. INDIVIDUAL PSYCHOTHERAPY FOR ROBERTA TERMINATED AND THE PARENTS TERMINATED A FEW MONTHS LATER. FOR THE FUTURE, ONE COULD EXPECT THAT:
1. Roberta will need a private school to fulfill her potential
2. Roberta's problems are just beginning
3. Roberta may develop anorexia at puberty and her ability to play will most likely be less than other children's
4. Roberta will have pseudocyesis, become frigid, have marked fluctuations in her weight, and be hospitalized for schizophrenia before she is 21
5. Roberta will get married and be free of emotional disturbances
6. Roberta's brain tumor will be discovered following an epileptic seizure in early adolescence
7. Roberta's problems may recur at puberty

Answer one does not pertain to the question. The second answer is too general and possibly incorrect. Answer three seems best to the authors. The fourth answer seems overly pessimistic, just as five seems overly optimistic. If Roberta's symptoms had resulted from a brain tumor, they would not have subsided gradually over two years of psychotherapy. The seventh answer is probably correct, but not as good as three.

REFERENCES:
1. Barbero, G.J., 1960: Cyclic Vomiting. Pediatrics 25:740

2. Berne, E., 1972: What Do You Say After You Say Hello? Grove Press, New York

3. Bruch, Hilda, 1962: Perceptual and conceptual disturbances in anorexia nervosa. Psychosomatic Medicine 24:187-195

CASE STUDY #20

4. Erickson, E. H. , 1964: Childhood and Society. Norton Press, New York

5. Groen, J. J. and Z. Feldman-Toledano, 1966: Educative treatment of patients and parents in anorexia nervosa. Br J Psychiat 112:671-681

6. King, Arthur, 1963: Primary and secondary anorexia nervosa syndromes. Br J Psychiat 109:470-479

7. Laybourne, P. C. , 1953: Psychogenic vomiting in children. Amer J Diseases of Children 86:726-732

8. Menking, M. , Wagnitz, J. G. , Burton, J. J. and R. D. Coddington, 1969: Rumination, a near fatal disease of infancy. NEJM 280:802-804

9. Satir, V. , 1967: Conjoint Family Therapy. Science and Behavior Books, Palo Alto

10. Warren, W. , 1968: A study of anorexia nervosa in young girls. J Child Psychology and Psychiatry 9:27-40

11. Winnicott, D. W. , 1971: Therapeutic Consultations in Child Psychiatry Basic Books, New York

CASE STUDY #21

A Model 12-Year-Old

Twelve year old Jimmy was referred to a child psychiatrist because his behavior had produced a community crisis. The psychiatrist admitted him to an adolescent unit for a thorough, three-month evaluation.

During this time he was a model patient, obeying every rule, and never participating in the "uprisings" which are common to adolescent psychiatric units. He participated in regular psychotherapy but related only superficially to his therapist, for whom it was very unusual not to feel close to his patients. Jimmy claimed that every patient on the unit was his friend, but that he had no "best friend." No staff member, nurse, attendant, or professional staff member felt close to Jimmy, although they could not identify any specific characteristic about him that irritated them. He participated in all group activities but never initiated anything. After three months no one, neither staff nor patient, knew much about Jimmy; he had not confided in anyone.

Jimmy was the older of two children. The second child was a girl one year his junior. When this girl was seen during the evaluation, she seemed to be more concerned about Jimmy than he was about her, but she had no specific complaints regarding his behavior.

Jimmy's parents had been married, after a three-year courtship, several years prior to his birth. His mother and father had much in common; they had been raised in the same small mid-western town, and both had fairly close ties with their family members. In fact, the mother had felt close enough to her brother that she had asked him and his wife to accompany them on their honeymoon. However, this close relationship diminished during the next 10 years as Jimmy's mother slowly withdrew from social contacts. For a year or two prior to Jimmy's admission, she had rarely been seen in public except at an occasional church supper. By this time, apparently as a result of the mother's decreasing ability to maintain close relationships, the parents had relinquished all contacts with family members, even though they were still living in the same community.

If Jimmy seemed to develop normally, it was mostly due to his father's interest rather than his mother's. She devoted herself, as best she could, to her daughter rather than to Jimmy. The father was active in 4-H Club activities where he enjoyed the contact with the children in the Club. The mother contributed to the Club only in those activities which could be done in her home, such as helping with the correspondence.

Jimmy's parents disagreed to some extent about how to handle his behavior. His mother tended to be more strict, and insisted upon school attendance despite minor somatic complaints, while the father tended to be more permissive. Despite such differences, the parents rarely argued. In fact, aggression was not expressed openly at all in the home.

In school, Jimmy did well throughout his entire scholastic career. The teachers described him as a model pupil, one on whom they could count when no other child knew the answer or had done the assignment. He was clearly a bright boy. Jimmy had one or two close friends in school.

QUESTION A:
WHAT IS THE FUNDAMENTAL PERSONALITY STRUCTURE WHICH JIMMY APPEARS TO BE DEVELOPING?:
1. Passive-aggressive personality
2. Hysterical personality
3. Sociopathic personality
4. Inadequate personality
5. Schizoid personality

CASE STUDY #21

QUESTION B:
THE CRISIS THAT PRECIPITATED REFERRAL TO A PSYCHIATRIST WAS:
1. Refusal to attend school
2. A suicidal attempt
3. Running away from home
4. An overtly aggressive act
5. Shoplifting

In this case it was necessary to reconstruct a great deal of the information, since we had no opportunity to interview Jimmy's mother. The crisis which resulted in Jimmy's referral was that he had murdered his mother. It is always difficult to evaluate a person retrospectively. However, it appears that Jimmy's mother gradually became more distant from her relatives and perhaps also from Jimmy, as she turned her attention almost exclusively to Jimmy's sister. The therapist entertained the hypothesis that Jimmy's mother became schizophrenic and was unable to provide Jimmy with a close affective relationship. As a result, Jimmy seems to be well on his way to developing a sociopathic personality disturbance.

Even though Jimmy seemed to relate well to school teachers and all of the nursing and professional staff during his three-month hospitalization, all these relationships were superficial. His therapist, who usually related well to other adolescent patients, was unable to form a close attachment with Jimmy. During all the discussions between Jimmy and his therapist about his mother's murder, Jimmy shed only one tear on one occasion; he seemed to feel little remorse about his act of aggression. He indicated that he was sorry he had killed his mother only because it resulted in his admission to a psychiatric unit for three months.

The actual deed was reconstructed thus: according to Jimmy, he awoke one morning and complained of a headache. His parents discussed the problem, and his father suggested that Jimmy stay at home, while his mother wanted him to attend school. They agreed that Jimmy should stay at home for an hour after the school bus had left, and then the mother would take him to school if the headache had subsided. After the father had left for work, Jimmy's mother still felt that he should attend school. There was an argument of sorts, but not an unusual one. Following the argument, Jimmy went up to his room, buckled a knife onto his belt, and went back downstairs. When he found his mother still angry at his refusal to attend school, he stabbed her 13 times. The mother, followed by Jimmy, ran from the house and attempted to hail a passing automobile. At this point, Jimmy fled into the nearby woods. His mother was dead upon arrival at a local hospital.

QUESTION C:
THE FOREMOST THERAPEUTIC GOAL IN THIS CASE SHOULD BE:
1. Getting Jimmy back to school
2. Developing a close relationship with Jimmy
3. Treating the depression with psychotherapy and/or antidepressant medication
4. Legal action
5. Treating his anxiety

With the information above, the therapist had the primary goal of attempting to establish a close relationship with the patient. He had to evaluate the patient's capacity to form close, positive relationships with others. In Jimmy's case this attempt was made for three months, but failed completely. While he was on the unit, his relationship to other children on the adolescent unit was closely observed in hopes that he would confide in one of them, but this did not occur. During the three months of hospitalization no other child found out the reason Jimmy had been admitted, which is an extremely unusual occurrence on such a close-knit unit.

Initially, it was expected that Jimmy would develop a deep depression after he had passed through a period of denial regarding the loss of his mother. The

CASE STUDY #21

therapist was prepared to deal with this depression. However, no such depression developed. Therefore, it seemed that this boy was truly sociopathic, that he felt little if any guilt about the murder of his mother, and that for some reason he had failed to develop the capacity to love another person. In retrospect, the therapist felt that this was due to his mother's possible schizophrenia, but this diagnosis was speculative, since the mother was not available for confirmation.

When the patient failed to develop a close relationship with the therapist or anyone else on the staff of the adolescent unit, the therapist was presented with another problem.

QUESTION D:
THE MOST APPROPRIATE DISPOSITION FOR THIS PATIENT WOULD BE:
1. Long-term residential treatment
2. No treatment, relying upon the father's close relationship with the boy to tide him over a developmental period
3. Intensive psychotherapeutic treatment for a period of up to six months
4. Long-term outpatient treatment
5. Psychopharmacological treatment

This decision is most difficult to make. If one were truly concerned about the possibility of a second murder by this boy, long-term incarceration would be indicated. How long it would take to make a real change in Jimmy's personality structure - six months of intensive treatment, years of residential treatment, or an even longer period of outpatient care - cannot be answered. To treat this boy as an outpatient would require much courage and optimism. At the present time, despite Adelaide Johnson's psychoanalytic study of murderers, we do not adequately understand such aggressive acts. The best answer appears to be one.

Jimmy was accepted in a residential treatment program designed for delinquent youths, where he remained for 11 months. Again he was a model patient. The other boys and some staff members never knew the reason for his admission and wondered why he was there. He never went through a depressive period that was discernible to the staff, but his individual psychotherapist reported that he had "worked it through." He was discharged with the recommendation that his family relocate in another state.

REFERENCES:
1. Aichhorn, A., 1935, 1963): <u>Wayward Youth.</u> Viking Press, New York, N.Y.

2. Freeman, L. and W. Hulse, 1962: <u>Children Who Kill.</u> Berkley Medallion Books, New York

3. Johnson, A.M., 1949: Sanctions for Superego Lacunae of Adolescents. In Searchlights on Delinquency. Eissler, K.R., (Ed.) New York Int. Univ. Press; reprinted in: Harrison, S.I. and McDermott, J.F., Eds.): <u>Childhood Psychopathology; An Anthology of Basic Readings,</u> New York, Int. Univ. Press, 1972

4. Lewin, B.D., 1949: Child Psychiatry in the 1830's: Three Little Homicidal Monomaniacs. <u>Psa St of the Child</u> 3/4:489-493

CASE STUDY #22

Obscene Letters to a Parish Priest

A 14 year-old white working-class ninth-grade boy was brought by his father on the suggestion of the police after he wrote two "obsc⸺ ⸺ers to one of his parish priests.

He had always seemed satisfactorily adjusted, with average school achievement, many friends, and occasional evidence of leadership. For four years he and his brother, one year younger, had played ball for the parish school and liked the priest who was coach. However, a year before referral, the boys became disenchanted with the priest because he stopped taking them so many places; he wished to spend more time with his own mother. The patient and his brother decided not to rejoin the team that year. Efforts by the priest to recruit the boys again resulted in more and more friction. About four months prior to the clinic visit, the patient worked off some of his anger by writing an "obscene" unsigned letter to the priest, "telling him that nobody liked him anymore." He admitted writing it after the police traced the letter to him through handwriting comparison.

He was forced to transfer to a public school, which he did not mind because he had a year previously asked his parents to let him transfer. However, he would rather have transferred under different circumstances because many people kidded him about the letter. Two or three weeks after the transfer he wrote a second "obscene letter," which he denied having written. At this point the police recommended psychiatric attention.

From that time until the clinic appointment things went smoothly. He passed all his subjects despite the difficulty of switching school in mid-semester. He had no further trouble and was not a discipline problem at home. He continued to enjoy time with his friends and was active in the "Y".

He was the third of six children. The father was a middle-aged "solid citizen" who discussed the boy's problem in a sensible, nondefensive fashion. He felt he had made a mistake in not letting the boy transfer when he originally asked. He did not believe that the patient wrote the letter merely to get transferred. He denied any problems in the marriage.

The patient was a lanky, well-developed, good-looking adolescent who appeared somewhat sheepish, occasionally avoiding eye contact, sometimes smiling. He was surprised and chagrined at the fuss made over the letters, which he expected the priest to forget about once he had looked at them. They were merely a way for him "to get back at him." He reported auditory hallucinations of bells ringing when he walked past the parish where the problem took place. Other people with him at these times did not hear the bells, and when he looked to see if anybody was ringing them, he saw no one there. The ringing usually stopped after he saw that no one was ringing the bells. He denied any other hallucinations, obsessions, compulsions, or suicidal or homicidal ruminations. He considered himself generally happy, crying only when he was hurt badly, such as with a sprained wrist. Though he was unable to interpret a proverb or detect a difficult absurdity, he was able to detect an easy absurdity and contrast a baby and midget adequately. He showed no evidence of thought disorder or bizarre mental content. He said with much embarrassment that the obscenities in the letters were terms like "son-of-a-bitch" which he called the priest.

QUESTION A:
THIS PATIENT'S HALLUCINATIONS OF BELLS RINGING WHEN HE WALKED PAST THE PARISH WHERE HIS TROUBLES OCCURRED IS PROBABLY:
1. Evidence of paranoid schizophrenia
2. Hysterical hallucination or "superego hallucination," probably indicating guilt about his part in the trouble
3. An organic hallucination
4. Evidence of Meniere's syndrome or some other otologic disease

CASE STUDY #22

5. Evidence of a temporal lobe lesion
6. Not a real hallucination, since it disappeared when the patient looked to see if anyone was ringing the bells

Though most of these possibilities should be at least briefly considered, various clinical facts make all but number two seem unlikely. He did not seem to present other signs or symptoms of psychosis, organic brain syndrome, or otologic disease. The termination of the bell ringing by reality checking does not disqualify it as a hallucination, but does help rule out a psychosis.

QUESTION B:
AT THIS POINT THE BEST DISPOSITION WAS:
1. Hospitalization for further evaluation and treatment
2. To tell the boy to "go and sin no more." Since he had been getting along so well the previous three months, (after the police referral), psychiatric intervention was not necessary
3. Family therapy and a tranquilizer
4. Electroencephalogram, neurological consultation, and the offer of psychotherapy
5. Psychological testing and the offer of group or individual psychotherapy

The presenting problem was of moderate concern and warranted further outpatient evaluation. Psychological testing could help elucidate the basic problem both in regard to its seriousness and need for treatment and in regard to the direction treatment should take. Neurological evaluation could be arranged later if the psychological testing raised questions about possible organicity, not likely on the basis of information thus far. Meanwhile, the boy could try group or individual psychotherapy to explore his feelings further and help prevent a future recurrence of the problem. In light of the previous three months' good record, such an offer of therapy need not be a firm recommendation until more evidence of the need is found. The best answer is five. Family therapy was not indicated in the absence of evidence of home disturbance.

QUESTION C:
WRITING THE SECOND LETTER AFTER A VISIT FROM THE POLICE CONCERNING THE FIRST:
1. Shows an impulsive inability to learn from experience, a forerunner of sociopathy
2. Shows an obsessive need to repeat
3. May indicate the intensity of the boy's anger and bitterness
4. May show the boy's trust in the priest: since the latter by then knew the source of the letters, he would probably not call the police again
5. May suggest the boy suffers hysterical amnesia and forgot he had already written the first letter

It does seem the boy had some difficulty learning from experience, but this one example hardly warrants prognosticating sociopathy. Also, he finally did learn, after the second police involvement. Answers two, four, and even five might be defended but do not seem nearly as good as three, the best answer. Undoubtedly the police involvement and forced transfer aggravated the boy's feelings of angry disappointment and helplessness, which seems the source of the urge to "get back at" the priest through a letter.

CASE STUDY #22

QUESTION D:
THE IMPORTANCE OF DETERMINING THE NATURE OF THE OBSCENITIES IN
THIS CASE WAS THAT IF THE OBSCENITIES HAD BEEN HOMOSEXUAL:
1. The case should have been disposed of without treatment
2. The boy should have been hospitalized for intensive treatment
3. The parents should have been informed so the boy could not seduce his brother
4. A different type of treatment might have been indicated
5. The boy could have been advised to "come out"

As they stand, the letters seem essentially angry outbursts with moderate
cause for concern. Though a homosexual content in the obscenities would lead to
more concern and would indicate a firmer recommendation for treatment, it would
not warrant hospitalization or alarmist warnings. It might, however, modify the
type of treatment offered. Though some authors report successful treatment of
homosexuality in heterogeneous adolescent groups, we feel an overt homosexual
problem is probably better handled in individual therapy because of the possible
disrupting effect on the rest of the group: most adolescents find it hard to em-
pathize with this problem because of their own tenuous defenses against it. Contrast this, however, with case 15, where group therapy appeared helpful for a
boy of the same age who had actually engaged in homosexual activity, but whose
main problem was a different one, acceptable for group discussion.

QUESTION E:
WHEN FACED WITH AN OBSCENE, THREATENING, OR ANGRY LETTER FROM
A KNOWN ADOLESCENT, CLERGY AND TEACHERS SHOULD:
1. Explore with the youngster why he wrote the letter and ask him to discuss
   future complaints in person. If this does not solve the problem, consider
   psychiatric referral
2. Ignore it as a passing, common adolescent phenomenon
3. Tell the adolescent's parents so they can take appropriate action, such as
   psychiatric consultation
4. Call the police to impress on the youngster the seriousness of what he did
5. Have a conference with the youngster and tell him he should get psychiatric help

Such a letter indicates intense feeling and should not be ignored. Ordinarily,
there is no need to bother the police. Parents should be told only after an attempt to work out the problem directly with the youngster. One is a better
answer than five because sometimes psychiatric referral is not necessary.

REFERENCES:
1. Berkowitz, I. H., (Ed.), 1972: Adolescents Grow in Groups, Brunner-Mazel,
   New York

2. Glass, S., 1969: The Practical Handbook of Group Counseling, BCS Publishing
   Co., Baltimore

3. Ollendorff, R., 1966: The Juvenile Homosexual Experience, Julian Press,
   New York

CASE STUDY #23

"I Could Pull My Hair Out"

Christopher had just turned nine when he was brought to the child psychiatry clinic by his white middle-class parents because of their concern about his pulling out his eyebrows and eyelashes for several months. Chris was a third-grader being treated by his pediatrician for hyperactivity with methylphenidate (Ritalin) 25 mg a day. The parents were also concerned about rituals, such as pulling up his socks, hitching up his pants, and walking almost on tiptoe.

Chris was born prematurely at eight months, the first child of the then 25 year-old parents. They felt that his developmental milestones had seemed normal and that he had a good attention span when doing things that he liked. When the time came for him to begin first grade at age six, they had kept him out until age seven because "he was too fidgety." After two months of the first grade, the teacher complained that he was making everyone else too nervous. He was also destructive at home. Therefore, the Ritalin was started when he was seven. By the time he was seen in clinic, the school had ceased complaining entirely about his behavior, and he was achieving well academically. Chris' sister, although two years younger, was only one grade behind him. This fact Chris repeated often to others within hearing of the parents.

The parents were still concerned that he was emotionally affected and had rather difficult discipline problems. Mother felt that she was "buffaloed" and no longer tried physically to contain him when he rebelled. Father used threats in order to achieve his goals. Father worked out of town frequently and the absences seemed related to Chris' behavior. Both parents had finished college and done graduate work.

Mother was a slightly overweight, worried, mousy, harrassed-looking woman who expressed her concern that she "could not handle Chris' temper tantrums." She was concerned over Chris' lack of friends and his withdrawn behavior, exemplified by his staying in his room for hours at a time. Because of her helpless-hopeless feelings, she requested a tranquilizer for herself. She stressed that Chris had been very upset for several years unless his report card was 100% A's. After several parent group therapy sessions and family sessions, she was able to begin talking about the resentment she felt towards her husband's apparent lack of feeling.

Father admitted that he was "working towards the Nobel Prize" in research, and felt that "if he pushed too hard he would never attain his goal." He was a rigorous bike racer and stated emphatically that he was proud of being able to "ride until complete exhaustion occurred" with resulting "retching at the side of the road." This had been observed by Christopher. He felt his "pain threshold, like all competitive bike racers" was extremely high. When asked if he ever let Chris have a feeling of being able to outdo him, he went into great detail about the method used to handicap himself and let Chris win at least half the time. In a family session, when Chris threw a plastic pillow in his face and almost knocked his glasses off, father vehemently denied irritation. He claimed he was not angry despite obvious tension in his face and voice.

Chris was a small, thin boy with prominent upper incisors and an odd appearance due to his clumsy gait and missing eyelashes, eyebrows, and frontal scalp hair. He was fearful, demanding, and either shy or verbally loud and abusive with few normal responses in between except when there was no social pressure.

QUESTION A:
CHILDREN WHO PULL OUT THEIR OWN HAIR ARE:
1. Usually suffering from a psychotic reaction
2. Usually obsessive-compulsive neurotics
3. Offspring of upper middle class intellectuals
4. Suffering diets deficient in vitamin E
5. Manifesting autoerotic mannerisms
6. Usually daydreaming children who do poorly in school

CASE STUDY #23

7. Trying to disfigure themselves so they will look odd and attract attention
8. Children with seizure disorders and the hair pulling is an epileptic equivalent
9. Trichotillomaniacs
10. Classified as overanxious reactions of childhood

Children who pull out their own hair have not been found to be specifically classifiable as having one set of dynamic problems relating to a specific diagnosis. The best answer for Question A should consider that these children are often obsessively neurotic as well as overanxious. The diagnosis is not limited to a certain social class nor has any evidence been found to indicate it is an organic disorder. The self-destructive elements of this disorder do not seem to be conscious. When Chris had pulled out most of the hair in the front of his scalp, he went to the barber shop on his own and had his hair cut quite short so that it would not be as noticeable. His parents were quite proud of this and felt he had been very resourceful. Answer nine, though correct, merely restates the symptom in scientific jargon. The best answer is two, although answer ten is possible.

QUESTION B:
WHEN CHRIS' FATHER SAYS THAT HE IS NOT ANGRY ABOUT CHRIS' SOCIALLY UNACCEPTABLE BEHAVIOR, THIS, IN LIGHT OF THE PREVIOUS HISTORY, MEANS THAT DAD:
1. Is an easy-going, tolerant man who is hopeful for the best
2. Is denying his real feelings of murderous rage
3. Needs practice using the Jacobsen relaxation exercises
4. Will never receive the Nobel Prize
5. Wants his son to fail so that he will feel better about himself
6. Has a poor self concept and must prove constantly to himself that life is worth living
7. Is an obsessive-compulsive neurotic who is afraid to make decisions
8. Cannot set adequate limits in order to support his son appropriately

This father seemed to have a great deal of difficulty getting in touch with his anger. The extreme limits to which he pushed himself in his athletic pursuits seemed to indicate his extreme need to stimulate and prove himself. He seemed to deny his feelings towards Chris and seemed doubtful of his own self concept. He was obsessive, but seemed to make decisions adequately enough at work in order to be promoted. He had difficulty in setting limits for Chris. Six is the best answer, but two, five, and three are also defensible.

Although methylphenidate (Ritalin), dextro-amphetamine (Dexedrine), and diphenylhydantoin (Dilantin) each proved helpful in controlling Chris' hyperactivity, explosive aggression, and temper tantrums, the worried parents felt that the drugs should be discontinued. His withdrawn behavior continued despite his father's efforts to spend more time with him in meaningful ways.

Individual therapy had seemed helpful for Chris in ventilating some of his frustrations. Group therapy was recommended and Chris came. He was initially shy and only talked to the male co-therapist, ignoring the other children and the female co-therapist.

After several group therapy sessions he refused to leave the waiting room and stated he would never return to the group. With his mother's and the therapist's assistance he entered the group room but immediately tried to leave. The co-therapist blocked his exit. Each week for several weeks he walked halfway down the hall, grinning and laughing, then bolted out of the area.

QUESTION C:
THE CO-THERAPISTS THEN RECOMMENDED THAT:
1. Father deny Chris his weekend bike riding sessions unless he enters group therapy voluntarily

CASE STUDY #23

2. Chris be dropped from group therapy
3. Another individual session per week be started
4. Chris be given a major tranquilizer
5. Chris wait in the waiting room during the group therapy session
6. Chris' parents should deliver him to the group therapy room
7. The other children in the group help Chris to come to the session
8. Chris be told that if he doesn't attend three sessions in a row, he will not be allowed to remain in the group

Chris was not dropped from the group therapy and no specific limits were recommended for him at home by the co-therapists. More individual sessions were considered, but at that time there was a shortage of therapists. It was not felt that it would be helpful for him to wait in the waiting room, since he came to the door, knocked, and turned the lights off and on just outside the group room in harassment. The members of the group wanted to help him come in but were not sure how they could help. It was finally agreed that one of the parents would accompany Chris to the group room and that if any help were needed, one of the co-therapists would be available. Within two weeks, when it seemed clear that his parents really wanted him to come, Chris was coming voluntarily. The third answer wasn't tried but could have helped.

QUESTION D:
CHRIS OFTEN HID UNDER FURNITURE IN GROUP THERAPY. HE SPOKE HESITANTLY AT FIRST. LATER HE SHARED INFORMATION ABOUT SCHOOL, BUT NEVER ABOUT HOME. THIS MEANT THAT HE:
1. Hated his family
2. Didn't trust the peers in the group
3. Didn't trust the co-therapists
4. Was only concerned with making good grades
5. Was lonely for his mother
6. Was frightened of his father
7. Could not allow himself to share information about which he had strong feelings
8. Wanted family therapy

Chris was proud of his family and seemed to show some trust in his peers in the group. His anger at the co-therapist might have indicated a lack of trust but this was not clear. Chris was very concerned about making good grades and spoke of this in the group. He did not appear lonely for his mother or frightened of his father. Whenever family dynamics for any of the children were discussed, Chris became upset. Therefore, the therapists felt that his failure to mention family issues meant that this was one of his greatest concerns. He seemed rather happy during most of the family sessions, but did not demand this instead of the group. Seven is the best answer.

QUESTION E:
CHRIS OFTEN SPUN HIMSELF AROUND ON CHAIRS AND STOOLS. HE DID NOT RECOVER "TERRITORY" FROM OTHER CHILDREN IN THE GROUP. WHEN PROVOKED, HE NEVER HURT ANYONE DIRECTLY BUT CAUSED OBJECTS TO HIT OTHERS IN THE GROUP. THE BEST THERAPIST RESPONSE WOULD BE:
1. "You enjoy hurting people indirectly"
2. "Anger is difficult for you to express"
3. "At times you appear confused"
4. "You feel unsafe at times"
5. "You don't defend youself"
6. "The group should express their feelings to Chris about his behavior"
7. "You seem to bring on accidents"

CASE STUDY #23

8. "You need support so I will hold you"
9. "Let your anger out directly"

It seems unlikely that Chris would have been able to understand what was meant by the first answer. The second answer was often used by the co-therapists, but it was not clear that Chris understood. The response that proved helpful to Chris was to mention his accident-proneness, which he then began to notice himself. The third answer concerning confusion probably would have been incorrect since it seemed that he almost knew what he was doing. It would be very difficult to apprise Chris that he didn't defend himself without this being seen as a put-down. Chris often needed support to maintain his control and seemed to enjoy the co-therapist's restraints. The last answer, similar to the first, was not helpful to Chris, because he had difficulty getting in touch with his anger. The best answers are two and seven.

QUESTION F:
CHRIS CONTINUED TO IMPROVE IN PEER RELATIONSHIPS IN SCHOOL, THE NEIGHBORHOOD, AND THE GROUP. HE OFTEN SHOWED ANXIETY ABOUT HIS GRADES, BUT OTHERWISE HE BEGAN TO SPEAK WITH LESS ANXIETY. THE PARENTS REQUESTED A CONFERENCE. THE CO-THERAPISTS MET WITH THE PARENTS, CHRIS, AND HIS SISTER. THE PARENTS EXPRESSED GRATIFICATION ABOUT CHRIS' IMPROVEMENT. THEY ASKED FOR SUG-GESTIONS, BUT SEEMED UNCONCERNED. FOR THE FUTURE, WE MIGHT SAY:
1. Father will win the Nobel Prize
2. Chris will begin pulling out his hair after treatment stops
3. Chris' isolation from peers will allow him to be deeply interested in the physical sciences and imitate his father
4. Chris will need residential treatment
5. Chris should continue in group therapy
6. Should Chris' hyperactivity recur, a stimulant should be used again
7. Chris will show symptom substitution

The long-term outlook for children who pull their hair out seems to be that they show symptom substitution, with tics or other neurotic behaviors later in life, unless the hairpulling is "eradicated" by treatment. However, it was not thought that there would be a recurrence of symptoms in this case. Children who isolate themselves from their peers have been found to develop skills in other specific areas, so the prediction in answer three is possible. Residential treatment was not recommended for Chris. The parents were very pleased to continue him in group therapy. They felt he was able to restrict his socially unacceptable behaviors to the group. It seemed that Chris' hyperactivity was decreasing, as is often seen in children approaching pre-adolescence. Five is the best answer. Six could be defended, but does not seem likely.

REFERENCES:
1. Alessi, S. L. and M. D. Kahn, 1972: Group Psychotherapy with latency age boys: research, training and practice in different settings. Paper presented at the Annual Meeting of the American Association of Psychiatric Services for Children, Washington, D. C., Nov. 5, 1972

2. Barcai, A. and E. H. Robinson, 1969: Conventional group therapy with adolescent children. Int J Group Psychotherapy 19:334-345

3. Berger, M. M., 1968: Nonverbal communications in group psychotherapy. Int J Group Psychotherapy 8:161-178

CASE STUDY #23

4. Clement, P. W. and D. C. Milne, 1967: Group play therapy and tangible re-inforcers used to modify the behavior of eight year-old boys. Behavior Res & Therapy 5:301-312, 1967

5. Delgado, R. A. and F. V. Manning, 1969: Some observations on trichotillo-mania in children. J Am Acad of Child Psychiatry 8:229-246

6. Eisenberg, L., 1972: The clinical use of stimulant drugs in children. Pediatrics 49:709-715

7. Frank, M. G. and J. Zilback, 1968: Current trends in group psychotherapy with children. Int J Group Psychotherapy 18:447-460

8. Gerard, M. W., 1949: The psychogenic tic in ego development. Psychoanalytic Study of the Child 2:133-161

9. Godenne, G. D., 1964: Outpatient adolescent group psychotherapy (Part I) Amer J of Psychotherapy 18:584-593

10. Godenne, G. D., 1965: Outpatient adolescent group psychotherapy (Part II) Amer J of Psychotherapy 19:40-53

11. Grotjahn, M., 1971: Laughter in Group Psychotherapy. Int J of Group Psychotherapy 21:234-238

12. Kimsey, L. R., 1969: Outpatient group psychotherapy with juvenile delinquents. J Dis of the Nerv System 30:472-477

13. Mahler, M. S., 1946: A psychoanalytic evaluation of tic in psychopathology of children. Psychoanalytic Study of the Child 3-4:279-310

14. Millichap, J. G., 1968: Drugs in management of hyperkinetic and perceptually handicapped children, JAMA 206:1527-1530

15. Senn, M. and C. Hartford, 1968: The Firstborn: Experiences of 8 amercan families, Basic Books, New York

16. Vargas, F. and E. Gratz, (Unpublished): Group psychotherapy for parents in the child guidance clinic

17. Wender, P. H., 1971: Minimal Brain Dysfunction in Children, John Wylie and Sons, New York

CASE STUDY #24

An Orphan Hears His Dead Grandmother

A 15-1/2-year-old, ninth-grade, black male orphan was brought by his aunt-guardian because of being very nervous and hearing voices of his grandmother calling his name since her death a year previously.

He had trouble getting to sleep, felt worse in the afternoon, and sometimes felt like he wanted to die, but denied suicidal ruminations. His sleeplessness had not been helped by two different kinds of tranquilizers, which he voluntarily discontinued because of the taste.

He presented as a tall, lanky, neatly dressed adolescent who at first appeared warm and friendly, but on sitting down appeared tired and sullen. Rapport was established with difficulty. He reported that the voices were getting worse and he had begun to hear them during the daytime as well as at night, though he never heard them when with someone else. They only called his name. When he turned around, no one was there. He appeared of dull normal intelligence. His fund of knowledge showed the ravages of cultural and educational privation. He had poor calculating ability and declined to attempt abstracting a proverb, but was able to detect an absurdity and to contrast similar things.

When he was 8 years old, his mother had died from alcoholic cirrhosis. He and his younger brother then lived with his grandmother for 6 years until she died. At that point he moved to a different city to live with his aunt, and his brother went to live with another relative. Since his grandmother had set no limits on the boys, he found it hard to adjust to the stricter environment of his aunt and uncle's home. He also found it hard to adjust to a school where he was not allowed to sass the teachers as he had in his home town. Because of his disruptive behavior, he was expelled from one school six months prior to the clinic visit. At the second school, he made a satisfactory adjustment and had a warm relationship with his guidance counselor. His aunt also noticed an improvement in his home behavior at that time.

He was started in group therapy and was given a prescription for chloral hydrate, which helped him sleep.

In group therapy he was at first hostile, somewhat bizarre, loose, and defensive. He tended to challenge the male co-therapist, but eventually accepted his authority when a firm limit was set. During eight months of group therapy he gradually became more relevant and appropriate, with gradual disappearance of the hallucinations and continued improvement in his social functioning. At about the midpoint of group therapy he was able to give up the chloral hydrate with continuation of satisfactory sleep.

QUESTION A:
THIS CASE ILLUSTRATES:
1. The sequelae of repeated object loss
2. The results of maternal deprivation
3. Organic brain syndrome
4. Normal grief reaction
5. Depressive neurosis
6. Psychotic reaction to object loss

This boy's tenuous grasp on reality and security suffered a severe blow on the death of his grandmother, the nearest thing to a mother that he had known for six years (perhaps 14), and his last surviving "caretaker" in the city where he grew up. We might deduce that he received rather poor mothering his first eight years from a severely alcoholic mother who was probably debilitated towards the end of that time. His grandmother did not seem able to provide the kind of limit-setting and structure that growing boys need, but apparently did provide some love and warmth. The result seems to have been a borderline personality who was pushed over the brink into a psychotic depression or a schizo-

CASE STUDY #24

affective psychosis by the combined loss of his grandmother and of his familiar neighborhood and friends. Answers one, two and six are correct.

QUESTION B:
INSOFAR AS THIS BOY ILLUSTRATES MATERNAL DEPRIVATION, MOST OF THE DAMAGE WAS PROBABLY DONE:

1. At birth
2. 0-6 months
3. 6-18 months
4. 2-8 years
5. At 8 years, when his mother died
6. At 14 years, when his grandmother died

The deaths were certainly serious psychological traumata--serious losses. They undoubtedly contributed immensely to the boy's problems. However, this does not fit the usual understanding of maternal deprivation. There is good reason to question the quality of his mothering from the very start. If it was deficient from infancy, most of the damage was probably done at 6-18 months, because that is the most vulnerable age, right after the infant becomes capable of distinguishing his mother from others.

QUESTION C:
THIS PATIENT'S CHALLENGE TO THE AUTHORITY OF THE MALE CO-THERA-PIST IN THE GROUP WAS PROBABLY:

1. A racial problem
2. Counter-transference
3. A reenactment of conflicts in his foster family, where he had difficulty accepting the limits set by his aunt, and especially by his uncle
4. A displacement of feelings of resentment for the teachers who thwarted his impulsive desire to do as he pleased
5. Evidence of schizophrenia
6. A sign of paranoia
7. An essential step in the resolution of conflicts which most boys work through earlier in life

This boy apparently had little chance to work through oedipal feelings prior to the time he was thrown as an adolescent into his aunt and uncle's family. His uncle seemed to be the father figure at this point, and many of his feelings about the uncle were undoubtedly transferred also to the male co-therapist, as representing authority and power. Teachers undoubtedly came in for similar transference phenomena, in addition to the problems their position of authority naturally elicited. There is nothing particularly racial, schizophrenic, or paranoid about such transference, which should not be confused with countertransference, a problem within the therapist. Answers three, four and seven are correct.

QUESTION D:
THIS CASE DEMONSTRATES THAT PSYCHOTIC ADOLESCENTS:

1. Can sometimes be adequately treated without major tranquilizers
2. Should be treated in group therapy rather than individual therapy
3. Can sometimes compensate with outpatient treatment
4. Should not be given tranquilizers
5. Can sometimes be helped even when they are at first hostile and resistant
6. 1, 3 and 5

Though tranquilizers are often useful in treatment of psychotic (and some nonpsychotic) adolescents, this patient did not appear to be helped by them and was unwilling to take them. It did seem useful, however, to help him get a good night's sleep by means of a more conservative drug, which he accepted. Likely the improved sleep pattern, as well as the psychological feeding this medication symbolized, contributed to the effectiveness of the group therapy, which was the more important treatment modality in this success. Six is the best answer.

QUESTION E:
THIS BLACK ADOLESCENT MALE'S SUCCESSFUL THERAPY PROBABLY TOOK PLACE IN:

1. An all-black all-male group with a black therapist
2. An integrated, co-ed group with co-therapists, representing both sexes and both races

CASE STUDY #24

3. An otherwise white all-male group with white leaders
4. An integrated, co-ed group with white co-therapists, one male and one female
5. An all-black co-ed group with black co-therapists

Much is presently bandied about the "necessity" of having black therapists for black patients. Though desirable, this is not always necessary. It seems more important for the therapist, of any race, to be warm, caring, perceptive, honest, and skilled. Occasionally, the clinical picture might even contraindicate a therapist of the same race, just as a therapist of the same sex or religion is sometimes contraindicated. Nevertheless, similarity of race or sex is usually an advantage in treating adolescents, for whom identification with the therapist is often an important part of therapy. The latter consideration makes male and female co-therapists highly desirable for adolescent group therapy, at least for co-ed groups. Actually, this patient was treated in a racially and sexually integrated group with white co-therapists (male and female). The therapists at first worried about race being a problem in the integrated group. However, race did not seem to be a problem for the patients, and it soon ceased to be a problem for the therapists.

REFERENCES:
1. Berkovitz, I. (Ed.): 1972: Adolescents Grow in Groups, Brunner-Mazel, Inc., New York

2. Bowlby, J., 1944: 44 Juvenile Thieves, Int'l J Psychoanalysis 25:107-128

3. Brown, R., 1965: Social Psychology, Free Press, New York, pp. 38-41

4. Clark, A. D. B., 1961: Some Recent Advances in the Study of Early Deprivation, J of Child Psychology & Psychiatry 1:26-36

5. Coleman, J. S., 1961: The Adolescent Society, Free Press, Collier-Mac-Millan, Ltd., London, Eng.

6. Comer, J. P., 1972: Beyond Black and White, Quadrangle, New York

7. Crumley, F. E. and R. S. Blumenthal, 1972: "Children's Reaction to Temporary Loss of Father" Paper 212, 1972 APA Convention Abstracts

8. Giovannoni, J. M. and A. Billingsley, 1970: Child Neglect Among the Poor: A Study of Parents' Adequacy in Families of Three Ethnic Groups, Child Welfare 49:196-204

9. Glass, S., 1969: Practical Handbook of Group Counseling, BCS Publishing Co., Baltimore, Md.

10. Grier, W. H. and P. M. Cobbs, 1968: Black Rage, Basic Books, Inc., New York

11. Kohl, H., 1967: 36 Children, Mentor & Plume Books, New York

12. Kozol, J., 1967: Death at an Early Age, Houghton Mifflin Co., Boston

13. Meeks, J. E., 1971: The Fragile Alliance, Williams & Wilkins Co., Baltimore, Md.

14. Spitz, R., 1945: "Hospitalism"..., Psychoanalytic Study of the Child 1:53-74

15. Wolins, M., 1969: Group Care: Friend or Foe, Social Work 14:35-53

CASE STUDY #25

A 6 Year-Old Terror

The parents of a six year-old girl requested placement in a residential center. They complained that she screamed with rage from morning until night. Her energy seemed endless. She threw food and furniture and wrecked their home. She refused to go to bed until 1 or 2 in the morning, and when her mother would try to get her up, she would vomit. They had kept her out of school for about four weeks, possibly because of the difficulty getting her up in the mornings.

She kept her little brother, age 2-1/2, "covered with bruises," had set the kitchen on fire, and had recently defecated in a drawer. Two large department stores had asked mother to leave because of the child's misbehavior. The parents feared eviction from their apartment because neighbors were complaining of the noise, the child's pulling up flowers, and stealing. The parents had also found her in the kitchen eating in the small hours of the morning. The only time she seemed happy was when her parents would take her to a coffee shop. She would then paint her nails, put on lipstick, and wear her mother's shoes.

One evening a neighbor, who could no longer tolerate the noise, came into their apartment and quietly put the child to bed. She immediately fell asleep.

Mother was a small, verbose, anxious woman who talked constantly and often lost the trend of what she was saying. She spoke of suffering "nerves," and said that she hated housekeeping and much preferred "being on the go." She had an older child by a former marriage who was now living with a relative.

Mother described Bonnie as born "bathed in pus" from an abscess within mother's body. She could give no further details other than that she and her infant were placed in isolation for a month following the birth. The baby was breast-fed for the first three months, but didn't nurse well and screamed most of the time. However, she took easily to the bottle, and at the time she was seen, she still insisted on having one daily. Although she walked at a year, parents were vague about her other milestones. They both agreed, however, that her behavior problems started about the time of the birth of her brother, when she was 3-1/2 years old. Parents had never allowed her to be alone with him because of her jealousy and violence.

Father appeared much older than mother. He had suffered from schizophrenia since adolescence, but claimed that he got along well as long as he remained on large doses of two major tranquilizers. He often smiled rather vacantly, but when he spoke, his ideation was appropriate. However, he had become violent on several occasions, requiring hospitalization.

On one occasion, when Bonnie was about three, mother found father sexually molesting her. When Bonnie was four years old, she insisted on sleeping with her father, and mother moved to another bedroom to allow this. She slept with him for a period of about six months.

Bonnie had never caused any trouble in the classroom. She got along well with the other first-graders and was well liked by her teacher. Her school attendance had always been erratic, but school personnel were puzzled by a letter from mother saying that the child wouldn't be back to school until she received psychiatric treatment.

A psychological evaluation indicated that she was a very precocious child who had strong feelings of isolation and depression. The projectives contained an unusual amount of sexual material, and several of the Children's Apperception Test (CAT) stories suggested that the child may have been sexually molested or have witnessed parental intercourse.

Bonnie was also concerned about her identity, she did not see herself as a little girl, but rather as an adult.

She mentioned food in eight out of the ten stories, which suggests that she may have felt very empty emotionally. She was of high average intelligence.

CASE STUDY #25

QUESTION A:
BONNIE WAS MOST LIKELY:
1. A school phobic
2. A pre-schizophrenic child resulting from heavy genetic loading
3. Suffering from a severe disturbance as a result of her parents' mental illness
4. Overly mature because the parents didn't relate well to infants or young children
5. Suffering from hypothalamic syndrome (with voracious appetite) due to the intrauterine infection

The first answer is incorrect because this child wanted to go to school. The fourth answer is wrong because Bonnie exhibits regressive behavior most of the time and pseudomature behavior only on trips to the coffee shop. There is no evidence to suggest the hypothalamic syndrome. The child was very disturbed, especially in the home situation. Her father was schizophrenic and the mother's description of the birth process sounds like the product of schizophrenic delusions. If both parents were psychotic, there was a genetic loading, but she didn't behave in a pre-psychotic manner in school. The most likely answer is three.

QUESTION B:
ALTHOUGH BONNIE APPEARED TO BE A HYPERKINETIC CHILD IN MANY WAYS, MINIMAL BRAIN DYSFUNCTION IS RULED OUT BY THE FACT THAT:
1. She was able to tell stories about the CAT cards
2. She was not hyperactive in school and got along well with teachers and peers
3. She liked to dress like a grown-up and to go to coffee shops
4. She was a precocious child
5. Her behavior was more like childhood schizophrenia

In general, the truly hyperkinetic child is hyperactive in the classroom whether or not he is at home. The child who gets along well in school while he is hyperactive and destructive at home, is usually responding to strained relationships within the family. Two is the best answer.

QUESTION C:
WE MAY SUSPECT MATERNAL DEPRIVATION BECAUSE:
1. Bonnie got along well in school, but was a behavior problem at home
2. She insisted on dressing like a grown-up
3. She got up in the night to eat and mentioned food in eight out of ten of her CAT stories
4. Her problems dated from the birth of her little brother
5. She refused to go to bed

The child who has suffered maternal deprivation often seems preoccupied with food. We see Bonnie trying to feed herself, to fill up the emotional emptiness, by keeping a bottle handy and by getting up in the night to eat. She substituted food for the emotional feeding, caring and love which she so desperately needed. The best answer is three.

QUESTION D:
ONE OF THE POSSIBLE PSYCHODYNAMICS UNDERLYING THIS LITTLE GIRL'S PRECOCIOUS MATURITY MAY HAVE BEEN:
1. That if she acted older she could go to the coffee shop
2. That mother would allow her to remain out of school because she was too "grown-up" for school
3. That mother may have encouraged her so that her daughter could baby-sit

CASE STUDY #25

4. That mother may have unconsciously encouraged the forced maturity in order to gain earlier relief from the responsibility of this disturbed child
5. That mother wanted her to grow up in order to look after father during his psychotic episodes

This may have reflected an unconscious rejection of the child by mother; one way of "getting rid" of her. However, the precocious behavior was probably overdetermined, with a number of psychodynamics contributing to it. It could have been a means by which Bonnie could deny that she was a little girl, separate from the adult mother. It also may have been a way of identifying with mother and competing with her for father's affections. The mother, who was also emotionally disturbed, had great difficulty coping with Bonnie. Therefore, she may have subtly encouraged Bonnie's adult dress, unconsciously hoping that it would facilitate her growth to adulthood. This case also illustrates the muddles that occur for children of mentally ill parents when the parents have difficulty in sorting out for themselves what's real and what's not real. The best answer is four.

QUESTION E:
BONNIE'S STEALING AND DESTRUCTIVE BEHAVIOR COULD HAVE BEEN ATTRIBUTED TO:
1. Hope
2. A desire to get even with father for sexually molesting her
3. The fact that her parents didn't give her an allowance
4. Her anger because she was kept out of school
5. Narcissism

Winnicott (1956) describes the relationship between antisocial tendencies and deprivation in children. He theorizes that the roots of antisocial behavior lie in the fact that the child has had something good (mothering) that has been taken away when the child could perceive that this was an environmental failure rather than an internal one. The withdrawal of the good went on over a longer time than the child could keep the memory alive. Hence, the stealing is a search for the child's previous relationship with the mother (before the interruption); the destructive behavior is a search for environmental stability that will contain his impulsive behavior, as mother did at an earlier time. Both the stealing and the destructiveness have an appropriate nuisance value: they call attention to the child's plight. This is exploited by the child and not necessarily unconscious. While hopelessness is one of the deprived child's outstanding features, antisocial behavior is an expression of hope. The best answer is one.

REFERENCES:
1. Anthony, E.J., 1969: A clinical evaluation of children with psychotic parents. Am J Psychiat 126:177-184

2. Bellak, L., 1954: The Thematic Apperception Test and the Children's Apperception Test in Clinical Use. New York, Grune and Stratton

3. Beres, D., Gale, C. and L. Oppenheimer, 1960: Disturbances in Identity Function in Childhood: Psychiatric and Psychological Observations. Am J Orthopsychiat 30:369-381

4. Bowlby, J., 1951: Maternal Care and Mental Health. Geneva, World Health Organization Monograph #2

5. Burke, H. and S. Harrison, 1962: Aggressive behavior as a means of avoiding depression. Am J Orthopsychiat 32:416-422

CASE STUDY #25

6. Dare, C., 1969: Your 6 Year Old. London, Corgi

7. Forrest, T., 1968: The family dynamics of the Oedipus Drama. Contemp Psychoanal 4:138-160

8. Fraiberg, S., 1972: On the sleep disturbances of early childhood in: Childhood Psychopathology. Eds: S. Harrison, and J. F. McDermott, New York, Int. Univ. Press pp. 310-339

9. Glaser, K., 1967: Masked depression in children and adolescents. Am J Psychother 21:565-574

10. Haworth, M. A., 1966: The CAT: Facts about Fantasy. New York, Grune and Stratton

11. Waelder, R., 1930: The principle of multiple function: observations on over-determination. Psychoanal Quart 5:45-62

12. Winnicott, D. W., 1958: The antisocial tendency in: Collected Papers through Paediatrics to Psycho-analysis. London, Tavistock, pp. 306-315

13. Winnicott, D. W., 1965: The effect of psychotic parents on the emotional development of the child in: The Family and Individual Development. London, Tavistock, pp. 69-78

CASE STUDY #26

"Intractable" Asthma

Sandra was six years old at the time of psychiatric evaluation. She had suffered from chronic intractable asthma since hospitalization at eight months of age. This was the history:

Though both her parents were very short, her slow weight gain and small size, with some diarrhea, had suggested the diagnosis of cystic fibrosis, and she was admitted for observation and investigation. The findings were unremarkable, but on the day of discharge the mother noticed something wrong with her respirations and called the physician's attention to it. Sandra wheezed daily from then on. Over the next five and one-half years she had many asthmatic attacks, often requiring hospitalization. At 10 months of age she was found to be skin-sensitive to many antigens and was treated with autogenous vaccine. At two years of age the hospital staff noticed an extremely interdependent relationship between mother and daughter and felt the mother was unduly concerned about the child's physical state from hour to hour. Consequently, the pediatricians considered transfer of the child to a convalescent home after she was over her acute attack.

QUESTION A:
THIS SEPARATION OF MOTHER FROM DAUGHTER, COLLOQUIALLY KNOWN AS "PARENTECTOMY," WAS PROBABLY:
1. Indicated because the mother's overprotectiveness made it difficult to treat the child in an acute attack
2. Contraindicated because the child was only a little over two years of age
3. Contraindicated because if this was a true symbiotic relationship there might be dire side effects
4. Indicated in order to make sure the child was given her medications properly
5. Inappropriate

Although there is some rationale for answer one, two, and three, the third is best. Actually, this mother was extremely able to give medications accurately and kept charts showing this. There is nothing really inappropriate with the idea of separating them (fifth answer), but on the other hand, there is no good indication for so drastic an action. If this is truly a symbiotic relationship between mother and child, it may be reasonable to separate them, but there is a real danger unless such a separation is approached properly. Both parties need tremendous support after the separation, for they will certainly suffer the loss of each other. This question is considered in detail by Jessner, et al., (1955).

The pediatricians decided to send Sandra to a convalescent home, where she spent three weeks. No help was given the mother in the meantime. Another acute attack of asthma ensued, and she was promptly readmitted to the pediatric unit, where she was reunited with her mother. When discharge was possible, the mother refused retransfer to the convalescent home since she had suffered so much during the 3-week absence from her daughter. She took the child home, vowing never to readmit her to the hospital.

She was able to maintain this promise for 28 months. Although the child had many episodes of asthma, she, with the help of the family physician, was able to handle them at home. During this two-year period the entire family structure altered to take care of Sandra. Not only was this psychologically detrimental to every member of the family, it was physically detrimental to Sandra. She developed pulmonary hypertension and cardiac failure and was finally readmitted to the hospital at the age of four and a half in severe congestive heart failure. She was hospitalized many times in her fifth year of life, often critically ill, and many people felt death would ensue in a matter of hours. On one occasion anesthesia was necessary in order to interrupt an attack of status asthmaticus. Once the parents were told she might not survive the night. The medical and nursing

CASE STUDY #26

staff continued to observe a pathological relationship between Sandra and her mother and insisted upon psychiatric help.

The severity of this illness can be illustrated by a consideration of the financial expenses attributed to it. As shown in the accompanying chart (Fig. 26.1), the average annual cost over a 6-year period was $3,825. This was in the late "50's", when the father earned $5,000 to $6,000 as a successful hairdresser. The major portions labelled "hospital" and "doctor" were paid by third parties, but the rest was "out of pocket" expense.

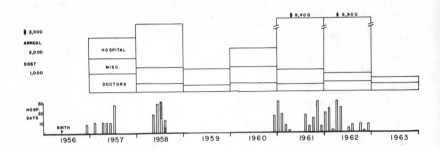

FIGURE 26.1 - Medical Costs Prior to Psychiatric Intervention

The psychiatric consultant had already seen Sandra on several occasions during the course of other visits to the pediatric unit, since she was so often there. When not acutely ill, she was a rather precocious, outgoing little girl who seemed to feel quite at home in the hospital. She'd run around the unit, often entering into a conversation the psychiatrist was having with another patient. She was at times demanding, at others whining, and at still other times a charming, sweet little girl. She was obese (secondary to steroid medication) and very short.

Her father was a somewhat effeminate man who was very proud of his experience in World War II as a Marine, pointing out the willingness of marines to "die for your buddy." Upon leaving the service he joined a family millinery but became dissatisfied in the working relationship with an uncle. He became a women's hairdresser and liked the work. There was considerable marital discord revolving around his role in the family. His wife (Sandra's mother) was highly critical of his habit of coming home from work, removing his trousers, and wandering about the house in his underwear. She saw him as unmanly and as failing to take enough responsibility. He had little interest in any form of psychotherapy.

Sandra's mother, on the other hand, had requested a psychiatric evaluation a year earlier; she was excited about the prospects of therapy. She wanted, and perhaps needed very much, to develop a strong, positive and dependent relationship with a psychiatrist. She felt that her family had forsaken her, that her husband didn't take his share of responsibility, and now the pediatricians who had once taken her child away were to be regarded with suspicion.

In this case family therapy was considered the treatment of choice, but the father's resistance, which turned into absolute refusal within three weeks, made it impossible. The mother was started in individual psychotherapy. Sandra should probably have had individual psychotherapy too, but no therapist was available at the time. She and her brother had occasional visits with the mother's therapist.

CASE STUDY #26

QUESTION B:
AS THE MOTHER'S THERAPIST, YOUR PRIMARY GOAL WOULD BE:
1. To support her and help her adjust to Sandra's disease
2. An analysis of her need to have a sick child
3. To enable her to permit both Sandra and herself to develop more independently
4. To help her accept her husband's inadequacies
5. To help her deal with her own body image problems

The first answer is very limited and suggests a rather pessimistic view of the value of psychotherapy. A thorough psychoanalysis would probably be necessary to achieve the goal stated in answer number two. The third is very realistic and by far the most important immediate goal. If the therapist succeeds at interrupting this symbiotic relationship, permitting each to grow in a more independent direction, he has achieved a great deal. Although this must be done with caution lest the mother become suspicious that he, too, is trying to take her daughter away, and although such a goal will require a lot of work, it is a very reasonable and realistic one. The goal stated in the fourth answer is inappropriate, since it would not be expected to be beneficial to Sandra. In fact, it would be more appropriate to do the opposite, namely, help her to get the father more involved in Sandra's care. Some mothers exclude the father when he really wants to be involved. The fifth answer is not pertinent to Sandra's problem.

The mother was begun in psychotherapy and two things happened. First, the child's asthma immediately and dramatically improved although no other significant changes were made in her treatment. Figure 26.1 shows that she had a few very brief hospitalizations in the beginning of her 6th year, but no further hospitalizations were necessary from that time until her current age of 16. The second thing that happened was that the mother's psychopathology became ever more evident as psychotherapy went on. When the termination of therapy was required because the therapist was moving out of town, Sandra's mother had a florid psychotic break and was hospitalized twice during the next year. This psychosis has continued over the past 10 years, but in spite of this, she has been able to maintain a degree of independence, working, living with her children, and providing considerable psychological support to them as they have grown. The marriage, however, has ended in divorce. Sandra continued to suffer from asthma and often tried to stay home from school because of "tightness" in her chest, but was continually encouraged by her mother to attend school.

QUESTION C:
IF YOU HAD BEEN ASKED TO BE SANDRA'S THERAPIST, YOU WOULD HAVE BEEN INTERESTED IN WHICH OF THE FOLLOWING GOALS?:
1. Helping her to express anger in other ways on the assumption that some of her asthmatic attacks represent internalized anger
2. Helping her to express feelings openly, including crying because the asthma may represent "internalized crying"
3. Helping her develop more trust in her physicians in order to minimize the element of anxiety in her attacks, thereby making them less severe
4. Helping her "desensitize" the bronchial tree through a deconditioning program on the assumption that her attacks represent a learned response
5. Helping her achieve more independence

Each of these goals has something to be said for it, but two is the best answer. This little girl never cried but appeared brave and "grown up" despite her life-threatening illness. (For another case of a child who couldn't cry see case 53.) Perhaps the father's admiration for brave marines encouraged her stoical attitude. This notion of psychodynamics has been described in the literature (Greenacre 1965) and was probably a factor in Sandra's case, but certainly not the whole story.

CASE STUDY #26

The goal stated in the first answer is all right, but is not so likely to be helpful in cases of asthma. The third too is good, but doesn't go far enough. The psychotherapist should aim for complete symptom relief, not simply the lessening of anxiety during attacks. The fifth goal is fine but too general. After all, Sandra's life has depended on her mother's care on many occasions; she is quite legitimately and realistically dependent and is much too young to be given full control of her medical treatment. The fourth answer may, in the future, be the most efficacious. Asthmatic-like wheezes have been induced in kittens by operant conditioning techniques (Turnbull, 1962), and attempts have been made recently to alter several physiological functions in humans in this way (Miller, 1969). However, the authors are unaware of any specific applications of such techniques to the treatment of asthma at the present time.

Sandra was never offered individual psychotherapy, but improved immensely when her mother alone was treated. The authors would like to point out, however, that they feel Sandra should have been treated, too. She continued to be symptomatic for many years, and later on had symptoms suggestive of a school phobia. She might have been helped in both of these respects. Furthermore, Sandra's treatment may have taken some of the pressure off the mother.

One additional point illustrated in this case is the occasional economic advantage of psychiatric care as compared to medical care. Even if the mother had been charged $35.00 an hour for her weekly psychotherapy and full rates during her psychiatric hospitalizations, it would still have been more economical than Sandra's pediatric care. Psychotherapy isn't always "too expensive."

REFERENCES:
1. Buffum, Wm. P., 1963: The Prognosis of Asthma in Infancy. Pediatrics 32:453-455

2. Greenacre, P., 1965: On the development and Function of Tears. Psa Study of the Child 20:209-219

3. Jessner, L., et al., 1955: Emotional Impact of Nearness and Separation for the Asthmatic Child and His Mother. Psa Study of the Child 10:353-375

4. Kluger, J. M., 1969: Childhood Asthma and the Social Milieu. J Am Acad Child Psychiatry 8:353-366

5. Knapp, P. H., 1963: The Asthmatic Child and the Psychosomatic Problem of Asthma: Toward a General Theory, in: Schneer, H. I. (Ed.) The Asthmatic Child: Psychosomatic Approach to Problems of Treatment, New York; Hoeber Div., of Harper & Row, pp. 234-255. Reprinted in: Harrison, S. I. and McDermott, J. F. (Eds.) Childhood Psychopathology, An Anthology of Basic Readings, New York, Int. Univ. Press, 1972

6. Knapp, P. H., et al., 1966: Asthma, Melancholia, and Death, II Psychosomatic Considerations. Psychosom Med 28:134-154

7. McLean, J. A. and A. Y. T. Ching, 1973: Follow-up Study of Relationships Between Family Situation and Bronchial Asthma in Children. J Am Acad Child Psychiatry 12:142-161

8. Miller, N. E., 1969: Psychosomatic Effects of Specific Types of Training. Ann of the N. Y. Acad of Sc 159:1025-1040

9. Turnbull, J. W., 1962: Asthma Conceived as a Learned Response. J of Psychosom Res 6:59-70

CASE STUDY #27

Little Joe Hears Judgmental Voices

Joe was an 8-1/2 year-old third-grade boy brought to the clinic in October by his mother for emergency evaluation because he had recently "become unable to stand any noise." He had attempted suicide by going to the bathroom and grabbing a bottle of pills, but his aunt prevented the ingestion. His mother also reported that he "seemed to be hard of hearing," had many tantrums, heard voices, grinned and giggled inappropriately, and had recently become overly attached to her. He had shown a change in his speech and a decrease in school performance. Previously, she stated, he had been a "sensible, loving, bright," serious boy, who "did good work in school."

Joe was the result of his mother's third pregnancy. She had previously delivered one stillborn and another baby who died after eleven hours. Following Joe's birth, she had undergone a hysterectomy for "cancer." Joe walked at 10 months and stuttered for a few months at 2 years of age.

The mother appeared very depressed and tearful. She frequently vacillated from saying on the one hand that the child "must have" severe emotional problems, to wondering on the other if a skull X-ray should not be done to rule out organic disease. Her 15-year marriage had been a stormy one, with frequent moves throughout the state. She divorced and remarried the same man, at which time a younger child was adopted.

The mother also seemed worried about her husband's family's mental problems: six out of eight of Joe's father's brothers and sisters had been hospitalized for mental illness. Their mother, the paternal grandmother, was hospitalized much of her life for mental illness. Joe's father was accident prone and experienced spells during which he turned white and looked wild.

Joe's teacher reported that Joe had been having severe difficulties with his work in school for about a year and a half, and was now hitting out at other children.

QUESTION A:
WHAT IS THE BEST ASSESSMENT AND MOST LIKELY CAUSE OF THIS BOY'S PROBLEM?:
1. The mother's loss of her first two babies and her feelings about her hysterectomy resulted in fear of losing her son and fostered an overdependent relationship. In addition, she is displacing angry feelings about the hospitalizations of her husband's relatives from the father to the son
2. The boy's recent hard-of-hearing spells are most likely due to a serious undiagnosed ear infection. Undoubtedly, his problems will improve
3. The family's transience has contributed to Joe's instability
4. Following the chronic stress of transience in the family, loss of loved ones, and difficulty in providing a stable family setting, it is likely that there has been some recent traumatic event
5. The mother's overprotection, the adoption of a younger sister at a time of stress with the parents' remarrying, and the family history of mental illness all contribute to the boy's present problems, including possible hallucinations
6. Joe's problems are typical of a third-grade child with minor family problems
7. The psychosis found in the boy's aunts and uncles has been inherited, and he is now having an early nervous breakdown

Item five is the best answer since it gives the best documented explanation. Answer one may be true, but it does not include the adoption of the sister as a dynamic factor. Answer number two is superficial and only considers a medical possibility. Answer number three, although probably true, is incomplete as five. Although there is some evidence to support a genetic inheritance of susceptibility to mental illness, we have to reject the last answer because it fails to incorporate the environmental factors mentioned above.

CASE STUDY #27

The mother was an obese, friendly woman, who had obviously worked very hard to present the children immaculately dressed. She stated that in her school conference she found out that the teacher had spent a "great deal of time trying to work with Joe to do his work." Joe's teacher was black and the mother stated that the father had voiced some negative feelings about that.

QUESTION B:
WHICH OF THE FOLLOWING STATEMENTS BEST DESCRIBES JOE'S FAMILY SITUATION?:
1. The mother and father, although immature, tried their best to provide a stable home for these children by remarrying
2. The mother and father's rather mild concerns about Joe can be easily checked out with a hearing test and a few sessions of parental guidance
3. The boy is probably manifesting an early onset of congenital neurologically degenerative disease
4. All of the boy's problems are due to the school's integration of teachers, to which Joe's parents object
5. The mother's pregnancy losses, her obesity, her compulsiveness, and her ambivalence will all have some bearing upon how she is likely to deal with her son. Her concern, along with her depression, indicates that she is going to suicide herself
6. The mother seems sincerely concerned and shares information concerning her family. Her anxiousness and ambivalence about Joe and herself, along with her overprotectiveness, are most likely related to her previous losses, family instability, and several recent stresses
7. More information is needed about the interaction between the mother and the father. The mother seems overprotective, and historically this is understandable

Answer six is the most complete. The first answer, although true, is an overgeneralization. Answer two denies the possibility of the boy's severe emotional disturbance, while three is an unlikely possibility, too organic. While some of the boy's problems may result from his parent's objection to the black teacher, this cannot be causing all his problems, since his troubles started before he was in this teacher's class. Answer five is partially true, but it would be an overinterpretation to state that she "is going to commit suicide herself." Answer seven is correct, but not as complete as answer six.

QUESTION C:
WHEN THE MOTHER SPOKE TO HER GENERAL PHYSICIAN DURING A VISIT FOR AN UPPER RESPIRATORY INFECTION, SHE MENTIONED THE BOY'S PROBLEMS AND EMPHASIZED THAT HE HAD RECENTLY BEEN CONSTIPATED. THE BEST COURSE OF ACTION FOR THE PHYSICIAN AFTER OBTAINING THE ABOVE HISTORY WOULD HAVE BEEN:
1. To prepare the parents and the child for future visits to discuss the problems
2. To tell the mother to call the school board and have the child's teacher changed so that he would not have to be in a classroom with a black teacher
3. To examine the child, give him a physical, obtain a barium enema, and hospitalize him for a complete neurological checkup
4. To immediately refer Joe to a child psychiatrist because of the temper tantrums
5. To tell the parents that there is nothing wrong with the child if the routine physical is normal
6. To give the child a routine examination, including a neurological workup. During this examination an effort could be made to interview the child in a friendly, supportive manner. Consider a telephone consultation with a child psychiatrist

CASE STUDY #27

7. Intensive treatment for the boy's constipation, which is highly correlated with the mother's obesity, the family's instability, the worry over the relative's mental hospitalizations, and maternal dependency

Number one, while not wrong, is an overgeneralization. Number two unfortunately may actually happen, but, of course, is incorrect, since there are other more important causes for the boy's problems. Number three also all too frequently happens and may reflect a particular physician's inability to do an adequate psychological exam, with only the organic aspects noticed. Temper tantrums are not enough for an immediate referral to a child psychiatrist. Number five is incorrect since even if the physical examination were normal, the boy certainly is not. The best answer is six. Answer seven puts too much emphasis on one physical symptom.

When he was brought in, Joe seemed very confused and frightened. He had garbled speech, sat in a slumped position, and frequently moved his eyes up, down, and sideways. After his mother left the office and he had been reassured, he spoke of hearing voices, which he thought were similar to his mother's and father's voices. Joe related that on the few occasions when his father, who was a truck driver, came home, he slept with Joe and sometimes "rolled over on him." Joe also stated that his father frequently talked about "hitting people." Joe then said that his paternal uncle "gives me a hard time" and "pushes me around," but if a woman would give him a hard time he would "pop her in the mouth."

QUESTION D:
THE MOST SIGNIFICANT MEANING OF THIS INTERVIEW WOULD BE:
1. Joe is afraid of the doctor, who reminds him of his father. His mentioning his father's aggression indicated his wish to leave the interview
2. His indistinct speech shows a need for a hearing test and a referral to a speech clinic. He is an anxious and inhibited child with displaced expressions of hostility
3. The boy seems depressed and not always in contact with reality. He is probably hallucinating and worrying about aggression in the family
4. The boy has ingested LSD at school and has a toxic psychosis
5. The boy is frightened, but following the reassuring supportive interview by a physician he should have no difficulty in school
6. The boy is obviously confused and needs help
7. The boy is mad at his uncle for pushing him around and is acting in a confused manner to gain attention

Number one assumes a transference that may not be there. Number two is only partly correct; indistinct speech is not necessarily an indication for a hearing test, but the second half of the answer is pertinent. The best answer is three. There is no evidence for answers four or seven. Answer five is too optimistic in view of all the problems of Joe and his family. The boy will continue to have difficulty despite reassurance; his symptoms are chronic as well as acute. Number six is obviously true, but is not specific enough.

QUESTION E:
THE BOY WAS ASKED TO DESCRIBE SOME OF HIS FREQUENT NIGHTMARES, BUT BECAME ANXIOUS, STARTED TO STUTTER, AND WAS NOT ABLE TO COMPLY. THE BEST WAY TO CONTINUE THE INTERVIEW WOULD BE TO:
1. Ask him to draw the picture of a person, a tree, and a house and then to leave Joe in the office alone
2. Take him for a walk through the "canteen" and buy him a treat
3. Tell him that you like him very much and that his nightmares and hearing of voices is a normal temporary phase that he will soon get over

CASE STUDY #27

4. Tell him that his inability to complete the story of his dream indicates that he is inhibited by his angry feelings towards his father
5. Tell him that his hearing is abnormal because of a recent ear infection and that the ear, nose and throat physician will see him
6. Tell him that the women's liberation movement is getting too strong and that women will have to be put in their place
7. Encourage him to tell a different dream. Suggest to him that he has been able to share a great deal of his feelings and continue to ask him questions about his life and family which he can easily answer

    Seven is the best answer. Six may be what his father would tell him, but, of course, is inappropriate. It is doubtful that his "hearing" problem is caused by an ear infection. Four is inappropriate because the boy will not be able to understand such an overly psychological interpretation. Three does not deal with Joe's feelings. Even though it may be helpful to establish rapport by taking the boy for a walk, it is not pertinent to this question. It may be helpful to have the boy draw some, but this will not necessarily allow him to feel better about himself; answer one is not appropriate at this point.

    Following the second interview, the patient had been given Thioridazine, 25 mg three times daily. He was much less anxious, and had been attending school. He stated that his terrific nightmares had subsided somewhat. During the third interview he again wore his heavy outside coat in the office. He talked about taking his father's .22 rifle and climbing into his treehouse from where he hoped that he could "shoot at things." When asked by the therapist what else he would buy if he could have money, he mentioned that he would like to "buy more guns to store up an arsenal." His speech had become more distinct. He now appeared to show an infantile, "functional speech pattern" of regression.

QUESTION F:
WHAT WOULD BE THE BEST LONG-TERM PLAN THAT COULD BE RECOMMENDED FOR JOE?:

1. The parents should be informed that the child needs no special treatment and that he will grow out of this phase in time
2. The boy needs immediate hospitalization in a residential treatment setting and the parents should move to the town in which the treatment center is located so that they can obtain intensive family treatment
3. The boy should be referred back to the general practitioner who should continue prescribing laxatives and manipulating the patient's environment
4. Joe should continue to take the major tranquilizer and should be seen in individual psychotherapy which will further clarify the psychodynamic factors. Both the mother and the father should be interviewed, and the possibility of marital counseling should be entertained
5. The patient should be referred to the speech clinic and receive speech therapy every afternoon after school
6. The parents should enroll in a behavior modification course and reward the boy only when he speaks distinctly and responds to their voices. They should also tell him that he will receive a new bike when his nightmares stop
7. The parents should be advised to seek continued treatment by a mental health professional for the boy and themselves

    The best answer is four. The boy will not outgrow his difficulties. Immediate hospitalization in a residential treatment setting may not be necessary, the parents often cannot afford it, and often there is not such a setting available. Laxatives will not be adequate treatment (number three). The boy's difficulty in speech is due to his acute psychosis rather than a functional speech disorder (number five). Number six seems too extreme an application of principles which would be more appropriate in other situations. Number seven is correct but too general

CASE STUDY #27

REFERENCES:
1. Adams, P. L. , Schwab, J. J. and Aponte, J. F. , 1965: Authoritarian parents and disturbed children, Amer J Psychiatry 121:1162-1167

2. Aug, R. G. and B. S. Ables, 1971: A clinician's guide to childhood psychosis, Pediatrics 47:327-338, 1971

3. Mahler, M. S. , 1952: On child psychosis and schizophrenia, Psychoanalytic Study of the Child 7:294-303

4. Rakoff, V. , Sigal, J. J. and S. S. Sanders: Patterns of report on the hearing of parental voices by emotionally disturbed children. J Psychiatry 8:43-50, 1970

5. Sabbath, J. , 1969: The expendable child. J Amer Acad Child Psychiat 18:272-289

6. Wilking, V. N. and C. Paoli, 1966: The hallucinatory experience. J Amer Acad Child Psychiatry 5:431-440

CASE STUDY #28

A 4-1/2-Year-Old Bullies for his Peace-Loving Father

A 4-1/2 year-old white, Protestant, middle-class boy was brought by his parents because of aggressiveness and hitting other children.

He was the oldest of three children of a couple who appeared insecure but sincere and well-motivated. They had attended a sensitivity group and were concerned about poor communications in their apartment complex. They were also concerned lest prohibitions put on children might result in inhibitions and problems later in life. This particularly worried the father, who complained that he felt guilty about having fooled his mother into thinking he was a perfect boy even though he was doing bad things she did not know about. He seemed unable to distinguish between entertaining prohibited thoughts and executing prohibited action. His difficulty distinguishing between speech and action extended to his assessment of his son's problems. Both parents were concerned about the child being able to develop his own self control rather than having to be controlled from without. They cited examples from the father's teaching experience where children would sometimes go wild when external controls were removed.

After normal gestation and delivery, with birthweight of over seven pounds, the boy showed normal developmental landmarks. The parents described him as having always been very intense and noted that he ran almost from the day he walked. They considered him more active for his age than his younger brother and perhaps more active than other boys in the neighborhood the same age.

He had successfully completed a preschool program in which his behavior was satisfactory. In fact, his teachers were surprised when they learned of his problems. He had friends, was often asked to come out and play, and much of the time seemed to get along well with other children.

His parents dated his problems to about three months previously. Prior to that time he had been so nonaggressive he would run home crying rather than fight. Then his father encouraged him to defend himself, after which he "went to the other extreme" and began hitting other children even for just saying things he did not like. This seemed to worsen progressively, but his parents did not know what to do about it.

They were not even fully aware of how serious it had become until two or three weeks prior to the clinic visit. At that time they learned his behavior had so bothered one of the other mothers in the apartment complex that she had begun to yell at him, correct him, and even shake him. She had not thought there was any use reporting his activities to his parents because he had told her that he was allowed to hit. Reportedly, other parents were also concerned about his behavior. After the patient's parents asked the other mother not to have anything to do with the boy except where her own child was involved, his behavior seemed to improve slightly.

The patient presented as a healthy youngster who made good eye contact. He was rather shy at first, but soon warmed up and answered questions. When seen with his parents, he tended to lean against one of them in an affectionate manner. At one point he stroked his hand up his mother's thigh somewhat under her skirt. His mother pulled her skirt down but made no other effort to correct him. This appeared to be part of a generally affectionate attitude. He also leaned on his father at times in an affectionate manner and at other times played quietly with toys. On one occasion he put his hands around his mother's neck in a choking fashion which his mother interrupted. Then he went to his father and socked him in the belly about four times with no paternal response or intervention. When his parents reported his rather cool, hostile reaction to a friend moving away, he participated in the discussion. He revealed that he thought the friend had moved away because of the fact that he had hit the friend. He separated from his parents easily and played with his younger brother, but complained when he was left alone for awhile. His Bender-Gestalt was unremarkable for his age. He was able to make a cross and a rather poor square.

CASE STUDY #28

QUESTION A:
THE PARENTS IN THIS CASE APPEARED:
1. Overprotective
2. Oversubmissive
3. Overcontrolling
4. Overindulgent
5. Seductive
6. Rejecting

The case presents nothing to suggest rejection, overindulgence, or overprotection. The mother's tolerance of the boy's thigh stroking seems more oversubmission than seduction. A case might be made for anxious overcontrol in the father's urging the boy to fight for himself, but we cannot conclude from one example. By contrast, the case presents many examples of oversubmission (lack of limit setting), the best answer. The parents also clearly expressed the anxious, guilt-ridden dynamics typically underlying parental oversubmission.

QUESTION B:
THIS BOY"S FIGHTING PROBABLY RESULTED FROM:
1. Antagonism to his father
2. Parental reluctance to set limits
3. His temperament
4. The interaction between his temperament and parental expectations and insecurity
5. Temporal lobe behavior disorder

This appears to be a child of rather high intensity who readily adapts to what his parents want. Because of his adaptability and eagerness to please his parents, he followed his father's instructions to hit back at other children. Because of his intensity, he naturally "went to extremes," as the parents reported. This would likely not have been a problem if the parents had felt comfortable in setting limits when they noted that he was going to such extremes. Their limit setting appeared to be paralyzed by a concern that they might interfere with his developing his own inner controls by setting such limits. Four is the best answer, with two also correct.

The parents were immediately seen for an additional hour's counseling, during which the father's feelings were further explored. The distinctions between thoughts and words on the one hand and action on the other were repeatedly explained. Both parents were assured not only that it would not hurt children to set limits firmly but also that they even needed it and would be aided in developing their internal controls by having rational, firm limits set for them. Tips were offered about how to set limits in a fair, reasonable way. The parents were advised not to let the children hit them or to engage in inappropriate fondling. If they were concerned about future inhibitions they could help prevent such problems by relating prohibitions to the time, circumstances, and age of the child. The parents seemed relieved by this counsel and appeared more confident of being able to handle the children's problems. They indicated that they would call and ask for another appointment if they felt further need for counseling after trying the things that had been discussed.

The therapist felt that the father may have been using the child's symptoms as a ticket of admission (Kanner, 1972) for himself for some therapy, and was prepared to refer the father for appropriate psychotherapy if the opportunity arose. However, the family did not call for another appointment, the problem apparently having been resolved by the therapeutic consultation.

CASE STUDY #28

QUESTION C:
THE BEST DIAGNOSIS IS:
1. Unsocialized aggressive reaction
2. Anti-social personality
3. "Difficult Child" in Thomas and Chess' terminology
4. Minimal brain dysfunction or hyperkinetic reaction
5. Explosive personality
6. Adjustment reaction of childhood

The problem is of too short duration to justify a personality disorder diagnosis, which is unlikely in preschool children anyway. The boy's problem is more "socialized aggression" than unsocialized aggression; he fought at his father's behest. He does not appear a "difficult child," being rather adaptable to parental instructions and eager to please (Thomas & Chess, 1968). For a discussion of why answer four is not correct, see question D. This is one case which is appropriately diagnosed in that overworked category, adjustment reaction. It fits the criteria of a transient situational adjustment in an otherwise normal child. Six is the right answer.

QUESTION D:
IN SPITE OF THE PARENTS' STATEMENT THAT THIS CHILD RAN FROM THE TIME HE WALKED AND APPEARED OVERACTIVE COMPARED TO HIS SIBLINGS AND OTHER CHILDREN THE SAME AGE, MINIMAL BRAIN DYSFUNCTION (HYPERKINETIC SYNDROME) CAN BE RULED OUT BY THE FACT THAT:
1. He is too young for it
2. Hyperkinetic children do not fight
3. He had no problems in nursery school
4. He did not show visual-motor deficits (Bender-Gestalt and drawing of square)
5. His presenting complaint seemed to come in response to parental instruction
6. There was no history of brain damage
7. He is the oldest in his family

"MBD" occurs more often in first-born boys, often with no history of brain damage. Such children tend to fight more than most. They often show symptoms from infancy. The absence of difficulties in school, even in nursery school, is an extremely convincing argument against the diagnosis. A useful guide is that if a child has trouble at school and not at home, he is probably hyperkinetic; if he has trouble at home and not at school, he is probably not hyperkinetic; and if he has trouble both places, he may be hyperkinetic. Four and five, though not conclusive in themselves, help to confirm the improbability of "MBD" in this case. Nevertheless, three remains the best answer. For hyperkinetic boys, see cases 1 and 32.

QUESTION E:
THE FACT THAT THIS BOY STROKED HIS MOTHER'S THIGH AND PUNCHED HIS FATHER'S BELLY COULD EASILY BE TERMED OEDIPAL BEHAVIOR. THE REASON THE THERAPIST DID NOT ATTEND TO THE OEDIPAL POSSIBILITIES IS THAT:
1. In the context of this case, it seemed more pertinent to interpret these observations in other ways
2. The boy was too young for oedipal problems
3. The boy was too old for oedipal problems
4. The therapist did not have time for the long, intensive psychotherapy which oedipal problems would require
5. The oedipal situation has been discredited as a psychiatric theory

CASE STUDY #28

Despite many recent criticisms of psychoanalytic theories, the oedipal complex remains a useful concept in trying to understand much childhood and adolescent behavior. This boy is just the right age to be involved in his first oedipal conflict, usually coming between ages 3 and 6. In fact, the sequence described might be considered acting out of normal feelings for a boy his age. Such oedipal feelings do not necessarily warrant long, intensive therapy. However, the parents' handling of the acting out warrants some advice. Therefore it is more useful to note the oversubmissive condoning of the boy's acts than to note their probable oedipal roots. One is the best answer.

REFERENCES:
1. Arnold, L. E., 1973: Is This Label Necessary? J School Health In Press, October, 1973

2. Freud, S., 1909: "Little Hans" in any collection of Freud's papers, e.g. in The Sexual Enlightenment of Children, Collier Books BS190V, New York, 1963

3. Kanner, L., 1972: Child Psychiatry, 4th Ed., Charles C Thomas, Springfield, Ill.

4. Missildine, H., 1962: Preventive Psychiatry in Emotional Development, Feelings 4, no. 10, Nov.-Dec., 1962

5. Missildine H., 1963: Your Inner Child of the Past, Simon and Schuster, New York

6. Thomas, A., Chess, S. and H. G. Birch, 1968: Temperament and Behavior Disorders in Children, New York University Press, New York

7. Thomas, A., Chess, S. and H. G. Birch, 1970: Origins of Personality. Scientific American 223:102-109

CASE STUDY #29

The Boy Who Tried to Be Perfect

Danny was a 15 year-old, thin, pale, fragile-appearing white boy who was huddled almost into a fetal position when he was transferred to the adolescent psychiatric unit from a general hospital.

He had been attending a boarding school for three years prior to admission. During the winter of the third year, at about the same time that his father married for the third time, Danny began to appear "strange." He spent considerable time doing such things as getting dressed or drinking water. He spent many hours sitting at his desk with a blank stare or sitting in the bathroom. When things became worse during the spring and summer, he was dismissed from the school.

He spent five days in the local public school but was dismissed because he was unable to participate. The family physician admitted him to a general hospital, where he was very depressed, obsessional, and delusional. He often cried hysterically. He was afriad that he would be punished by God for doing bad things. He was in the general hospital psychiatric unit for approximately one month prior to the transfer.

Danny had always been considered a "nervous" child, and he was enuretic. His mother, the father's first wife, died of breast cancer when Danny was 9 or 10 years old. He seemed to feel responsible for his mother's death, ruminating over this during his three years at the boarding school. Gradually, he tried to compensate by doing everything "perfectly," becoming very obsessive in the process. When he discovered that he could not do everything perfectly, he decided to do everything a little "imperfectly." He became compulsive in doing things first perfectly and then undoing them slightly so they were slightly imperfect. He developed many compulsive rituals, such as counting to unknown numbers prior to standing up or sitting down. He became very concerned about the way in which he put on or took off his clothes. He developed habits such as making a complete 360° turn before sitting down, after arising, and upon leaving a room to go down a corridor. He tried to always place his bicycle exactly parallel to the wall of the garage and would become anxious if the front wheel turned.

There was no history of mental illness in the family. Interestingly, both of the father's subsequent wives were women who already had diagnosed cancer of the breast. This made three wives with breast cancer. A divorce occurred about a year after the second marriage.

Physical examination revealed a rather thin boy, small for his age, but otherwise within normal limits. Psychological testing could not be accomplished at the time of admission because he would not or could not cooperate. He was reported by the school to have an IQ of 116, a probable underestimation.

His ambivalence was very marked, manifested throughout his daily life by a drive to do things and drive not to do them. He would step back and forth across the threshold of a room as if trying to decide whether or not to enter, paralyzed by his obsessiveness. He was very depressed, expecting to die, and at times attempted to bring about his own death by lying on his bed and refusing to eat, waiting for death to come. At times he was delusional about who he was and seemed very paranoid. He was unable to talk without counting, unable to get dressed without his rituals, and unable to participate in ward activities or psychotherapy because of his obsessive thinking. He also showed primary process thinking. For example, he felt that he and his therapist were one, undifferentiated being and was furious when she would not urinate for him. He feared annihilation.

The severity of Danny's illness cannot be overstated. He was originally felt to be schizophrenic and catatonic, but the most prominent picture was that of a severe obsessive-compulsive neurosis. He had considerable difficulty handling anger. He felt that he should either lie down and prepare to die if he felt angry toward someone, or he should attack that person. On many occasions in the early hospital months he did attack nurses. Tranquilizing medication and isolation were necessary on many occasions.

CASE STUDY #29

It was very difficult for Danny to participate in either individual or group psychotherapy. He was initially seen daily by his therapist, but these visits were gradually diminished to three times a week. Medication was discontinued after the first 4-5 months, when he reached a point where he could profit from individual psychotherapy. Although he participated in group activities, he never seemed to profit much from group therapy. Gradually he improved to the point where he could use his intelligence in fairly deep insight psychotherapy, and was able to give up his compulsive rituals. At times of anxiety he still resorted to some of the rituals, but not to such an incapacitating extent.

QUESTION A:
THIS CASE ILLUSTRATES WHICH OF THE FOLLOWING MENTAL MECHANISMS OF DEFENSE?:
1. Denial
2. Undoing
3. Sublimation
4. Suppression
5. Rationalization

Two very prominent features in this case are Danny's anxiety, which was truly overwhelming, and his depression, which was so great that on many occasions he wished to lie down and die. So, whatever defense mechanisms he was utilizing were not very effective. If he could have denied what he felt to be his responsibility in his mother's death, he would have been much better off. Sublimation means the channeling of psychic energy, such as hostility, into some more socially acceptable endeavor, such as athletics. It was not prominent in this case. Neither was suppression, consciously pushing down psychic material into the unconscious.

Danny did use some ineffectual rationalization. For instance, his mother told him and his younger brother that she had pain in her breast and warned them not to tell their father for fear he would make her go to a doctor. Therefore, Danny, being the oldest, felt he should have taken the responsibility for obtaining medical care, thereby saving her life. On the other hand, he reasoned that he was always a "nervous" boy anyway, and his mother had no right to rely on him this way.

In this case, undoing was the most prominent defense mechanism of those listed. This is illustrated by his attempts at undoing his previous bad or sinful behavior by becoming perfect, even by his attempts to be imperfect, undoing part of a finished task, and by all of his obsessive deliberations. Such undoing is characteristic of obsessive-compulsives.

QUESTION B:
THIS BOY WAS PARANOID ON OCCASION. WHICH OF THE FOLLOWING MECHANISMS OF DEFENSE USUALLY RESULT IN PARANOID THINKING?:
1. Repression
2. Displacement
3. Identification
4. Introjection
5. None of these

Repression, the unconscious process by which threatening or unpleasant notions are pressed into the unconscious (as opposed to suppression, a conscious mechanism described in the previous paragraph would not by itself result in paranoid thinking. Displacement usually refers to the transfer of symbolic meaning from one part of the body to another as in hysterical conversion or transfer of feelings from one person to another. Although Danny has undoubtedly used identification and introjection, they do not ordinarily result in paranoid thinking.

CASE STUDY #29

Projection is the process by which specific impulses, wishes or other aspects of self are attributed to some other person. Projection is preceded by denial, of which it might be considered a specific form. Danny, feeling he had caused his mother's death, hated himself. He denied this hatred and instead accused others of hating him. Even this paranoid projection, though, was not effective in avoiding his tremendous feeling of guilt and its resultant anxiety and depression.

QUESTION C:
THE REFERENCE TO "PRIMARY PROCESS" MEANS DANNY:
1. Has regressed to an infantile level
2. Is intellectually dealing with fundamental issues
3. Is most likely psychotic
4. Is functioning at a mentally retarded level
5. None of these

Primary process refers to the most fundamental psychological level of "thinking," characteristic of unconscious mental activity. This is contrasted with secondary process thinking, a conscious activity, which obeys the laws of grammar and formal logic. Primary process is exemplified in dreaming, the secondary process by thought. Danny's feeling of "oneness" with his therapist and expectation that she could urinate for him indicates marked regression to an infantile level of psychic organization. Answer one is the best, but three is also correct.

QUESTION D:
THE BEST FINAL DIAGNOSIS IS:
1. Schizophrenia
2. Manic-depressive illness, depressed type
3. Obsessive-compulsive psychoneurosis
4. Obsessive-compulsive personality
5. Withdrawal reaction of adolescence

Danny appeared to be schizophrenic and catatonic on admission, but the obsessive-compulsive features and response to psychotherapy led to the diagnosis of obsessive-compulsive psychoneurosis. After the initial improvement during the first year in the hospital, he decompensated a year later to a psychotic level of organization and became clearly schizophrenic. The obsessive-compulsive features which might lead to a diagnosis of psychoneurosis, as happened in this case, or an obsessive-compulsive personality disorder, are also very common in schizophrenic patients. It is sometimes very difficult to tell whether a patient is suffering from schizophrenia or a severe obsessive-compulsive neurosis. The diagnosis of a personality disorder is less tenable than either psychoneurosis or schizophrenia because Danny, although nervous and enuretic prior to his mother's death, became much worse thereafter. He was manic sometimes, attacked the nurses, and was certainly depressed much of the time, but manic-depressive psychosis is unlikely at this age and does not include obsessive-compulsive symptoms.

REFERENCES:
1. Berman, L., 1942: The Obsessive-Compulsive Neurosis in Children. J Nerv Ment Dis 95:26-39

2. Despert, J. L., 1955: Differential Diagnosis Between Obsessive-Compulsive Neurosis and Schizophrenia in Children. In Hoch, P. H. and Zobin, J. (Eds.): Psychopathology of Childhood, New York, Grune & Stratton, 240-253

CASE STUDY #29

3. Hall, M. B. , 1935: Obsessive-Compulsive States in Childhood. <u>Arch Dis Childhood</u> 10:49-59

4. Nagera, H. , 1970: Children's Reactions to the Death of Important Objects: A Developmental Approach. <u>Psa St of the Child</u> 25:360-400

5. Rycroft, C. , 1968: <u>A Critical Dictionary of Psychoanalysis.</u> Basic Books, Inc. , New York, N. Y.

CASE STUDY #30

Home Angel and Fourth-Grade Tyrant

Rebecca was a 10 year-old, fourth-grade girl of Jewish heritage. Her mother brought her to the clinic because of severe learning difficulties, being teased at school, and having no friends.

The mother recalled that at the time Rebecca was to enter kindergarten, the public school felt she was not mature enough. She consequently spent a year in a private kindergarten before starting first grade in an upper-class school at age 6-1/2. It seemed ovbious that Rebecca would have to repeat the fourth grade. With each succeeding year she became more demanding and had occasional temper tantrums while in class. Some personnel in the school system wanted to transfer her to another school outside her district because of her low IQ and "sassing" the teacher. Various IQ scores, including the Stanford-Binet and the Peabody Picture Vocabulary test, ranged from 65-75.

Rebecca had been the product of a difficult labor. Her development had been slow when contrasted with her only sibling, an older sister. Frequent trips to developmental clinics had yielded a variety of diagnoses: mild cerebral palsy, hyperactivity, and brain damage. These were difficult for the mother to accept and she resisted Rebecca's attendance at anything other than the neighborhood public school. It was not clear if Rebecca's academic problems were primarily a function of emotional problems completely or also due to an intellectual deficit. The mother was very proud of the fact that Deborah, the sister (age 13) was attending a private school, even though she was doing only fair.

Rebecca's mother was an immaculately dressed, rather assertive woman who was proud of her own achievements and, as one might imagine, held high ideals for her daughters. It was very difficult for her to admit to Rebecca's intellectual limitation. She hoped that by devoting herself to the child she could overcome the deficit. Furthermore, she seemed to feel that the birth of a defective child somehow reflected on her own capacity as a woman. It was only after considerable therapeutic support that she was able to reveal the fact that she had had two miscarriages, one early and one late in the course of pregnancy.

There was another interesting facet of this woman's life; she was exceedingly close to her own mother. The two left their families for annual vacations together. Actually, the pregnancies, births and infancies were difficult times with many unhappy associations.

Father was a nice-looking business man whose job demanded long hours daily. During initial family evaluation sessions he usually maintained a bored, depressed attitude as if he had heard it all before. Frequently, he and his wife put each other down; each then withdrew into a shell of anger.

Maternal grandmother came to two family sessions and insisted defensively the Rebecca was the only problem the family had. Between tirades against doctors, she often mentioned her high social status.

Rebecca was an average-sized, black-haired girl who smiled a great deal. She walked in a rather odd fashion with her head bobbing up and down and her left leg slightly dragging. The head bobbing had started abruptly following the change in kindergartens. She wore glasses and had a slight strabismus. She spoke mostly in a whiny, babyish, poorly articulated, demanding voice.

She frequently raised her voice in pitch to say, "Leave me alone" after she provoked other children.

QUESTION A:
IN WHICH OF THE FOLLOWING ANSWERS IS THE BEST EXPLANATION OF REBECCA'S PROBLEMS FOUND?:
1. Her birth defect with a central nervous system lesion easily accounts for all her hyperactivity, demandingness, abnormal gait, temper tantrums, and school failure
2. Rebecca's problems are caused by her mother's difficulty in relating

CASE STUDY #30

3. Although Rebecca has difficulty in public school with children whose intellect is greater than hers, she would do well in a special education class with children of her own level, where her behavior difficulties would cease
4. Rebecca's problems are related to her mother's narcissism and the father's lack of assertiveness
5. Rebecca's head bobbing is a sign that she is searching for someone who feels she is worthwhile. The limp is a means to gain attention. While hating her mother and feeling indifferent about her father, Rebecca has withdrawn into a feeling of self pity
6. Rebecca's central nervous system difficulty is handicapping. The mother unconsciously rejects the child. Rebecca hungers for a father relationship. Her demandingness may result from parental oversubmission related to guilt that the parents feel for the birth of a defective child
7. Rebecca's difficulties arise from the parents' guilt over their anger towards this defective child

Answer one implies that organic lesions account for all behavioral problems. Answer two is too narrow. Answer three is overoptimistic and gives no explanation. Answer four is correct but incomplete. Answer five overstates Rebecca's problem psychologically, ignoring the obvious physical handicap. Answer six, the best, describes a common dynamic found when parents have to face the problem of a defective child. Answer seven overlooks the central nervous system problem and other family dynamics.

QUESTION B:
AT REBECCA'S THERAPY SESSIONS, HER MOTHER FOLLOWED REBECCA AND THE THERAPIST TO THE PLAYROOM AND SAT JUST OUTSIDE THE DOOR DESPITE STRONG SUGGESTIONS THAT SHE WAIT IN THE WAITING ROOM. AT ONE POINT, SHE ENTERED THE SESSION EVEN WHEN TOLD THAT IT WOULD NOT BE HELPFUL. WHEN THE THERAPIST AND REBECCA LEFT THE PLAYROOM FOR VARIOUS ACTIVITIES, THE MOTHER COULD BE SEEN FOLLOWING AT A DISTANCE. MOTHER WAS MOST LIKELY TRYING TO:
1. Make sure that the therapist did not rape her daughter
2. Keep her daughter from dealing with anger, since she herself could not deal with angry feelings about her expectations of Rebecca
3. Let Rebecca know that her mother cared about her. By keeping distance, she was not really interfering with the individual psychotherapy
4. See what goes on in therapy since she felt that by learning play therapy technique she could relate better to Rebecca at home. By keeping Rebecca within her sight or hearing she knew that she would not die and she wouldn't have to feel guilty about not protecting her
5. Bug the therapist in her frustration about not knowing what was going on. In her own demanding, narcissistic way she was angry that she had not been able to deal with Rebecca's learning problems and peer relations herself
6. Make sure that Rebecca wore her coat during cold days when the therapist and the patient might go outside
7. Understand what the therapist was trying to do
8. Give the therapist a message about her own feelings

Answer one seems very unlikely even for a mother this disturbed. Answer two may be correct, but is incomplete. Answer three is naive and superficial. Answer four is overinterpretive. Answer five sounds possible, but not as good as eight. Answer six sounds like something mother would give as the correct answer. Answer seven is overgeneralized. Answer eight's correctness became more obvious after mother admitted her own difficulties later in therapy.

CASE STUDY #30

A three-generation symbiosis seemed obvious in this difficult case. The mother was consistently overprotective, and at the same time she childishly, like a sibling rival, would not bring Rebecca for visits unless the therapist gave her equal time.

QUESTION C:
REBECCA HAD BEEN TAKING METHYLPHENIDATE (RITALIN) FOR SEVERAL YEARS. IT SEEMED TO HELP HER, ALTHOUGH THIS WAS NOT DOCUMENTED. IT SHOULD BE RECOMMENDED THAT:
1. Rebecca be given diphenylhydantoin (Dilantin) in addition to the Ritalin since the temper tantrums are most likely epileptic
2. The Ritalin be stopped. Rebecca does not need the medication any longer. By now with adequate support from the teacher she will be able to pass the fourth grade without medicine
3. Rebecca's family relationships be studied
4. Rebecca be seen in therapy at least once a week
5. Rebecca have a trial of group therapy for her peer difficulties. Additional information from her physician, school, and birth records should be obtained. A family meeting to familiarize the psychiatrist with the relationships is necessary
6. Rebecca be placed out of the school so that she won't have to compete. Perceptual-motor training will make her less frustrated
7. The parents have therapy; they need it much more than Rebecca. They should be told that their rejecting, hostile attitudes towards their daughter are the result of their own wounded narcissistic pride. Father should work only eight hours a day, five days a week, so that he can spend more time with Rebecca and make up for time that he has lost

Temper tantrums are unlikely to be confused with true seizures. There is no present evidence that supports a definite time limit for stimulants to be given. Answer three overgeneralizes the problem. Answer four is all right as far as it goes, but the best answer is five. Answer six does not address the worst problems. Answer seven would seem to be an overreaction.

QUESTION D:
REBECCA WAS SILENT WHEN SITTING WITH HER MOTHER. SHE SEEMED TO SMILE AT HER MOTHER AND OTHERS ALL THE TIME. FREQUENTLY MOTHER SAID THAT REBECCA FELT UNHAPPY ABOUT COMING TO THE CLINIC. REBECCA WOULD ASK FOR A COKE EVERY FEW MINUTES AND SULK IF SHE DID NOT GET IT. WHICH OF THE FOLLOWING STATEMENTS IS MOST CORRECT?:
1. Rebecca was bored and needed sleep since she was up watching TV too late the night before
2. Mother and daughter had a communication problem
3. Mother consistently stated how Rebecca felt rather than asking her
4. Mother's symbiotic relationship with Rebecca meant that she could not be separated from Rebecca. She expressed Rebecca's feelings as if they were her own. Rebecca was showing mother's unconscious feelings by acting bored and being demanding
5. While mother had difficulty perceiving Rebecca's feelings, she spoke as if she could read her mind. Indirectly Rebecca showed some anger towards her mother by constantly smiling and making frequent demands. Probably few limits had been set for her in the past
6. Rebecca was an early diabetic and needed extra fluids to prevent acidosis
7. Mother had known her daughter a long time and could accurately read her mind. Rebecca's needs were common and frequently found in children of this age

CASE STUDY #30

Answer one may be true but does not look at the dynamics between mother and daughter. Answer two is correct but overgeneralized. Answer three is incomplete. Answer four could be correct but seems an overstatement. Answer five sounds the best. Answer six is irrelevant and incorrect. Answer seven seems to be how some mothers feel about the children whose feelings they overlook.

QUESTION E:
USUALLY REBECCA CAME TO THERAPY WITH A BIG SMILE ON HER FACE AND RAN RAPIDLY AWAY FROM MOTHER TO THE GROUP THERAPY ROOM. AS SOON AS SHE WAS AROUND THE OTHER CHILDREN, SHE PROVOKED ANGER WITH A LOUD, WHINY, DEMANDING VOICE. RATHER QUICKLY SHE STATED THAT SHE HATED THERAPY AND WOULD NEVER COME AGAIN. WHENEVER SHE ASKED ONE OF THE CHILDREN TO QUIT HARASSING HER, SHE GRINNED AND GIGGLED. ONE COULD INTERVENE BY:
1. Suggesting to Rebecca that her smile and her tone of voice were somewhat inconsistent. It might be helpful to remind her of how she provoked the other children's retaliation. The fact that she eagerly started into the therapy room was possibly an indication that she was gaining from it
2. Suggesting that Rebecca's grin was further evidence of her cerebral lesion
3. Rebecca was inconsistent in her behavior
4. Pointing out that Rebecca's difficulty in the group was related to the other children's vicious attacks. Without them, she would be able to cope adequately
5. Allowing Rebecca to hear herself. Ask her to reflect on her statements
6. Stating that Rebecca would be isolated from the group whenever she provoked them into retaliation
7. Interpreting that the smile on Rebecca's face during the provokation and retaliation were evidence of a thought disorder. The giggles and the gain indicated that she was probably hallucinating. The other children in the group should be made more aware of their retaliation through a rise in the therapist's voice

Answer one incorporates accurate observation and a gentle statement that may be acceptable to Rebecca. Answer two is too "organic." Answer three is too global. Answer four belies Rebecca's past history. Answer five has some merit, but is not as good as one. Answer six is poor technique at this point. Answer seven is both incorrect and overinterpretive.

QUESTION F:
SCHOOL REQUESTS FOR PARENT CONFERENCES ELICITED PANIC FROM THE MOTHER. SHE SEEMED AFRAID THAT THEY WOULD BANISH REBECCA FROM THE SCHOOL. REBECCA'S FUTURE THERAPY SHOULD INCLUDE:
1. A further neurological workup, including EEG, brain scan, skull X-rays, and pneumoencephalogram to delineate the exact nature of Rebecca's cerebral lesion. A trial of additional tranquilizers seems indicated
2. More intensive psychotherapy with Rebecca. Five-day a week psychoanalytic therapy both at school and at home might be indicated, since the parents could afford it
3. Allowing for the mother's apparent symbiosis with her own mother
4. Long-term plans
5. Prolonged individual and group therapy, a trial without the stimulant drug, and a trial of a major tranquilizer to handle some of the overt anxiety
6. Termination, because as soon as Rebecca moves into the fifth grade she'll feel so good about herself, she will stop her head bobbing.
7. Electroshock therapy to try and correct the cerebral lesion which occurred at birth

CASE STUDY #30

Answer one would be of little help. Answer two is an unusual option, not readily available in today's clinics, and probably not indicated. Just because parents can afford intensive therapy is not an indication for it. Answer three is correct, but incomplete. Answer four is not specific enough. Answer five is the best. Answer six is unlikely; the head-bobbing is unconsciously determined and not likely to leave without treatment. Also, this ignores the rest of her problems. Answer seven is obviously incorrect.

REFERENCES:
1. Alessi, S. L. and M. D. Kahn, 1972: Group psychotherapy with latency age boys: Research, training and practice in different settings. Paper presented at the Annual Meeting of the American Association of Psychiatric Services for Children, Washington, D. C. , Nov. 5, 1972

2. Barcai, A. and E. H. Robinson, 1969: Conventional group therapy with adolescent children. Int J Group Psychotherapy 19:334-345

3. Berger, M. M. , 1968: Nonverbal communications in group psychotherapy, Int J Group Psychotherapy 8:161-178

4. Chandler, C. , Norman, V. and A. Bahn, 1962: The mentally deficient in outpatient psychiatric clinics. Amer J Ment Deficiency 67:218-226

5. Chess, S. , 1962: Psychiatric treatment of the mentally retarded child with behavior problems. Amer J Orthopsychiatry 32:863-869

6. Frank, M. G. and J. Zilback, 1968: Current trends in group therapy with children. Int J Group Psychotherapy 18:447-460

7. Gerard, M. W. , 1946: The psychogenic tic in ego development. Psychoanalytic Study of the Child 3-4:279-310

8. Godenne, G. D. , 1964: Outpatient adolescent group psychotherapy (Part I) Amer J of Psychotherapy 18:584-593

9. Godenne, G. D. , 1965: Outpatient adolescent group psychotherapy (Part II) Amer J of Psychotherapy 19:50-53

10. Mahler, M. S. , 1949: A psychoanalytic evaluation of tic in psychopathology of children. Psychoanalytic Study of the Child 3-4:279-310

11. Menaloscino, F. J. , 1968: Parents of the mentally retarded. J Amer Acad Child Psychiatry 7:589-602

12. Menaloscino, F. J. , 1970: Psychiatric Approaches to Mental Retardation Basic Books, New York

13. Potter, H. W. , 1965: The needs of mentally retarded children for child psychiatry services. J Amer Acad Child Psychiatry 3:352-374

14. Solnit, A. J. and M. H. Stark, 1961: Mourning and the birth of a defective child. Psychoanalytic Study of the Child 16:523-537

CASE STUDY #31

Mother Shipped Out

A Child Welfare social worker brought in a thin, nine year-old shabbily dressed boy to discuss placement for him. He was sullen and suspicious. He expressed lack of interest in why he was brought to the clinic and insisted on remaining in the waiting room.

He was living with his mother in a small walk-up fourth floor apartment in a tough tenement section of the city. His behavior alternated between withdrawal, when he would lock himself in his room, refusing to come out, and frenzied violence when he would destroy furniture and his own possessions. He would even physically attack his mother. He played with matches and frightened himself and others by hanging as far as he could stretch out of the fourth floor window. He was also given to compulsive eating and drinking and had no friends.

The patient and his ten year-old brother were the issue of the mother's second marriage. She also had two sons by her first marriage who by this time were in their late teens. However, her second husband refused to have these boys around, so mother had sent them to live with their father. She maintained no contact with them.

The mother described the father of the patient as an "alcoholic psychopath." He deserted her when Robert was born. About two years later he was killed in an accident.

The mother never wanted children and placed the patient and his brother in residential nurseries when they were about eighteen months old. However, she occasionally had them with her on weekends. When Robert was about seven, his mother sent him to a boarding school and had his older brother placed in a foster home. She then obtained work as a maid on an ocean liner and left on a world cruise. She maintained no contact with her sons. When she returned about eighteen months later, the patient had been placed in a children's hospital following a seizure. He was adjusting well to the residential routine and the attending psychiatrist had diagnosed the seizure as related to emotional problems rather than to epilepsy.

The mother refused to discuss her son's problems with the psychiatrist and had the boy discharged against medical advice. She then immediately flew to another country with him. However, he was so violent and destructive during the flight and subsequently at home that within a week the mother took him to court and charged him with being incorrigible. He was then placed in a children's home where once more he quickly settled in under firm and kindly discipline. After several months he was returned to his mother and she then placed him in a Catholic boarding school. However, she didn't pay his fees and he was again sent home to her. He was very subdued when he arrived home on this occasion and refused to leave the apartment. During the three month period prior to the referral, he had again become violent and anti-social.

Following the interview with the social worker, the mother was persuaded to come in to discuss her son's problems. She was painfully direct as well as completely lacking in insight into his behavior. She stated that she had not wanted children and had no maternal feelings whatsoever. She suspected that both of her sons had their father's traits. She added that she despised the patient more and more and said that she felt "chained" to him. She also accused him of wanting to get "familiar" with her, i.e., to kiss her. In contrast to his attempts to obtain physical contact with her, she awakened one night to find him stabbing her bed with a knife. She threatened that if her son were not removed from her, she would have a "breakdown." She spoke again and again of her "nerves," and said that she prescribed her own medications because she did not trust physicians. She also mentioned that she had a broad knowledge of psychiatry. Finally, she presented a vague threat that she would "disappear" if her son were not removed.

A psychological evaluation indicated that the patient was functioning at the low average level of intelligence at that time. He felt very rejected and seemed to find his world a frightening, undependable place in which he could gain a niche for

CASE STUDY #31

himself only through physical prowess. The paranoid quality of some of the material, together with his lack of control over his aggressive impulses, could only have led to further conflicts and unhappiness. Although in some ways he was quite withdrawn, he was also open to contact and was able to relate well to the psychologist.

QUESTION A:
THROUGH HIS BEHAVIOR THE PATIENT SEEMED TO BE SHOUTING TO HIS MOTHER:
1. That he wanted her to know how angry he was with her for leaving him too many times and that he needed limits in order that he might be able to control his aggressive behavior
2. That most of all he wanted her to get rid of him
3. That he wanted his father back
4. That he could not stand the proverty-stricken conditions in which she made him live
5. That he hated her for cruising around the world while he had to remain in drab institutions

We see in this lad's behavior increasingly desperate attempts to elicit some affection and control from his mother which she seemed completely unable to give him due to her own emotional problems. Hence, he seemed to escalate his behavior to the point of becoming dangerous both to himself and his mother. She was still unable to respond to his needs. The best answer is one.

QUESTION B:
IN THIS CASE AN APPROPRIATE INTERVENTION WOULD HAVE BEEN:
1. To leave the boy with his mother and to provide individual psychotherapy for each of them
2. To leave them together and provide individual psychotherapy for the mother
3. To place the boy under court custody in a foster home or in residential treatment and to provide psychotherapy for him
4. Residential treatment for the boy
5. Family therapy

In most instances when the patient was placed in a structured setting, where he felt contained and that those around him were concerned about his well-being, he settled down and made a fairly adequate adjustment. Short term individual psychotherapy might have been considered in order to help him better understand and accept his mother's limitations. This boy certainly needed the protection of long term relationships with people he could trust in a setting that mother could not suddenly move in and destroy. Court custody was necessary to prevent the mother from capriciously moving him again. Three is correct.

QUESTION C:
THE FACTORS IN THIS BOY'S LIFE WHICH MAY HAVE PREVENTED HIM FROM BEING EVEN MORE SEVERELY EMOTIONALLY DISTURBED MAY HAVE BEEN:
1. That his two older half-brothers left early in his life
2. That he had a chance to see much of the world early in life by traveling with his mother
3. That his mother kept him with her until he was eighteen months old and his brother remained with him in the residential nursery
4. That his alcoholic father left
5. That his mother occasionally had him with her on weekends during his early years and he may have found kindly, firm people with whom he could relate during his many placements

CASE STUDY #31

Although this case is a dramatic example of maternal deprivation, the patient still had the capacity to make attachments. Although he was emotionally damaged, his needs for affection and containment suggested there was still the possibility that he could make an adjustment if an appropriate setting could be found for him. The best answers are three and five.

QUESTION D:
WHEN ROBERT HUNG OUT OF THE FOURTH FLOOR WINDOW, HE WAS:
1. Expressing his ambivalence
2. Showing off
3. Trying to commit suicide
4. Practicing gymnastics
5. Trying to get mother to express concern about him

While this is a good example of the extremes to which this boy would go to arouse feelings of concern in his mother, his acts of precariously hanging out of the fourth floor window demonstrated, on a deeper level, Robert's ambivalent feelings, i.e., his wish to live and his wish to die. Another example of his ambivalence or co-existent feelings was apparent in his efforts to kiss mother and to stab her bed while she slept, i.e., his love and his hate. The best answers are one and five.

QUESTION E:
THIS BOY'S COMPULSIVE EATING SHOWED:
1. That his mother starved him
2. His obsessive-compulsive traits
3. His feelings of affective starvation
4. Oral aggression
5. A normal, healthy appetite for a growing boy

This boy was certainly starved for affection. Consequently, his compulsive eating was probably a constant effort to assuage the feelings of emptiness in his inner world. The best answer is three. (See Case 6, Question B and Case 32)

REFERENCES:
1. Bowlby, J., 1958: The nature of the child's tie to his mother. Int J Psychoanal 39:350-373

2. Bowlby, J., 1953: Some pathological processes set in train by early mother-child separation. J Ment Sci 99:265-272

3. Burkes, H. and S. Harrison, 1962: Aggressive behavior as a means of avoiding depression. Am J Orthopsychiat 32:416-422

4. Earle, A. M. and B. V. Earle, 1961: Early maternal deprivation and later psychiatric illness. Am J Orthopsychiat 31:181-186

5. Frank, G., 1965: The role of the family in the development of psychopathology. Psychol Bull 64:191-205

6. Herzog, E. and C. E. Sudia, 1969: Fatherless homes: a review of research. In: Annual Progress in Child Psychiatry and Child Development. Eds., S. Chess and A. Thomas, New York: Brunner/Mazel pp. 341-351

CASE STUDY #31

7. McCord, V., McCord, W. and E. Thurber, 1962: Some effects of paternal absence on male children. J Abnorm Soc Psychol 64:361-369

8. Redl, F. and D. Wineman, 1952: Controls from Within. Glencoe, Illinois, The Free Press

9. Wolff, S., 1969: Children Under Stress. London, Penguin Press

CASE STUDY #32

Whom Can You Trust When Your Father is Wanted for Murder?

A seven year-old, white, Catholic, second-grade boy was brought to the clinic by his mother because of school misbehavior and suicide threats since his father had become a fugitive from the law a year before. Despite an IQ of 130, he was not reading at age or grade level.

Though psychological testing showed evidence of visual-motor dysfunction, it was felt that his behavior disturbance was mostly associated with the abandonment by his beloved father, who was wanted for murder. This boy had been a much desired child who was born eight years after the couple's only other child, a girl. He had been spoiled and doted upon, especially by his father, who spent a lot of time with him. A year earlier, the father allegedly killed a man who had been dating his niece, and then disappeared. During this time the boy had many fantasies relative to the television program, "The Fugitive," which was popular about that time. He became overly sensitive with friends and classmates. Though at first charming, he tended to wear on the nerves of those who had to put up with his inability to conform to the requirements of a given situation. He tended to tease and test. For instance, knowing the doctor had been informed of his suicide threats, he asked where the windows were and how many floors up he was.

His symptoms tended to worsen whenever his mother would be temporarily ill. At such times he wanted to sleep in her bedroom and verbalized fears about her health.

He was seen in a twice-a-week therapy for almost three years. His first two therapists saw him for only six months each before rotating off the service. At first he tended to avoid treatment. He spent a lot of time out of the therapy room wandering around and trying to set up triangles with various secretaries and his first two therapists. When the third therapist, starting a two-year fellowship, accepted his invitation to accompany him on the wanderings, the boy soon developed an attachment. This attachment was then used as leverage to keep him in the therapy room: the therapist gradually refused to wander the halls with him, and the boy preferred to stay in the room with the therapist rather than wander off. He started bringing in snacks and treats which he and the therapist shared. He repeatedly expressed satisfaction that he could have this therapist for "four times" (two years) rather than only a six-month rotation. (See cases 12 and 52 for discussions of therapist rotations).

In the second month with this therapist (after about a year of treatment), his father was captured. His reaction to this was to begin verbalizing a lot of anger, resentment, and even desire to kill his father. He repeatedly acted out trials and executions in which he revelled in hanging, shooting, or beating to death the puppet defendant, and could hardly wait to get the trial over to begin the execution. Eventually, he was able to tolerate a visit with his father and fell into his arms in tears. He began to talk about how "we" were going to "get a lawyer and fight it."

From the beginning, there had been strains of suspiciousness and sensitivity, catalyzed by his fantasies about the questions detectives had asked him. After his father's capture, these began to crystalize into definite paranoid tendencies. He began accusing the therapist of conspiring with the police and the school officials, of "tailing" him, and even of actually being an undercover police agent rather than a doctor. At one point, the therapist was asked to prove his legitimate role by showing his hospital identification card. The boy related stories of people sneaking in his bedroom at night and injecting medicine into his veins. He brought knives and other weapons to treatment, with which he sometimes attempted to attack the therapist. He also brought matches and wanted to light fires. As firm limits were set on these aggressive acts by interpretation and prohibition, he began to open up more and more about the intensity of his paranoid fears. For several sessions, it was necessary for the therapist to restrain him physically to prevent attacks. It was during these times that the boy was able to share his fear that he might kill someone. He pleaded for a tranquilizer.

CASE STUDY #32

The therapist was inclined to try to work this through without medication, until he received a request from the school for consultation on how they could manage him there. A visit to the school (with the boy's prior knowledge and consent) revealed that he had been very disorganized, hyperactive, and misbehaving there. He seemed ambivalent about his role as a psychiatric patient, worrying that people would find out but then impulsively announcing to the whole class that he was leaving for an appointment with his psychiatrist. It was decided to honor his request for a "tranquilizer," and several medications were tried: Thioridazine (Mellaril®) made him too drowsy and d-amphetamine (Dexedrine®) made the light hurt his eyes, but methylphenidate (Ritalin®) seemed to help his behavior, his school performance, and even his paranoid symptoms as seen in therapy.

During the next year, observation with and without methylphenidate seemed to indicate that he should continue taking it for a while. As his father's trial was settled, and as he developed a relationship with his sister's fiance, his paranoid symptoms disappeared. When he indicated a desire to have therapy interfere less with school, the sessions were reduced in frequency to once a week, during which time termination feelings were successfully worked through.

QUESTION A:
PARANOIA DURING LATENCY AGE:
1. Is rather common
2. Is rather unusual, but can result from the right confluence of circumstances
3. Is always associated with minimal brain dysfunction
4. Should be suspected in a boy who claims that somebody else attacked him when it is well known that he himself started the fight
5. Tends to occur in dull children
6. Should be suspected in a child who says others pick on him

True paranoid symptoms are rather rare during the elementary school age, even among the high risk groups, such as schizophrenics and handicapped. In fact, when this case was presented to Dr. Leo Kanner, the dean of American child psychiatrists, he stated that he had never personally seen a child whom he believed to be truly paranoid, though he agreed that this boy was. Apparently the right confluence of circumstances operated to convince this rather precocious boy that the world was conspiring to wreck his life: 1) sudden abandonment by a beloved, loving father, whom the public was suspecting of murder (whom can you trust?), 2) periodic illness of his mother, 3) failure experiences at school, and 4) notoriety as the son of a fugitive, all of which he was expected to handle with 5) a nervous system that in retrospect appeared slightly impaired. The frankly paranoid suspicions and delusions (e.g. that the therapist was an undercover police agent) are easily distinguished from the defensive lying commonly engaged in by many children when confronted with their misbehavior. Two is the right answer. When a latency age child says he's being picked on, the chances that he really is picked on are greater than that he is paranoid. (Of course, this does not mean he's an innocent victim. He may be picked on because of things he does).

QUESTION B:
THE RELATIONSHIP BETWEEN PARANOIA AND MINIMAL BRAIN DYSFUNCTION (HYPERKINETIC SYNDROME) IS:
1. Most hyperkinetic children are paranoid
2. Paranoia is more common than minimal brain dysfunction in latency
3. Minimal brain dysfunction is more common than paranoia in adults
4. Hyperkinetic children are more vulnerable than most to develop paranoia because of their sense of having been injured, vague anxiety that the world may be a dangerous place, and tendency to annoy other people enough to elicit hostile social feedback

CASE STUDY #32

5. Hyperkinetic children, because of their intellectual impairment,are less likely to develop paranoia
6. None

The prevalence relationships in two and three are reversed. One is incorrect, but some hyperkinetic children eventually drift toward either a sociopathic or paranoid adjustment. Though adult psychotics seem to show a correlation between paranoid symptoms and intelligence, the slight average intellectual impairment suffered by hyperkinetic children seems to be outweighed by the considerations listed in answer four, the correct answer.

QUESTION C:
AN OEDIPAL ELEMENT IN THIS BOY'S PSYCHOLOGICAL PROBLEMS IS SUG-GESTED BY:
1. His murderous rage towards his father as shown in puppet executions of a defendant who represents his father
2. The crucial age at which his father left, the incestuous overtones of his father's murder of a niece's suitor, his feeling of murderous omnipotence, and his fear of retaliation
3. His desire to sleep in his mother's room
4. His transference tendency to arrange triangles with his male therapists and clinic secretaries
5. Nothing in the history as presented
6. His precocity
7. His concern for his mother's health
8. None of the above

The rage towards his father could be explained as well by the sudden abandonment as by oedipal feelings. His desire to sleep in his mother's room, coming only when she was ill, seems connected with his concern about her health. Both of these seem related to fear of losing his sole remaining parent. Number four is a correct answer, but two is more complete and the best answer.

QUESTION D:
WHEN THIS CHILD BROUGHT FOOD TO THERAPY AND OFFERED IT TO THE THERAPIST:
1. He was probably attempting to appease the therapist to ward off anticipated danger
2. He was cementing the relationship, expressing positive feelings nonverbally, and perhaps trying to bribe the therapist not to abandon him
3. He was trying to distract the therapist away from painful examination of feelings, and therefore the therapist should not eat the food
4. The therapist decided it would be best to eat it in this case to prove he trusted this paranoid boy not to poison him, but ordinarily the therapist should not accept such gifts from children
5. The therapist should accept the food, but not eat it, at least not in the child's presence
6. The therapist should eat with gusto and ask for more to show appreciation

In contrast to the more critical attitude appropriately taken with adult patients, food offered by a child may be accepted with gratitude and immediately eaten with pleasure. Such gifts are a natural expression of feelings for many children, especially in a positive transference. The meaning of the food offering can usually be ascertained and dealt with in the context of the rest of the session and in light of the child's affect during the offering and eating. The best answer is two. Number

CASE STUDY #32

one is correct as far as it goes, but incomplete. Three, five and six are correct in their first clauses, but are rendered incorrect by their endings.

QUESTION E:
THIS BOY'S PROPENSITY FOR PLAYING WITH FIRE BOTH AT HOME AND IN THE CLINIC WAS SO GREAT THAT HE MADE ROUNDS OF CIGARETTE MACHINES TO OBTAIN MATCHES. SUCH FIRESETTING BEHAVIOR:
1. Often relates to sexual, aggressive, and power conflicts
2. Often also occurs in teenagers, where it has the same psychological meaning as in younger children
3. Is a normal developmental phase of most boys
4. Should be allowed as a means of promoting therapeutic expression of feelings
5. Tends to occur more often than chance in children with minimal brain dysfunction
6. Never results in serious fires

Though most children are fascinated by fire and many go through a stage of playing with matches, most soon learn to channel this interest into parentally supervised activities, such as helping light the fireplace. Continued firesetting indicates some disturbance. It needs to be firmly limited, though the usual acceptable channels may still be allowed if the child seems capable of making such distinctions. Firesetting in prepubertal children seems more related to impulsiveness, fascination with the fire, difficulty with controls, and inability to learn from experience, often with minimal brain dysfunction. In adolescents a more neurotic acting-out picture emerges, with sexual excitation or revenge as prime motivaters. Adolescents are more likely to set "serious" fires, but even latency-age "fireplaying" can result in catastrophes. Both one and five are correct.

QUESTION F:
UNPROVOKED ATTACKS ON THERAPIST (OR PARENT, OR TEACHER) BY A CHILD:
1. Should always be firmly stopped
2. Sometimes need to be tolerated in order to bring out the child's true feelings
3. Are an indication for immediately terminating treatment (or other relationship)
4. Can be motivated by a variety of conscious and unconscious things
5. Are always related to oedipal conflicts

Although a child's attacks on an adult may be an acting out of oedipal feelings, they may also be a means of asking for limits, a means of acting out hostility, an attempt to set up a sado-masochistic relationship, angry retaliation for a real or fantasied deprivation either in the past or present, a game, a means of expressing feeling, or an introduction to expressing feeling, among other things. Such attacks should be firmly limited by whatever means are necessary (interpretation, prohibition, reassurance, even physical restraint). To allow such attacks to continue does not promote either true communication of feeling or any other therapeutic goal. On the contrary, assisting the child in controlling himself will promote the kind of security that will allow him to communicate feelings in a constructive way. In this case, for example, the youngster was only able to share his fear that he might kill someone when he was being physically controlled by the therapist. Where interpretations and other means fail to stop such attacks and where the adult in charge is not able physically to control the child, the adult must either obtain help in controlling the child or transfer the child to another therapist (or teacher, or foster parent). One and four are correct.

CASE STUDY #32

REFERENCES:
1. Biller, H. , 1970: Father absence and the personality development of the male child. Developmental Psychology 2:181-201

2. Crumley, F. E. and R. S. Blumenthal, 1972: Children's reaction to temporary loss of father. Paper 212, 1972 APA Convention Abstracts

3. Kurlander, L. R. and D. Kolodny, 1965: Pseudoneurosis in the neurologically handicapped child. Amer J Orthopsychiat 35:733-738

4. Vandersall, T. A. and J. M. Wiener, 1970: Children who set fires. Archives of General Psychiatry 22:63-71

5. Wender, P. H. , 1971: Minimal Brain Dysfunction in Children, John Wylie and Sons, New York

CASE STUDY #33

"Tell Me About Death"

A child psychiatrist was asked to consult with a pediatrician regarding Connie, a 13 year-old, white, Protestant girl. Suffering from cystic fibrosis, she had been admitted to the pediatric unit monthly for the previous year. The pediatrician, who had followed her for years, felt she was not physically sick enough to require such frequent hospitalizations. Hence there must be a psychological issue. Since Connie's mother was not in the hospital at the time of consultation, the first interview involved Connie alone.

She had been followed in the Cystic Fibrosis Clinic since infancy. She seemed a reliable historian, describing her treatment regimen accurately. Three of her mother's siblings had died during childhood, two in infancy and one at the age of 10, from muscular dystrophy. Connie stated that the latter child had died in a body cast.

The psychiatrist was curious about Connie's interest in death, in light of the reason for consultation. He wondered if this interest represented a fear of impending death or some distortion of reality somehow connected with the excessive hospitalizations. He examined the entire medical chart (3 volumes) and found no documentation of the three deaths. The pediatric resident was asked to confirm or refute the information by checking with the mother. A few days later he said that he had been too busy to see the mother. The medical director of the Cystic Fibrosis Clinic denied any knowledge of this family history, although he had known Connie for several years.

QUESTION A:
SINCE CYSTIC FIBROSIS IS GENETICALLY DETERMINED, IT WAS RATHER SURPRISING TO FIND NO ORGANIZED FAMILY HISTORY IN THREE VOLUMES OF CONNIE'S MEDICAL RECORD. THE LATTER FACT, COMBINED WITH THE DIRECTOR'S IGNORANCE AFTER KNOWING THE CHILD SEVERAL YEARS AND THE RESIDENT'S INABILITY TO TALK WITH THE MOTHER EVEN WHEN ASKED TO INDICATES:
1. Pediatricians' disinterest in family histories
2. The inhibitions that physicians have in talking about death
3. The sympathy that physicians have in dealing with chronically ill patients
4. The over-reaction of the psychiatrist to this small amount of information
5. The limited intelligence of the patient and her family

The mother was interviewed by the psychiatrist and confirmed Connie's history, which was distorted. Two of her siblings did die as infants, but probably not from cystic fibrosis. One died during birth. The third dead sibling, the 10 year-old who Connie said had died from muscular dystrophy in a body cast, had actually died from polio in an "iron lung." The psychiatrist felt that this latter distortion might have been because Connie knew a girl with cystic fibrosis down the hall, who was in an iron lung. If it were too threatening for her to consider death in an iron lung, she might change her recollection from an iron lung to a body cast. It was quite clear that Connie and her mother were more interested in talking about death than were the pediatricians. Connie, a bright girl, had suffered from this disease for 13 years, had seen children whom she had met disappear from the clinic group, and had read much about cystic fibrosis. She wanted to talk about the possibility of death in her own case. Two is the best answer.

CASE STUDY #33

QUESTION B:
CONNIE'S FREQUENT, MEDICALLY UNNECESSARY HOSPITALIZATIONS IN-
DICATED THAT SHE:
1. Was unduly concerned about death
2. Had some insight that death was imminent
3. Was contemplating suicide
4. Had become seriously psychologically disturbed and had developed a morbid
   curiosity
5. None of these

Connie died six months after consultation. Therefore, the second answer
seems best. Connie may have known she was about to die, and may even have
brought on her own death by feeling hopeless, in the manner of a "voodoo death."
She could also have suicided by refusing to take some necessary medication, but
there was no evidence of that serious a psychological disturbance.

"Voodoo death" refers to observations by many anthropologists who have
found that in many primitive tribes, when a healthy man loses hope for life, he
dies. For example, when a young, healthy man has committed a tabooed act and
the witch doctor points a bone at him, everyone in the community knows the result
will be death; accordingly, he dies.

QUESTION C:
"VOODOO DEATH" MIGHT STILL OCCUR IN OUR MODERN INDUSTRIAL
SOCIETY BECAUSE:
1. Our society is becoming decadent
2. Our society is overly suspicious
3. Many people in our society are still very primitive
4. People still can feel hopeless and helpless
5. People are overly concerned about psychological factors

The correct answer is four. People can still die in our technological society
if they lose hope and feel they are unable to help themselves or obtain help. A
very common case in point is the "will to live" known to every surgeon. The
chances of a patient without the will to live recovering from a major procedure
are much less than if he had a strong desire to survive.

Curt Richter (1957) placed rats in a jar of water in such a way that they could
not survive. He measured the time the rats struggled to keep alive and found a
great variation, from a few minutes to 40-60 hours. After studying physical
variables, such as water temperature, he discovered that it was something akin
to hopelessness that disposed some rats to swim immediately to the bottom of the
tank and die within a few minutes. Furthermore, wild rats, in contrast to domes-
tic rats, sometimes died from the handling prior to immersion. When he taught
these "hopeless" wild rats that they might be able to survive by letting them out
of the tank once, they gained hope and survived longer.

During World War II, young merchant seamen died in torpedoings more often
than the older, more experienced men. In direct response to this, Kurt Hahn
developed a training program which put young men through a series of experiences
designed to "develop in them the strength of character and will needed to survive."
This "natural experiment" succeeded, and from this the Outward Bound Schools
evolved. (Schulze, 1971) The Schools emphasize the development of increased
self-knowledge and hopeful realization of inner resources through a program of
wilderness survival and group living.

CASE STUDY #33

For an excellent discussion of handling the dying patient, the reader is referred to Dr. Elizabeth Kubler-Ross (1969). She has delineated five stages, or psychological phases, which the dying patient goes through: denial, anger, bargaining, depression and acceptance. These "stages of dying" are normal coping mechanisms. They are not static; they can follow each other in sequence or exist side by side. One thing, however, persists throughout: the need for hope. This is required by even the most realistic and accepting patient.

QUESTION D:
CONNIE WOULD APPEAR TO BE IN THE PHASE OF:
1. Denial
2. Anger
3. Bargaining
4. Depression
5. Acceptance

With the limited information, the answer has to be somewhat speculative, but it would seem that she is in the acceptance, or preparation stage. The physicians seemed to be denying the full extent of her illness if, indeed, she was preparing for death. The physician's denial is a commonly encountered limitation on his effectiveness in dealing with this problem.

QUESTION E:
THE 9-10 YEAR-OLD CHILD VIEWS DEATH IN TERMS OF:
1. A "bogey-man" or some other form of outside intervention
2. A permanent biological process
3. Separation from loved objects
4. Mutilation (against body integrity)
5. A temporary happening

Generally speaking, the very young child views death as separation, the 3-6 year-old as mutilation and a temporary happening, and the 6-9 year-old as a "bogey-man" or some other form of outside intervention. Children over 9 are beginning to think of death as a permanent biological process. The second answer is correct. This knowledge can serve as a guideline to management of the dying child or the child of a dying parent. Connie had been sick a long time and was aware that other children with the same disease occasionally died. She needed to talk realistically to someone able to discuss this emotionally charged subject.

REFERENCES:
1. Cannon, W. B., 1942: Voodoo Death. Amer Anthropologist 44, No. 2. Reprinted in: Psychosom Med 19:182-190, 1957

2. Friedman, J. B., et al., 1963: Behavioral Observations on Parents Anticipating the Death of a Child. Pediatrics 32:610-625

3. Gartley, W. and M. Bernasconi, 1967: The Concept of Death in Children. J Gen Psychiatry 110:71-85

4. Green, M., 1967: Care of the Child With Long Term Life Threatening Illness. Pediatrics 39:441-445

5. Kubler-Ross, E., 1969: On Death and Dying. MacMillan, New York, N.Y.

CASE STUDY #33

6. Lurie, R.S., 1963: The Pediatrician and the Handling of Terminal Illness. Pediatrics 32:477-479

7. Norton, J., 1963: Treatment of the Dying Patient. Psa Study of the Child 18:541-560

8. Richter, C.P., 1957: On the Phenomenon of Sudden Death in Animals and Man. Psychosom Med 19:191-198

9. Schulze, J.R., 1971: An Analysis of the Impact of Outward Bound on Twelve High Schools. Outward Bound, Inc., Reston, Va. 22070

CASE STUDY #34

A Hippie and His Home Are Soon Parted

A 16 year-old, white, Catholic, suburban 10th-grade boy was brought to the clinic by his mother because of truancy, "rebelling," including refusal to attend classes he did not like, participating in protests, and lighting a match in class to weld back together the nylon strand on which his love beads were strung.

He presented as a long-haired but clean, appropriately dressed, likable youth who dated his troubles to the beginning of high school. Prior to that time he had been a straight-A student and safety patrol boy. Now he believed in "complete freedom" for everyone. He seemed to have rather high ideals and a devotion to principles which he had not clearly thought out. He used marijuana and sometimes "acid," and had experienced flashbacks. In some ways he presented as a "martyr" for causes and for family. He had thought about leaving home so that his mother could pursue her job instead of looking after him. He felt that she liked money more than him. He saw his father as being unhappy in his job and drinking a lot because of it.

His mother was a well-groomed, restrained matron who appeared obviously concerned about him and worried that his 29 year-old "hippie" brother had been influencing some of his thinking. She was reported by the patient to drink quite a bit. She said his two younger sibs were doing well in school.

A Minnesota Multiphasic Personality Inventory (MMPI) was invalid because of a high "lie" score.

The father failed to cooperate with the recommendation for family therapy. Therefore, the patient was seen individually and his mother in a parents' group.

During the course of therapy, an interesting family pattern of running away in the late teen years came to light. First, the 29 year-old brother had left home, then the patient's older sister. When she "ran away," the parents drove her to the airport. In similar overt and covert ways, they seemed to be communicating to this patient the expectation that he also would run away.

The importance in the family dynamics of this disposition for the teenagers of the family soon became apparent. Though this boy had made no effort to run away, the father began insisting on the following arrangement "to keep him from running away": the mother took him to work with her during the day, and he had to remain in the same room with the father during the evening. With the support of his therapist, the patient submitted gracefully to this surveillance and assured his father that he wouldn't run away. Within a few days the father became severely depressed, for which he treated himself with heavier alcohol intake.

It began to appear that the father would soon be forced to consider the need for some more appropriate form of therapy, such as psychotherapy or family therapy. However, the father's and the family's maladjustment was saved by the timely reappearance of the 29 year-old brother, who persuaded the patient to run away with him. The family was so relieved at this narrow escape that they refused to return for further treatment even after the patient was located. One encouraging fact, however, was the mother's telephone report that the father traveled to another state to retrieve the patient, a marked contrast to his response when the older children had "run away."

QUESTION A:
THE TRANSACTIONS WITHIN THIS FAMILY:
1. Might be called "the run-away game"
2. Seemed to be a result of drug use
3. Seemed to be tied in to some neurotic need of the father
4. Exemplified a schizophrenic family
5. Seemed to be influenced by the mother's interest in money

This family's preoccupation with running away seems to contain the essential elements of one of the "Games People Play" as described by Eric Berne

CASE STUDY #34

(1964), with negative "strokes" on all sides. (Strokes are packets of interpersonal attention: "If you don't get strokes, your spinal cord will shrivel.") In fact, the game seemed to be developing even into a script, with interchangeable parts for various members of the family. In the limited state of our knowledge, it appears likely that the game was originated by some neurotic conflict or need of the father, and was maintained because of its continuing value in that regard. This did not seem quite the same as a schizophrenogenic family, because even though there were conflicting verbal and nonverbal messages, the children were not really forbidden to respond to the nonverbal message, and they were certainly allowed to escape from the situation. The drug use in the family seemed more a result than a cause. One and three are both correct, one being a transactional answer and three a psychodynamic answer.

QUESTION B:
THIS BOY'S USE OF DRUGS:
1. May be partly identification with his alcoholic father, partly a manifestation of "logopathology" as described by Victor Frankl, and partly a symbol of rebellion
2. Has severely damaged his health
3. Is entirely explained by an obvious need to escape from an intolerable family situation
4. Is not unusual among middle-class suburban youth
5. Might have been prevented or ameliorated if the father had been able to admit his own use of alcohol as a drug dependence and share his feelings about it more frankly with his son
6. Manifests a constitutional need for excessive oral gratification inherited from his alcoholic father

No evidence was presented that drugs had yet harmed this boy's health. Though the family situation undoubtedly could have driven him to drugs, this did not appear the sole determinant. There is nothing in the case to suggest a genetic inheritance of the drug problem. One, four, and five are correct answers.

QUESTION C:
THIS BOY'S CLINICAL PICTURE CLEARLY SHOWS:
1. Usual adolescent drug abuse
2. Masked schizophrenic syndrome
3. Sociopathy
4. Adolescent adjustment reaction
5. None of the above

Drug abuse does not account for most of this boy's problems. There was not good evidence for two or three. A case could be made for answer four, which is used as a diagnostic wastebasket anyhow, but five is the best answer here. The boy did not clearly show any one diagnostic syndrome, though he did seem mildly to moderately disturbed.

QUESTION D:
THE PATIENT'S "FLASHBACKS":
1. Are a common result of marijuana use
2. Probably resulted from LSD ("acid")
3. Would not recur if he never uses drugs again
4. Probably resulted from adulterants with which his drugs had been "cut" by enterprising pushers
5. Were probably pleasant

CASE STUDY #34

Flashbacks are a common aftermath of potent hallucinogen use, but are rare after marijuana. They are usually unpleasant, and may occur months after ceasing all drug use. In contrast to the expensive, commonly "cut" heroin, hallucinogens are not usually cut, though a cheap one like LSD or STP may be sold under the name of an expensive one like mescaline. Two is correct.

QUESTION E:
THE PROGNOSIS FOR THIS BOY IS:
1. To progress to amphetamine use and then heroin, or perhaps directly to heroin, within 10 years
2. Rather poor
3. Very good
4. That he may spontaneously give up drug use, or switch to legal drugs like his father
5. That he may develop into a useful citizen after working through his conflicts with his parents
6. That he will probably become a lifetime hippie like his 29 year-old brother

Though most hard narcotic users started with marijuana, most marijuana users do not progress to hard narcotics. This boy's biggest obstacle to a decent life is his problem with his family. The prognosis is fair, with four and five defensible answers. Five is possible even if he continues occasional "social" marijuana use.

REFERENCES:
1. Berne, E., 1964: Games People Play. Grove Press, New York

2. Coddington, R.D. and R. Jacobsen, 1972: Drug Use by Ohio Adolescents: an Epidemiologic Study. Ohio State Med J 68:481-484

3. Distler, L.S., 1970: The Adolescent "Hippie" and the Emergence of a Matristic Culture. Psychiatry 33:362-371

4. Frankl, V., 1970: Man's Search for Meaning: An Introduction to Logopathology. Simon & Schuster, New York

5. Harris, T.A., 1967: I'm O.K., You're O.K. Harper & Row, New York

6. Johnson, A., 1952: Genesis of Antisocial Acting-out in Children and Adults. Psa Quarterly 21:323-343

7. Rosenthal, R. and L. Jacobson, 1968: Pygmalion in the Classroom. Holt, Rinehart & Winston, New York

8. Sabbath, J., 1969: The Suicidal Adolescent - the Expendable Child. J of Amer Acad of Child Psychiatry 8:272-289

9. Snyder, S.H., 1971: Uses of Marijuana. Oxford Univ. Press, New York

CASE STUDY #35

A Child Who Couldn't Settle Down

A rather sad-appearing, skinny, ten year-old girl was brought to the clinic by her parents because she was unhappy and they found it difficult to communicate with her. They described her as not having friends, being awkward, and lacking in self-confidence. Occasionally she acted mean and spiteful to her 14 year-old and 7 year-old brothers, who seemed to be well-adjusted boys. She sometimes was obstinate and negative, sulked for long periods, and stole small sums of money.

Her parents' greatest concerns were her unhappiness and her uncommunicativeness. The latter was apparent when she remained almost silent throughout most of the interview and spoke only in monosyllables. Both parents were from strong religious backgrounds and did not allow negative feelings to be expressed in the family.

The child had been an ordinary, healthy, full-term baby, breast-fed for the first four months. She was then easily switched to the bottle, which she had until she was fifteen months old. There had been some difficulty with vomiting solids, but this quickly passed. She was a large infant for her age, and she walked at eleven months. In contrast to her siblings, she seemed completely fearless.

Father's work as a news correspondent took the family to another country and another culture every few years. The child was born in Spain. When she was four years-old, the family moved to Hong Kong. From there, father's work took them to many foreign capitals, where the family always lived in American colonies. Hence, the child spoke both English and Spanish fluently. Shortly before the first clinic visit, the family had started speaking English in the home; previously, only Spanish had been spoken. The child's live-in baby sitter, who had been with the family for six years, was returning to Spain. Each time the family moved, their pets were left behind.

A Wechsler Intelligence Scale for Children (W. I. S. C.) obtained a verbal I. Q. of 86, a Performance I. Q. of 117, and a Full I. Q. of 101. The discrepancy between the verbal and performance scales was due to the child's reticence: she used as little speech as possible. Hence, the Full I. Q. of 101 was probably a low estimate.

QUESTION A:
THE ROOTS OF THIS CHILD'S PROBLEMS COULD HAVE BEEN:
1. That she was an unwanted child
2. Too strong an oedipal attachment to her father
3. Subtle brain damage
4. Repetitive attachments and losses brought about by frequent moving, together with the parents prohibition of the expression of negative feelings
5. That she didn't speak the language of some of the countries in which she lived

In many ways this little girl was a very angry, controlling child. Her uncommunicativeness was one way of expressing negative feelings as well as passively controlling other members of the family. Her jealousy of her brothers was manifested in her spiteful behavior towards them. Although the family constellation remained constant and there was no maternal deprivation, this little girl was forced several times to give up her peer relationships and her pets to start over again in a new school with new language and customs. The fact that she so often felt the "outsider" may have contributed to her lack of self-confidence. The best answer is four.

QUESTION B:
APPROPRIATE INTERVENTION IN THIS CASE WOULD HAVE BEEN:
1. Family therapy
2. A tranquilizer for the child

CASE STUDY #35

3. A behavior modification program for the child
4. Individual psychotherapy for the child and counselling for the parents
5. To advise the parents to settle down and to stop moving every two years

Though no one could doubt the advantage of settling down, this would not be sufficient intervention here, and would undoubtedly be rejected by the parents. Answers two and three might be helpful, but in themselves do not do justice to the gravity of the problem. This child was seriously disturbed and needed intensive individual psychotherapy. The parents also needed help in working through some of their problems, such as their inability to accept negative feelings. They also needed the opportunity to gain more insight into their daughter's needs. The best answer is four, with one a desirable adjunct, at least later in therapy.

QUESTION C:
A DIAGNOSIS IN THIS CASE COULD HAVE BEEN:
1. Elective mutism
2. An adjustment reaction of childhood
3. Withdrawing reaction of childhood
4. Overanxious reaction of childhood
5. Childhood schizophrenia

In this situation, the child's tendencies towards withdrawal had not yet stabilized, and although she was seclusive, she was certainly not detached. She had been able to form relationships in school situations, but each time they were terminated by moving. All of this would help to rule out childhood schizophrenia. Although the child was not an elective mute, she was possibly using her uncommunicativeness as a defense against expressing her angry, aggressive feelings, which occasionally were manifested though mean, spiteful behavior. There is, of course, the possibility that without therapeutic intervention, she could have drifted into elective mutism because of the secondary gains; increased concern from her parents, the passive-aggressive frustration of others, and control of others. The best answer is three.

QUESTION D:
WHEN THE EXPRESSION OF NEGATIVE FEELINGS IS FORBIDDEN IN A FAMILY:
1. The children are guiltless and pure in heart
2. There are no quarrels nor unhappiness
3. There are only pleasant thoughts
4. There are no negative feelings
5. Communication may become unclear (or absent)

One of the basic tenets of object theory is that the individual seeks communication and that the neuroses constitute his failure to do so. Thus, the child who is forbidden to express his negative feelings verbally must adapt by the use of defense mechanisms. In this case, we see the defense of uncommunicativeness doubling as a sort of hostile passive-aggressive communication, which the parents cannot control as well as active communication. The best answer is five.

REFERENCES:
1. Bowen, M., 1966: The use of family therapy in clinical practice. Comp Psychiat 7:345-374

2. Bower, E. M., 1967: American children and families in overseas communities, Am J Orthopsychiat 37:787-796

CASE STUDY #35

3. Bowlby, J., 1969: Attachment and Loss, Vol. 1 Attachment, New York: Basic Books

4. David, H. and D. Elkind, 1966: Family adaption overseas - some mental health considerations. Ment Hyg 40:92-99

5. Frank, G., 1965: The role of the family in the development of psychopathology. Psychol Bull, 64:191-205

6. Freud, A., 1936: The ego and the mechanisms of defense. New York: International Univ. Press., rev. ed. 1966

7. Levy, D., 1972: Oppositional syndromes and oppositional behavior. Childhood Psychopathology. (eds.) S. Harrison & J. F. McDermott, New York, Internat. Univ. Press

8. O'Shaughnessy, E., 1969: Your 10 Year Old. London, Corgi

9. Pustom, E. and R. W. Speers, 1964: Elective mutism in children. Am J Child Psychiat 3:277-279

10. Reed, G. F., 1963: Elective mutism in children: a re-appraisal. J Child Psychol Psychiat, 4:99-107

11. Spitz, R. A., 1957: No and Yes. On the Genesis of Human Communication. New York: International Univ. Press

12. Wechsler, D., 1949: Manual: Wechsler Intelligence Scale for Children. New York, Psych Corp.

CASE STUDY #36

From Glue to Eternity

Kathy was a 13 year-old white girl living with her divorced mother when she first began to sniff glue. This occurred shortly after her father married another woman, who also had teenage children. Kathy felt this not only as the loss of her father, but also as losing out to another adolescent, namely the new step-daughter.

Kathy was the fourth of five children and the first girl in the family. In school she had always done average work. She excelled in her dancing lessons, which she had taken great pride in for seven years. It gave her considerable pleasure when her parents watched her at the regular recitals.

Apparently no one was aware of the glue sniffing, even though it became very frequent. At 14, Kathy and a friend began to frequent the campus hangouts at the nearby university and became acquainted with other drugs, such as marijuana, LSD-25, cocaine, mescaline, and the amphetamines. By this time, her friend had begun psychotherapy and asked her therapist to see Kathy, who felt she was too involved with drugs.

Psychotherapy was begun. Kathy's mother gave permission, but seemed disinterested and did not participate in it herself. At one point family therapy was attempted, but the mother soon terminated. Kathy was so heavily involved with drugs that she had to be admitted to a psychiatric hospital on seven occasions, much as an alcoholic needs to be admitted in order to "dry out." She also had difficulties with bronchitis and malnutrition, which resulted from the life she lived during these years of drug abuse.

Even though Kathy developed rapport with the psychotherapist, she did not like to delve deeply into unconscious material and ran away from therapy whenever it became too threatening. One significant area, for instance was sexuality. Kathy was a very attractive adolescent, and between the ages of 5 and 12 she excelled in a dancing program which she enjoyed very much. By age 15, however, she was reluctant to wear short skirts or bathing suits and wished that the long dresses her grandmother had worn were fashionable again. While at an earlier age she had enjoyed the exhibitionism involved in the dancing program, now, in adolescence, she resisted the suggestions of her friends to develop a modeling career. During her drug escapades she often spent the night or several days in an apartment occupied by boys - sometimes with other girls and sometimes alone - but she never engaged in sexual behavior during those mid-adolescent years. She often had bad dreams about some kind of physical injury, with a suggestion of rape, and being rescued by a male bystander. Clearly, she looked upon her therapist as a substitute father rather than a physician and often asked him to act in a parental way: she asked him to drive her home, to lend her money, and to accompany her on her first job interview.

Much has been said about the home environment of drug abusers, including the suggestion that drugs are also used by the other members of the household. Kathy invited her therapist to visit her home and to meet her mother and brothers one Saturday afternoon. When they arrived at the house at 4:30 PM, all the blinds were drawn, and it was clear that the family was not prepared for visitors, but Kathy insisted that the therapist come in. On the outside the house was a small neat ranch house in a suburban area, but inside it was dark, disarrayed, and dirty. Kathy's mother had stayed out late the night before and was just arising. Her younger sister was napping, and one brother was asleep in the living room. Another brother was talking on the kitchen telephone, apparently about drugs. Every inch of counter surface in the kitchen was covered with dirty dishes, pots, and pans, many of them still containing left-overs. Although this was a middle-class neighborhood, the conditions within the house were appalling. In talking with the family, the therapist learned that all three of Kathy's brothers had used drugs. Her mother occasionally used sedatives and tranquilizers, but she was not a heavy user and did not drink excessively.

At the age of 15-16 years, Kathy could be characterized as 1) feeling very inadequate, 2) being overly dependent on her therapist as well as on drugs, and

CASE STUDY #36

3) being rather infantile in her need to receive instant gratification rather than postponing satisfaction to a later date. She had many somatic complaints, such as abdominal pain, for which she wanted some sort of drug. On many occasions she also suffered from sleeplessness and bad dreams, for which she demanded sedatives. Whenever she was given a prescription for any specific medication, she always seemed to require greater than average dosages. It seemed that her tolerance for all drugs was much higher than that of other people.

QUESTION A:
KATHY IS CLEARLY DRUG DEPENDENT, BUT WHAT IS THE BASIC UNDER-
LYING DISORDER?:
1. Psychoneurosis, hysterical type
2. Psychoneurosis, hypochondriacal type
3. Personality disorder, passive-dependent type
4. Personality disorder, antisocial type
5. Drug dependence with no underlying disorder

There are certain hysterical features in this girl, such as the nature of the bad dreams and the anxiety over exhibiting her legs in short skirts, but this is not her primary personality type. Nor are her physical complaints prominent enough to diagnose her as hypochondriacal. She is antisocial in many ways, and she is certainly depending on drugs at the present time, but one can clearly see that she also depends on people, such as the therapist and friends. The clue to the diagnosis is her dependent inability to postpone gratification in a manner consonant with her age. The best answer is number three; she is suffering from a personality disorder, passive-dependent type. She cannot fend for herself and needs to rely upon other supports, whether they be drugs, friends, "therapist," or employers.

Despite her therapist's efforts to provide her with the needed psychological support, Kathy began using hard narcotics. She continued to run from therapy, sometimes to a distant city, only to call the therapist a couple months later and ask his help in returning home. She was treated with methadone detoxification on several occasions, but usually reverted to heroin, at least on a weekly basis. By age 19 she had held several jobs, leaving some after a few months simply because she didn't enjoy them. She liked being hostess in a restaurant, but would get into difficulties with the waitresses which would cause her either to quit or be fired. The longest she held a job was when she worked as a bartender. During this time she began to drink regularly, though not heavily. Eventually, she dated regularly and became sexually active, but she derived little pleasure from it.

The three-year supportive psychotherapy provided for Kathy in terms of personality growth and maturation cannot be called successful since time alone may have permitted Kathy to develop as much as she did. On the other hand, Kathy claims that she would have overdosed and been dead by now if it had not been for the therapist's support. She felt depressed on many occasions. She said that the knowledge that her suicide would hurt her therapist's feelings was a major preventive factor. This insight may explain the apparent relative rarity of suicides among adolescents actively involved in treatment as compared to those not in active treatment. See Drye and Goulding (1973) for a discussion of suicide prevention by patient-therapist contract.

QUESTION B:
SHOULD "METHADONE MAINTENANCE" HAVE BEEN USED WHEN SHE BEGAN
USING HEROIN AT THE AGE OF 16?:

Methadone maintenance is illegal for minors, because the method is still too new to use it indiscriminately. Guidelines established by the Food and Drug Administration suggest limiting its use to persons over 18 who have been narcotic

CASE STUDY #36

addicts for at least two years and with whom incarceration, Methadone withdrawal, and psychotherapy have been tried unsuccessfully. Although these guidelines are changing, they are becoming more strict rather than more lenient.

QUESTION C:
REPEATED, REGULAR USE OF TWO OR MORE DRUGS AMONG HIGH SCHOOL STUDENTS IS:
1. Confined, for the most part, to about 15-20% of the students
2. Spread fairly among 60-80% of the students
3. A problem in urban areas only
4. Found mostly in the middle class, suburban areas
5. None of these

Three large epidemiologic studies have attempted to answer these questions, one in Pennsylvania (6,969 children) (Anonymous, 1972), one in Ohio (4,615 high school students) (Coddington and Jacobson, 1972), and one involving the entire Dallas, Texas school system (56,745 students) (Gosset, et al., 1971).

Marijuana was found to be the most widely used illicit drug (excepting alcohol and tobacco) and was used "at least a few times" by 17-26% of Pennsylvania youths, at least once by 13-15% of students in the Ohio study, and by 11-17% of the Dallas school children. Estimates of heroin use ranged from 3-10% in the three studies.

Use of 2 or more drugs other than alcohol was found to be confined to 15-20% of high school students in the Ohio study. The first answer is best.

All three studies showed that drug abuse was present in urban, suburban, and rural populations as well as among all social classes, though it is somewhat less prevalent in rural areas.

QUESTION D:
ADOLESCENT DRUG ABUSERS COME FROM FAMILIES:
1. Who are too strict, causing the children to rebel
2. Who are too lenient, setting no limits on their children
3. In which the parents are overly dependent on drugs themselves
4. In which there are no other children
5. Who are poor

Sometimes the families are too strict and sometimes too lenient; these traits are not specific for the development of drug abuse in the children. The parents themselves are often heavily dependent on drugs, at least such drugs as prescribed or over-the-counter preparations, alcohol, tobacco, and caffeine. They are not necessarily poor. In fact, they often belong to the middle class. Although drug abuse is common in the ghetto, the reason for this may be availability rather than the people's low socioeconomic standing. The best answer is three.

This case study pretty well fits the stereotype for drug abusers and alcoholics. The reader is cautioned, however, from relying too heavily upon such stereotypes. The following vignette is given to illustrate an exception.

> John came from a black, lower middle-class, urban family
> and was raised according to the Christian work ethic. While
> he was attending high school, he was introduced to drugs,
> but he did not become heavily involved until he was stationed
> in the Panama Canal Zone while serving in the U.S. Army.
> Upon discharge he was addicted to heroin, but he used the
> drug in a pattern very much like other members of our society
> use cocktails.

CASE STUDY #36

John never missed work and never used drugs at work. He made his "buy" after work and took the entire dose in one injection in his own apartment. Afterwards he went to sleep while watching T.V. He maintained two separate circles of friends, one of whom knew nothing of his illicit activities.

When his father suddenly died, John became depressed and over a two-month period increased his dose from 2 to 7 "bags" daily. He still took them all in one shot and did not let his drug use interfere with his work. It was at this point that he sought help, for he knew that he could not continue this way.

A Methadone detoxification schedule was set up, to which John strictly adhered. He has now been free of heroin for a full year.

REFERENCES:
1. Anonymous, 1972: Drugs and Youth. Pennsylvania Health 33:2-3 (Fall)

2. Coddington, R.D. and R. Jacobsen, 1972: Drug Use by Ohio Adolescents; An Epidemiologic Study. Ohio State Med J 68:481-484

3. Coles, R., Brenner, J.H. and D. Meagher, 1970: Drugs and Youth Psychiatric and Legal Facts. Liveright Publishing Corp., New York, N.Y.

4. Drye, R.C., Goulding, R.L. and M.E. Goulding, 1973: No-suicide Decisions: Patient Monitoring of Suicidal Risk. Am J Psychiatry 130:171-174

5. Glasscote, R., Sussex, J.N., Jaffe, J.H., Ball, J. and L. Brill, 1972: The Treatment of Drug Abuse. The Joint Information Service of the APA and NIMH

6. Cossett, J.T., Lewis, J.M. and V.A. Phillips, 1971: Extent and Prevalence of Illicit Drug Use as Reported by 56,745 Students. JAMA 216:1464-1470

7. Grinspoon, L., 1972: Marijuana Reconsidered. Harvard Univ. Press, Cambridge, Mass.

8. Harris, R.T., McIsaac, W.M. and C.R. Schuster, Jr., 1970: Drug Dependence. Advances in Medical Science II. Univ. of Texas Press, Austin, Texas

9. Snyder, S.H., 1971: Uses of Marijuana. Oxford Univ. Press, New York

CASE STUDY #37

Environment-Contingent Symptoms

A 6-1/2 year-old, white, Protestant, lower-class girl was brought by her mother the summer between her kindergarten and first grade years because of "getting upset real easily."

Her mother had noted for the previous three years these symptoms: 1) enuresis, increasing to almost nightly and intractable to maternal attempts to stop it, 2) nightly crying out during sleep, 3) "dry heaves" on awakening each morning, 4) vomiting "when she's really upset," about three or four times per month, and 5) crying a lot. The symptoms did not appear when she stayed with her grandmother, and they seemed to lessen when her five year-old brother was not home.

Her twice-divorced mother appeared anxious, overprotective, and guilt-ridden. She often answered for the patient. She stated she couldn't stand seeing the girl upset, and admitted giving in to her many times because of this. She characterized herself as very inconsistent. She allowed the girl to sleep with her when she became upset at night. The girl never wet the mother's bed, even though she wet her own bed almost nightly.

When the patient would get upset, she would call her grandmother and ask to stay with her for awhile. At the grandmother's house she would become even more withdrawn than she had become in the new neighborhood to which the family had recently moved. She had no friends there and mainly read books and watched TV. Despite all the problems, the mother characterized the girl as "very obedient."

The patient was born out of wedlock with no complications of pregnancy or delivery. She seemed to be an "easy" baby, sleeping through the night with no feeding problems. She enjoyed normal developmental milestones and was toilet trained by one and one-half.

The patient took her surname from a man whom her mother married after her birth. This marriage ended in divorce when the patient was 2-1/2. This stepfather was, at the time of the clinic visit, continuing to visit both her and the five-year-old brother who was a product of that marriage.

The mother's second marriage was to an alcoholic who "constantly abused" the patient and twice wrecked the car in what the mother saw as a deliberate attempt to "wipe the whole family out." The mother dates all of the girl's symptoms to the beginning of this marriage. However, even after the second divorce, the patient was further frightened in the kitchen of their home by a man trying to break in. Even though they moved to a new home, the patient was still afraid to enter the kitchen.

The patient looked her stated age. She smiled when spoken to but did not reply, tending to cling to her mother. One time she almost fell asleep on her mother's lap with her thumb in her mouth. She appeared rather depressed.

Though play therapy and parent counseling were originally recommended, the family did not manage to keep any appointments. By telephone, the mother was advised to set up a ledger sheet for the patient to keep track of her "wet" and "dry" nights for her own benefit. It was emphasized that this should be seen as something for the patient to do for herself and the main gratification should be the child's sense of mastery over herself, with the mother's involvement being at a minimum except for when the child wished to show her the record. With this program, the nightly enuresis ceased immediately. Within a week the improvement had "spilled" into other areas, with diminution of crying, nightmares, and desire to climb into the mother's bed. In short, the child appeared generally more mature.

QUESTION A:
THIS CASE ILLUSTRATES:
1. Traumatic neurosis
2. Psychophysiologic reaction, gastrointestinal and genitourinary types
3. Unsocialized aggressive reaction

CASE STUDY #37

4. Interaction of child's symptoms with parental guilt, anxiety, oversubmission, and overprotection
5. Hyperkinetic reaction
6. Minimal brain dysfunction as shown in behavior problem, enuresis, and restless sleep pattern

A tenuous case could be made for answer one since the problems dated back to psychologically traumatic experiences with the second stepfather and with the burglar. A case could also be made for two. However, the best answer is four. The main problem seems to have been the child's reaction to maternal feelings of inadequacy, guilt, anxiety, and possibly identification with the child. This impression is confirmed by the mother's admissions that she tended to give in to the girl because she couldn't stand seeing her upset and that the girl did not show her symptoms at all when staying with the grandmother. This interaction might be restated in these behavioral terms: the mother reinforced the child's symptoms by giving in to her or allowing her to get into mother's bed when she was upset. The mother's reinforcement for thus giving in was the relief of her own anxiety by thus ending the child's crying. Reinforcement of the child's symptoms naturally resulted in their increased frequency, providing an even more frequent reason for the mother to reinforce them inadvertently by giving in to them.

QUESTION B:
AMONG OTHER THINGS, THIS CASE ILLUSTRATES ENURESIS, WHICH MAY BE DEFINED AS:
1. Involuntary discharge of urine after the fourth birthday
2. Loss of urinary control and automatic passage of urine
3. Daytime pants-wetting
4. Nocturnal wetting
5. Involuntary discharge of urine after the second birthday

The exact age at which wetting becomes abnormal and merits the label "enuresis" is open to some debate, but age two is clearly too young. Ages three, four, or even five are more acceptable. Certainly, the persistence of bedwetting or pants-wetting into the school years deserves evaluation and treatment. Answer two defines incontinence, such as in a neurogenic bladder, which accounts for only a small percentage of childhood wetting. Daytime wetting without bedwetting accounts for not more than 5 percent of enuretic children. A much larger proportion wet both day and night, while at least half wet only at night. The best answer is one, but some question could be raised about the term "involuntary" in cases where the child does not appear motivated to control the wetting.

QUESTION C:
THE INCIDENCE OF ENURESIS AS DEFINED IN QUESTION B IS:
1. 5% or less
2. 5-10%
3. 10-20%
4. 20-30%
5. Over 30%

Enuresis has been reported to occur in over 25% of some nonrandom samples, but better estimates for the whole child population are in the neighborhood of 10 to 15%. This makes it one of the commonest childhood problems.

CASE STUDY #37

QUESTION D:
ETIOLOGICALLY, ENURESIS:
1. Is often physiologically or neuropathologically based
2. Is emotionally based
3. In this case seemed emotionally based because it appeared under psychologically traumatic circumstances two years after successful toilet training
4. Can often be helped by psychosocial therapy or habit training even when it has some physiological basis
5. Does not require pediatric examination to rule out urogenital pathology when it persists from infancy

Though some authors would support answer two (e. g. , MacKeith, 1972) we feel that enuresis is just as likely to be a cause of secondary emotional problems as a result of primary emotional problems. Sometimes the secondary problems form a neurotic cluster which perpetuates the enuresis even after the child matures neurophysiologically enough to achieve continence. In the present case, of course, the emotional problem seems primary. However, even here relief of the enuresis seemed to result in a clearing up of other problems, almost as if the immature behavior were being perpetuated by the girl's knowledge of her own enuresis. In "primary" or "essential" enuresis, persisting from infancy, a pediatric evaluation will in a small percentage discover frank urogenital pathology or other medical-surgical problems. This is even a possibility in "secondary" ("acquired," "onset") enuresis, occurring after a successful dry period. In the latter circumstance, however, pediatric evaluation can be postponed during a trial of psychiatric treatment if 1) the child appears in good physical health and 2) there seem obvious precipitating psychosocial factors, as in this girl's case. One, three, and four are correct answers, with three most pertinent to this case.

QUESTION E:
THE THERAPEUTIC INTERVENTION IN THIS CASE:
1. Is the treatment of choice for enuresis
2. Is an unusual approach which is not applicable to most cases of enuresis
3. Succeeded probably because it gave the mother permission to allow the child to take more responsibility for herself, gave the child the message that she was able to take care of herself, gave both the child and the mother something to focus on besides their anxiety, gave both of them some concrete, tangible hope of success, and provided immediate ego-enhancing reinforcement to the child for more mature behavior
4. Would be incompatible with psychotherapy because it involves a type of behavior modification or operant conditioning.
5. Is a good way of handling poorly motivated patients who fail to keep appointments

There are many therapeutic approaches to the problem of enuresis. Though all of them enjoy some success, none could be appropriately labeled the treatment of choice. The one used here works well for many cases where the child is old enough to understand, has enough competitiveness or collecting instinct to like accumulating "good marks, " and is not handicapped by obvious urogenital pathology. There is no conflict in the child's psychotherapist or play therapist simultaneously advising the parents on behavior modification techniques. Three is the only correct answer. See case 41 for behavior therapy of encopresis, and case 52 for more on behavior modification.

QUESTION F:
OTHER ACCEPTABLE TREATMENTS FOR ENURESIS INCLUDE ALL OF THE FOLLOWING EXCEPT:
1. Imipramine and other anticholinergic and adrenergic drugs

CASE STUDY #37

2. Operant conditioning apparatus, such as a buzzer which rings when the sheets are wet
3. Daytime forcing of fluids to stretch the bladder, and fluid restriction at bedtime
4. Urological surgery, such as circumcision
5. Psychotherapy and parent counseling
6. Habit training, e.g. with the child in charge of his own alarm clock to wake himself in time

The only intervention above which does not enjoy wide acceptance for enuresis is circumcision. This makes answer four correct, though other urological surgery is sometimes indicated, as in bladder neck obstruction.

QUESTION G:
WHICH OF THE FOLLOWING FACTS ABOUT THIS PATIENT DID NOT INCREASE HER CHANCES OF BEING ENURETIC?:
1. Being first-born
2. Being lower class
3. Having other behavior and habit disturbances
4. "Getting upset real easily"
5. Her generally immature behavior
6. Her sex

The first five answers all have a higher correlation with enuresis than randomly expected. The correct answer is six, because boys have much higher incidence of enuresis than girls.

REFERENCES:
1. Agras, W. S. (Ed.), 1972: Behavior Modification: Principles and Clinical Applications, Little-Brown, Massachusetts

2. Arnold, S. J., 1972: Enuresis, Amer J Dis Children 123:84

3. Campbell, W. A. III, Lupp, J. and M. Weissman, 1970: Bender Gestalt test and the urodynamics of enuresis. J of Urology 54:934-939

4. Edvardsen, P., 1972: Neurophysiological aspects of enuresis. Acta Scandinav 48:222-230

5. Gerard, M. W., 1939: Enuresis, Amer J Orthopsychiat 9:48-49

6. Graziano, A. M. (Ed.), 1971: Behavior Therapy with Children, Aldine-Atherton, Chicago, Ill.

7. Hallgren, B., 1957: Enuresis: A clinical and genetic study. Acta Psychiatrica et Neurologica Scandinavia Supp. 32:114

8. MacKeith, R. C., 1972: Is maturation delay a frequent factor in the origins of primary nocturnal enuresis? Develop Med Child Neurol 14:217-223

9. McKindry, J. B. J., Stewart, D. A., Jeffs, R. D. and A. Mozes: Enuresis treated by an improved waking process, CMA Journal 106:27-29

10. Missildine, H., 1962: Preventive psychiatry in emotional development, Feelings 4: no. 6, Nov.-Dec.

CASE STUDY #37

11. Missildine, H., 1963: Your Inner Child of the Past, Simon and Schuster, New York

12. Patterson, G. R. and M. E. Guillion, 1971: Living with Children, Research Press, Champagne, Ill.

13. Poussaint, A. F. and K. S. Ditman, 1965: A controlled study of imipramine (Trofranil) in the treatment of childhood enuresis. J of Pediatrics 67:283-290

14. Ritvo, E. R., Ornitz, E. M., Gottlier, F., et al., 1969: Arousal and non-arousal enuretic events, Amer J Psychiat 126:77-84

15. Starfield, B., 1972: Enuresis: Its pathogenesis and management. Clin Pediatrics 11:343-350

16. Thomas, A. and S. Chess, 1970: Origin of Personality, Scientific American 223:102-109

17. Thomas, A., Chess, S. and H. G. Birch, 1968: Temperament and Behavior Disorders in Children New York University Press, New York

CASE STUDY #38

"Cooling Out" Carla

Carla, a 15 year-old, black girl, was referred by an inner city school nurse because of fighting, profanity, and refusal to obey the principal. The nurse stated that Carla had considerable potential but was not working anywhere near her capacity. She felt that Carla's anxiety was the cause of her impulsive behavior, such as sassing teachers and hitting peers.

Carla's parents had been divorced for eight years, but both of them accompanied her to the clinic and seemed willing to cooperate. The divorce had apparently been caused by the father's alcoholism. Although he professed a continued, active interest in the family, Carla claimed that he was unreliable. He did provide the transportation for some of Carla's visits, but never missed an opportunity to point out that he had to do this because he felt one could not count on his ex-wife. Evidently both mother and father were continuing the marital battle eight years after the divorce. However, they both agreed that Carla was rather disobedient; they had been worried about her behavior, but had not known where to go for help. They themselves had only finished elementary school, but they wanted Carla and her sister to graduate from high school.

Carla's mother seemed quite ambivalent about the psychiatric referral. She showed considerable resistance to a psychotherapeutic program. Although she superficially cooperated, she was uneasy in the physician's office and apparently reluctant to become personally involved in therapy.

Carla also seemed to feel out of place in the psychiatrist's office. She spoke so quietly that she frequently had to be asked to repeat what she had said, and she fidgeted uneasily in her chair while she described the racial strife at school.

QUESTION A:
WHICH OF THE FOLLOWING IS AN APPROPRIATE WAY TO CLOSE THE FIRST INTERVIEW WITH CARLA AND HER PARENTS?:
1. Encourage her to come for a second visit
2. Recommend family psychotherapy
3. Refer her to the school guidance counselor
4. Set some limits for her and call the school principal in order to get him to enforce them
5. Refer her to the juvenile authorities in an attempt to teach Carla the consequences of her behavior

If there was ever a place for the cliche "play it by ear," this is it. Perceiving the discomfort of Carla and her family in his office, the middle-class psychiatrist may be tempted to put them at ease by referral elsewhere. But some of the discomfort may be his own, projected onto them. Adams and McDonald (1967, 1968) have described "cooling out" techniques used too often with the poor. These two articles are "required reading" for psychotherapists dealing with people from other cultures or subcultures. "Playing by ear" really means "let your conscience be your guide." When in doubt about what to do, encourage the patient to come another time in an effort to understand his feelings, as well as your own, more clearly. The first answer is correct.

If we take Carla or other patients from her subculture into treatment, however, we must be prepared to alter our usual treatment procedures. Carla was not only afraid of a white middle-class physician, but also of committing herself to weekly appointments, so that she would only accept one appointment at a time. However, she always came on time, and while steadfastly refusing to admit she was mentally ill, she missed only one appointment out of twelve. Although she sat as far away from the therapist as possible and had considerable difficulty talking, she was able to talk some in every session.

She described some paranoid ideation about the white assistant principal who had threatened her with a paddling and suspension from school. She had become

CASE STUDY #38

incensed at this idea and had flown into a rage dramatic enough to result in a consultation with the school nurse and the subsequent referral. Carla spoke infrequently about her relationship with her parents. Apparently her older sister was more important to her. About school she was rather casual and commonly shrugged off all questions about it.

As therapy progressed, it became clear that her relationship with the therapist was more important to Carla than the manifest content in any of the sessions. Her practice of choosing a seat as far from the therapist as possible might be interpreted as either suspicious distancing or reluctance to invade the therapist's personal space, his territory.

Every week Carla would say that she was getting along better at home and at school and suggest that this visit should be the last one. From this the therapist deduced that she could not believe that a high-status, white faculty member would really be interested in seeing her again. A little ritual evolved which was staged at the receptionist's desk after each session:

Carla: Well, good bye, I won't see you next week. ·
Therapist: I want you to come. (Turning to the receptionist) Marcia,
      give Carla an appointment card for 11 a.m. next Tuesday.
Carla: (Standing coyly in the far end of the reception room, smiling)
      I'm not coming.
Marcia: Here's your card, Carla.
Carla: Oh, all right. (Exits with card).

Carla did, in fact, improve, and good reports were sent by the school nurse and the mother at Carla's suggestion. Therefore a joint agreement was made to terminate after the 12th visit.

During the last appointment, when the therapist was explaining how he had enjoyed working with her, Carla seemed rather sad. While the therapist was expressing his positive feelings towards her, she suddenly grasped her abdomen as if in acute pain and stood up near the therapist. He thereupon also stood up, and she swooned into his arms and slowly sank to the floor. When her knees touched the floor, she regained her strength and stood up, only to swoon a second, third, and fourth time within two minutes. She did not say anything, but nodded that she was all right and headed for the door, walking very slowly. The therapist, worried about Carla, sent someone to follow her out of the building and make sure she was all right; he had no chance to talk with her at this point. A day or two later he received a letter from her, in which she apologized for her behavior in his office. The letter was written with such an obvious air of depression, that the therapist felt prompted to call her.

QUESTION B:
WITH THIS INFORMATION, WHAT IS THE BEST DIAGNOSIS?:
1. Pseudoneurotic schizophrenia
2. Psychoneurosis, hysterical type
3. Borderline schizophrenia
4. Psychoneurosis, obsessive-compulsive type
5. Unsocialized aggressive reaction

This girl was raised in a black urban ghetto with its cultural heritage. Her suspiciousness regarding the white school and medical authorities was cultural, not pathological. There was no evidence of a psychotic process. If she was more aggressive than other children in her school, it was a defense against her anxiety. The cause of her anxiety, i.e., the underlying conflict, was never determined, but it seemed that her capacity to develop a relationship with the therapist was helpful to her and resulted in a decrease in her acting-out behavior. Carla suffered from a neurosis, and the final dissociative incident suggests that it was of a hysterical type, not unusual for a girl with an alcoholic father.

CASE STUDY #38

QUESTION C:
IN THE TELEPHONE CONVERSATION WITH CARLA, HOW WOULD YOU INTER-
PRET THE SWOONING INCIDENT?:
1. Simply accept it as a fainting episode, probably caused by the heat and stuffi-
    ness of the office, and pass it off as insignificant
2. Say that her apology was unnecessary and that you thought that this was her
    way of saying goodbye
3. Explain hysterical dissociative episodes to her and suggest that she return
    for further treatment
4. Don't make any interpretation but simply suggest referral to a pediatrician
    for a physical examination
5. Don't make any interpretation but ask her to come in for another visit

We feel that any interpretation over the telephone is risky and inadvisable
because one can't observe the non-verbal communication.   Denial of any emotional
significance of the incident (answers one and four) is not in Carla's best interest.
The therapist chose to provide her with a rationalization by acknowledging that he
understood that it was her way of saying goodbye, which is, in fact, an interpretation, but a very simple and superficial one, designed to relieve her anxiety and
depression rather than provide any insight.   The option to return to psychotherapy
was considered and the decision left up to Carla.

Carla was much relieved by the phone call and elected not to make another
appointment.   She has maintained contact, however, by calling the therapist every
3-6 months over the following two years.   The nature of these contacts is friendly
rather than professional.   Carla always calls the therapist at home, identifies
herself only by her first name, and always just wants to chat for a few minutes.
She never has a complaint or a symptom.   She always agrees to stop in for a visit
at the office, but never does.   She apparently depends on this friendship and seems
to profit from it, for she has continued to do well.

REFERENCES:
1. Adams, P. and N. McDonald, 1968: Clinical Cooling Out of Poor People.
    Amer J of Orthopsychiat 38:457-463

2. Benedict, R., 1949: Continuities and Discontinuities in Cultural Conditioning.
    In: A Study of Interpersonal Relations; Mullahy, P. (Ed.) Heritage Press,
    New York. Reprinted in: Harrison, S.I. and J. F. McDermott (Eds.) Child-
    hood Psychopathology, An Anthology of Basic Readings; International Univ.
    Press, New York, 1972

3. Grier, W.H. and P.M. Cobbs, 1968: Black Rage. Basic Books, New York

4. McDonald, N. and P. Adams, 1967: The Psychotherapeutic Workability of
    the Poor. J Amer Acad Child Psychiatry 1:663-675

5. Meers, D.R., 1970: Contributions of a Ghetto Culture to Symptom Formation:
    Psychoanalytic Studies of Ego Anomalies in Childhood. Psa Study of the Child
    25:209-230

6. Minuchin, S., et al., 1968: Families of the Slums. Basic Books, New York

7. Proctor, J.T., 1958: Hysteria in Childhood. Amer J Orthopsychiatry 28:
    394-403. Reprinted in: Harrison, S.I. and J. F. McDermott, (Eds.) Child-
    hood Psychopathology, An Anthology of Basic Readings. International Univ.
    Press, New York, 1972

CASE STUDY #39

A Short-Tempered 5-Year-Old

Five-year-old Karen was referred to the Child Psychiatry Clinic by her mother's psychotherapist because of behavior problems at home and in nursery school. She was an only child, adopted at one month of age. Growth and development were normal. She had no medical problems except congenital strabismus, which was treated with corrective lenses.

Both parents described Karen as an easy infant to care for except for being a "picky eater." At approximately fourteen months, Karen began having tantrums, consisting of throwing herself on the floor, kicking, and yelling. These tantrums continued at the rate of one to three per day and caused Karen's dismissal from two nursery schools. They usually occurred after she had been denied some request. It also seemed to both parents that the smallest request from them would precipitate a tantrum. Karen often refused to comply with requests to keep her glasses on, stay in the neighborhood, or put away toys. She was not known to steal. Both parents had high expectations for Karen, with behavior goals beyond her age.

Karen's mother seemed to be the scapegoat for her hostility. For example, after being corrected by her father, Karen would run to her mother and shout at her. The father reacted by spanking, the mother by trying to hold Karen and talk to her. By the time the parents came to the clinic, Karen's mother was so afraid of the tantrums that she would not take Karen into stores or call her in from outdoor play.

The father was a 32 year-old fireman. He stated that he had always wanted a large family. He was expecially disappointed when, a month prior to Karen's adoption, his wife was told that she would be unable to conceive. They immediately applied for an adoptive child and within one month received Karen.

The adoptive mother was a 29 year-old woman who was still angry about having to stop work as an executive secretary. Her husband insisted on her remaining at home after Karen was adopted. This caused considerable disagreement and was a major issue at the time of the interview. He had numerous complaints about his wife's housekeeping and her persistent desire to return to work. She felt defeated and at Karen's mercy. She wanted to return to a field where she had received recognition and satisfaction. This marital discord was the reason Karen's mother had sought psychiatric help herself.

QUESTION A:
THIS PATTERN OF CHILD REARING COULD BE BEST CHARACTERIZED AS:
1. Overindulgent
2. Oversubmissive
3. Abusive
4. Neglectful
5. Autocratic

The parents' pattern of child raising can best be described as oversubmissive. They were not neglectful; they provided food, shelter, and clothing, and had repeatedly sought help to control Karen's behavior, which was handicapping her in school, with peers, and in receiving a normal amount of affection from her parents. Karen's father at times wanted absolute obedience from Karen, but on the whole parents only wanted control over reasonable safety and health rules. They were willing to allow Karen freedom in other areas. Karen was an oversubmitted-to child: the parents complied with her unreasonable requests. The mother, especially, would rather give in than suffer another tantrum. Neither parent indulged Karen with unrequested gifts or services. (See cases 5, 9, 28, 37, 48 and 55 for other examples of parental oversubmission).

During the interview, Karen played appropriately for her age, following directions and limits. Intelligence testing showed an IQ of 115.

CASE STUDY #39

QUESTION B:
WITH THIS INFORMATION, THE BEST DIAGNOSIS IS:
1. Habit spasms
2. Petit mal seizures
3. Schizophrenogenic parents
4. Hysterical psychoneurosis
5. Unsocialized aggressive reaction

No evidence has been presented that would support an organic diagnosis. In fact, we have support for a psychogenic process. By age five, one could consider psychoneurosis, but in Karen's case the process dates from 14 months, too early for neuroses. These are not schizophrenogenic parents by any stretch of the imagination. They may be oversubmissive and lacking in confidence, but not schizophrenogenic. The best diagnosis is unsocialized aggressive reaction.

QUESTION C:
THE MOST LOGICAL FORM OF THERAPY UNDER THESE CONDITIONS IS:
1. Family therapy
2. Individual play therapy
3. A behavior modification approach
4. No therapy since the mother is already in treatment
5. A trial of amphetamine

Both parents needed therapy. The mother was especially unable to set limits for Karen. Exploration of their feelings was needed, and this was being carried out, at least in the mother's case, by her therapist. However, resolution of the parents' conflicts would take considerable time and the parents needed more immediate help.

If Karen were older and in danger of expulsion from regular school, a trial of amphetamine could easily be justified. Fish (1971) reports that it is helpful with unsocialized aggressive reactions. However, we are reluctant to medicate pre-schoolers with stimulants until other means of management have been exhausted. The best intervention at this point is behavior modification. Behavior modification provides explicit guidelines for parents who have lost confidence in their ability to raise a child.

Setting up a behavior modification program requires noting what reinforcers maintain the undesirable behavior, and what competing acceptable behaviors are available to be reinforced instead. In Karen's case, her tantrums usually resulted in upsetting her mother, getting attention from her, and getting what she asked for. Karen's good behavior rarely got results because the parents rarely felt anything but anger or fear with her. The strategy would be to reinforce her acceptable behavior by whatever reinforcers were important to Karen. These vary with each child and family. At the same time, Karen's unacceptable behavior was not to be reinforced with attention or submission.

Together the therapist and the parents charted Karen's acceptable and unacceptable behavior and discussed what things were reinforcing to Karen. The program began with low requirements so that Karen would be rewarded immediately for her acceptable behavior and experience some success. Karen usually made her own bed. She was given a star for each day she completed this task. After receiving four stars in a five-day period, she could choose a small toy or a trip for ice cream. The stars thus became secondary reinforcers by their association with the primary reinforcers; they took on the quality of money, which is reinforcing because it can be used to buy primary reinforcers. After a successful five-day period, the requirements for a star were raised to bed-making plus putting away her toys. As Karen ascended to this level, another star was added for keeping her glasses on for the entire day. Other stars were added for other

CASE STUDY #39

activities. At the same time, Karen's parents enforced a "time out" period in her bedroom for every tantrum. The parents, of course, were instructed to ac-company the star-dispensing and other reinforcers with praise and physical af-fection. By this association, the latter were strengthened as reinforcers, antici-pating the eventual phasing out of the "star system. "

Within one month, Karen was earning her praise for every five-day period, and her tantrums had decreased to not more than one per week. At three months, both parents were very pleased with her improved behavior, and it had spilled over into other areas outside of the "star system. " They were pleased at their own success and became more confident as parents.

QUESTION D:
AN APPROPRIATE PLAN FOR THE FUTURE WOULD BE:
1. A shift to a major tranquilizer since the current behavior won't last
2. Discontinuation of therapy since things are going so well
3. An intensified program with the addition of negative reinforcements
4. A broadened program requiring a greater variety of good behavior over longer periods with less intensive reinforcements
5. A shift to individual psychotherapy

The best answer is the fourth, a broadened program. Introducing intensive negative reinforcement at this stage is contraindicated. A shift to individual psychotherapy could be elected but didn't seem necessary. The mother remained in therapy, and was encouraged to do so. What was accomplished was the relief of symptoms, and some therapists might elect a more thorough analysis of the child's intrapsychic organization. However, we saw no reason to posit complex neurotic dynamics behind the opportunistic behavior of a pre-schooler so obvi-ously reacting to parental mismanagement. (See cases 13, 37, 41, and 52 for other examples of successful behavior modificiation).

REFERENCES:
1. Agras, W. S. (Ed.), 1972: Behavior Modification: Principles and Clinical Applications. Little-Brown, Mass

2. Blom, G. E., 1972: A Psychoanalytic Viewpoint of Behavior Modification in Clinical and Educational Settings. J Am Acad Child Psychiatry 11:675-693

3. Carrera, F. and P. Adams, 1970: An Ethical Perspective on Operant Con-ditioning. J Am Acad Child Psychiatry 9:607-623

4. Fish, B., 1971: The "One Child, One Drug" Myth of Stimulants in Hyper-kinesis. Arch Gen Psychiatry 25:193-203

5. Graziano, A. M. (Ed.), 1971: Behavior Therapy With Children. Aldine-Atherton, Chicago, Ill.

6. Missildine, W. H., 1963: Your Inner Child of the Past. Simon & Schuster, N. Y.

7. Missildine, W. H., 1962: Preventive Psychiatry in Emotional Development. Feelings 4, No. 10, Nov. -Dec.

8. Patterson, G. R. and M. E. Gullion, 1968: Living With Children. Res. Press Co., Champaign, Ill.

CASE STUDY #40

(A) Anxiety, (B) Hyperkinesis, (C) Double Deprivation, or (D) All of the Above

Jimmy and John were 5-1/2 when their mother, Barbara, and a welfare worker brought them because of their hyperactivity. They were dizygous twins who had been living with Barbara for only one month. For the previous three years they had been in foster homes. Three months previously the foster mother's concern about the boys' hyperactivity and behavior problems had led to a visit to another clinic. There, a trial of dextroamphetamine (Dexedrine) apparently yielded no benefit and was discontinued.

Mother at first had no complaints about their behavior. She was very frightened that they would be taken away from her, as had happened with Matt, one of her other children. However, she was eventually able to admit concern about the boys' vicious attacks on one another and their constant bouncing from one end of the room to the other. She stated that this seemed to be happening much more in the office than it usually occurred at home.

Barbara's feelings about the children seemed contradictory. In the midst of their tearing the interview room apart, she seemed alternately frightened, anxious, and blase about their behavior. Eventually it became obvious that she was afraid to say what was really on her mind.

The boy's hyperactivity and distractability continued through the second and third visits. Specifically, when asked to do an interesting task, they remained interested for only 20 seconds before being distracted. By the third visit, after they started a major tranquilizer, this had increased to about 30 seconds. John was the more handsome of the twins, with a baby face and blond hair. Jimmy, whose features were not as fine, seemed less hyperactive. They called each other names, threw sharp objects at each other, and alternately laughed, smiled and cried.

During the third visit, the therapist mentioned that he had no interest in taking the children away from Barbara. This seemed to reassure her a great deal. She then felt comfortable enough to discuss details of their destructive behavior at home and how this concerned her. She had been married for a year to a carpenter and felt that she had now stabilized her life well enough to have her children back with her. When rapport was established and upon finding her interviewer empathetic, she began pressing for advice. An older son, Matt, a half-sibling of the twins, was in foster care, and she hoped that he could come home for Christmas, which was four weeks away.

The twins were born when mother's third marriage was ending. In fact, she had been separated from their father the last few months of gestation. Following the delivery she developed complications of diabetes and hyperthyroidism. During this illness the twins were placed with her estranged husband and custody was transferred to him. Later in psychotherapy she revealed anger that her own mother had gone to court to help transfer the custody. Though the father subsequently remarried, child welfare had to place the boys in foster homes because of neglect. They were separated in one of the three foster homes.

When initially seen, they were attending a well-organized pre-kindergarten nursery school. Through a scholarship provided by the welfare service, these two lower-class boys were enabled to attend school with middle-class peers. The teachers were somewhat concerned about the boys' hyperactivity. They felt that John's was worse than Jimmy's. They felt that the boys brought chaos with them from their erratic home life.

The boys' gross coordination was quite good. There was no history or hard neurological sign of brain damage. Their person drawings were markedly immature for their age. Their abilities to hold and use a pencil were poor.

CASE STUDY #40

QUESTION A:
CONSIDERING THE BOYS' PAST HISTORY, WHAT IS THE BEST DESCRIPTION
OF THEIR DIFFICULTY?:

1. The boys exhibited an unsocialized aggressive reaction of childhood manifested by hyperactivity, destructiveness, distractibility, and wide swings in mood. These problems probably resulted from a lack of consistent mothering. Both maternal deprivation and cultural deprivation need to be considered
2. The cause of the boys' hyperactivity, destructiveness, and aggression is a lack of separation of their egos. One ego mass, immaturely developed, is shared between them
3. The family's history of transience and intermittent foster care all speak of maternal deprivation
4. The boys are suffering from intermittent hypoglycemia, which accounts for their chaotic behavior. Perhaps they are also cretins, due to treatment of their mother for hyperthyroidism during pregnancy
5. It is to be expected that any two healthy 5-1/2 year-olds would be destructive, distractable, and constantly in movement, since their nervous systems have not yet matured
6. The boys' behavior is the result of their chaotic interaction prior to this time
7. Whenever children are in more than two foster homes they always exhibit an unsocialized aggressive reaction of childhood because of the lack of consistent mothering

The first answer given is the most comprehensive and therefore the best. The second answer, although sometimes a problem with twins, does not seem to be paramount in this case. The third answer is correct but incomplete. The fourth answer relates medically to mother's illness but the boys' behavior did not fit these two conditions. Normal 5-1/2 year-olds are not overly destructive, distractible, and hyperactive. The sixth answer is too general. Answer seven is not universally true.

The boys' mother, Barbara, had some difficulty keeping regular appointments. She frequently mentioned the welfare worker's visits, implying they were distasteful. Over the months, data was pieced together about her previous chaotic life. Her first child was born illegitimately when she was 17, and she did not finish high school. Since that time she had children by each of three husbands. Two of the older boys had been adopted by her mother and father in another state. She talked with an aura of circumstantiality, and elicited a feeling that one was not getting the complete story. Her older brother was a homosexual. Her older sister, whom she had idolized, died in an automobile accident four years previously. She talked at length about her profound grief. She had gone into a severe depression during which Matt was taken away from her because it was reported to the welfare department that she had left him alone without a baby sitter. She was angry and bitter over this. Because of these events she had begun drinking heavily, worked as a barmaid, and thought very little of herself.

QUESTION B:
FROM THIS HISTORY, ONE COULD EXPECT WHICH OF THE FOLLOWING
FROM THIS MOTHER?:

1. She will most likely abandon the three children that she has and return to an alcoholic life
2. She will continue to be unreliable
3. She will work through the boys' "phases," showing love and affection to the three boys who have missed her. Their hyperactivity and school difficulties will cease. She will miss no future appointments
4. Her hyperthyroidism and diabetes will require such prolonged hospitalization that her three children will have to be returned to foster homes
5. The amount of information that she shares will continue to increase

CASE STUDY #40

6. She will develop a strong transference relationship with the therapist involved. Because of her immaturity, sociopathic personality, and "super-ego lacunae," she will suggest to her children that they do not like their therapist and stop treatment
7. She will continue to miss a few appointments now and then. She will need continued support and reassurance that her behavior is more in question than she herself. Her feelings of anger toward herself for abandoning her children will continue to produce profound guilt and need to be worked through in treatment

There is little evidence for answer one since the history indicated that Barbara had worked very hard to obtain custody of her children. The second answer is not specific enough. The third answer seems overly optimistic, considering the severity of the family's difficulties. The fourth answer ignores the possibility of the present stepfather (the carpenter) continuing to provide a home for his stepchildren even if the mother's medical problems exacerbate. The fifth answer is correct but not very comprehensive. The sixth answer is partially correct since the patient did develop a transference relationship. However, she did not try to stop treatment. The seventh answer was the best prediction of Barbara's behavior.

When the twins came for therapy, their two inexperienced therapists had a great deal of trouble keeping them in separate rooms. They stated that they wanted to be together during the therapy hour. Although their hyperactivity subsided as their home became more stable, they continued to be destructive both at home and at school. Small doses of thioridazine (Mellaril) decreased their anxiety.

QUESTION C:
THE TWINS COULD BE FURTHER HELPED BY SUGGESTING TO THE MOTHER THAT SHE:
1. Focus on the anxious, angry feelings that seem to spark the boys' destructiveness. Suggest that they will need some help in differentiating themselves from each other, as many twins do
2. Stop dressing them alike since this is stunting their sense of self identity. They should be brought at separate times for their therapy hours to help in the separation
3. Provide needed support for the boys to handle their angry destructive feelings
4. Bring the twins for further hospitalization and neurological evaluation of their minimal brain dysfunction. EEG, brain scan, pneumoencephalogram, should be ordered
5. Let the twins finish out the year in their nursery school and go on to kindergarten next year. Mother should be told to be more tolerant of their destructiveness
6. Realize that the boys are angry and that they feel they should let someone know about it
7. Send the boys back to the foster home because she is an inadequate person to be handling their very difficult behavior disorder

The first answer seems the most logical and was helpful in this situation. The second answer may be a couple of good ideas, but it was impossible for this impoverished mother to make extra trips to the clinic each week so the boys could be seen at different times. Therapeutic strategy may also contraindicate separate appointments; the issue of separateness could be used as "grist for the psychotherapeutic mill." The third answer is correct, but not specific or comprehensive enough. The fourth answer would subject the boys to morbidity risks and the parents to financial strain for procedures that the authors feel were not indicated. The "soft neurological signs" of hyperactivity, distractibility, and

CASE STUDY #40

impulsiveness are not reasons enough for a pneumoencephalogram. The mother was in fact encouraged to allow the children to continue in nursery school, but at times she seemed to be too tolerant of their destructiveness and had difficulty setting limits. Answer six is not specific enough. Answer seven is inappropriately judgmental and presents two errors: the boys had already had behavior problems in foster homes, and to send them back would only further reinforce this mother's feelings of inadequacy.

At the clinic, each twin frequently searched out where the other was. They demanded the same toys and the same rewards from their therapists. During the year, their attention span increased from 20 seconds to over a minute on given tasks that they seemed to enjoy. The birth of another sibling, Judy, was followed within a few months by patchy hair loss on Jimmy. The pediatrician diagnosed "alopecia areata secondary to emotional stress." John had breath-holding spells when he was provoked to intense anger. At certain times each became quite engrossed in finger painting and seemed to forget the other twin.

QUESTION D:
THE TWINNING REACTION:
1. Indicated that two egos are irrevocably malformed and that they will become schizophrenic under stress
2. Makes it difficult for the parents to separate out their feelings from one boy or the other
3. Creates difficulties for parents and siblings concerning behavior
4. May be lessened because these boys are dizygous. It is manifested by their constantly seeking each other and it is probably further enhanced by mother dressing them the same
5. Will cause both boys to manifest diabetes at an early age
6. Will not occur because these boys do not look exactly alike
7. Only occurs when the twins are identical (monozygous) and are reared together

Although there is some evidence to indicate that schizophrenia is more common among twins, the prediction in answer one is not warranted. The second answer is correct but incomplete. The third answer is also correct as far as it goes, and new evidence to support this has recently been reported. (Cohen, 1972). The fourth answer is the most comprehensive. The offspring of diabetic parents have an increased risk of diabetes. However, answer five does not relate to the question since it is not twinning that causes diabetes. Although identical twins have greater difficulty with the twinning reaction, it still may occur in fraternal (dizygous) twins to a significant degree. Therefore, answers six and seven are incorrect.

Barbara, Jimmy, John, and Matt each had individual psychotherapy. When Jimmy's therapist was ill at the last moment, Barbara brought him to her interview. He appeared sad and quiet. When given a paper and pencil, he was able to draw for ten minutes without intervention by the mother or her therapist. This was a marked contrast to his behavior one year previously.

QUESTION E:
WHICH WAY COULD ONE INTERPRET JIMMY'S NEW ABILITY TO CONCENTRATE ON THE GIVEN TASK?:
1. Jimmy is hungry and tired since it is almost noon. His lethargy allows him to concentrate on the task for the given period of time
2. After coming to the clinic for almost a year, Jimmy is more trusting than he used to be
3. Jimmy is much less anxious about the security of his home life. He is also one year older and therefore more mature. A few months of regular kindergarten has allowed him practice in being quiet for short periods of time
4. Jimmy has developed a strong transference to mother's therapist. He is doing his best to satisfy him by drawing

CASE STUDY #40

5. Jimmy is much less hyperactive than he used to be because of maturity
6. Jimmy loves to eavesdrop and was not really doing the drawings. Likely he was remembering what was said in the interview with his mother so that he could report it to his twin brother
7. Any child of 6-1/2 years visiting the doctor will be able to sit still for at least ten minutes, as long as he is not distracted

Most children become more irritable and have less ability to concentrate when hungry, weak and tired. The second answer seems correct but is not complete enough. The third answer is the most comprehensive. No evidence has been given to suggest a strong transference reaction to the mother's therapist. Answer five may be correct, but is rather simplistic and incomplete. Answer six, if verbalized by a patient, would likely be taken as evidence of paranoia. The seventh answer is incorrect, unrealistic, and indicates a lack of appreciation for individual differences

QUESTION F:
THE WELFARE WORKER CONTACTED THE FAMILY'S COORDINATING PSY-
CHIATRIST AND ASKED FOR A LETTER TO USE IN COURT REGARDING THE
TRANSFER OF CUSTODY FROM THE COUNTY TO BARBARA AND HER HUS-
BAND. THE THREE BOYS HAD BEEN LIVING WITH THEM FOR A YEAR AND
CONTINUED TO SHOW SOME SIGNS OF EMOTIONAL DISTURBANCE. AL-
THOUGH THE MOTHER'S JUDGMENT SEEMED IMPROVED, HER ANXIETY
LESS, AND HER MOOD CHANGES LESS FREQUENT, SHE CONTINUES TO HAVE
DIFFICULTY MAKING DECISIONS REGARDING HER FOUR CHILDREN'S BE-
HAVIOR. AT THIS POINT:
1. The welfare worker should continue to search for more adequate foster homes since this family's inability to allay their children's anxiety within a full year will lead to serious psychological disturbances in the future
2. Because the family remains somewhat unstable, the welfare worker should intensify her role as a psychotherapist and keep the family in the county's custody
3. The family should continue to be under surveillance
4. The coordinating psychiatrist should continue to foster communication be-tween agencies
5. Because of mother's illnesses, including thyroid insufficiency and diabetes, the boys should have routine medical checkups every three months to insure that their diabetes is caught early
6. Now that the family has become stable, the welfare worker and the psychia-trist should reassure Barbara of her ability to mother her four children, and drop out of the picture
7. Continued mental health support should be given to this family. A recom-mendation should be made to return custody to Barbara and her husband. For continuity of care, the welfare worker should be encouraged to maintain a relationship with the family even though she is not legally bound to

The first three answers are unduly pessimistic. It is not obvious that this family will be unable to care for the children. The second answer assumes that the family has not improved and that the welfare worker will be a psychotherapist; also it would be untherapeutic by putting down the mother. The fourth answer is a part of the correct answer. The fifth answer neglects the psychological prob-lems. The sixth answer does not take into account the future needs of the family. Answer seven, the best, includes a preventive philosophy.

CASE STUDY #40

REFERENCES:

1. Arnold, L. E., In Press, 1973: Is This Label Necessary? J of School Health

2. Bowlby, J., 1969: Attachment and Loss, Basic Books, New York

3. Cohen, D. J., et al., 1972: Personality development in twins: Competence in the newborn and preschool periods. J of Amer Acad of Child Psychiatry 11:625-644

4. Leaverton, D. R., 1968: Pediatrician's role in maternal deprivation. Clinical Pediatrics 7:340-343

5. Leaverton, D. R., 1972: How to Establish Rapport. Humane Social Psychiatry Edited by P. Adams, Tree of Life Press, Gainesville, Florida

6. Sussman, K. E., 1971: Juvenile-type Diabetes and its Complications, Charles C Thomas Publisher, Springfield, Ill.

7. Winestine, M. C., 1969: Twinship and psychological differentiation. J Amer Acad of Child Psychiatry 8:436-455

CASE STUDY #41

An Encopretic 8-Year-Old - A Family Affair

Bruce was an 8 year-old boy who had soiled his pants with feces almost daily for about three years. Initially his toilet training had proceeded uneventfully. Although his parents made no special effort to train him early, his training was essentially completed by the age of three. Between ages 3 and 5 he had only soiled his pants occasionally. When the soiling increased to daily frequency at age 5, Bruce underwent several medical examinations, which were normal. When Bruce was seven years old, his parents consulted a psychiatrist about the problem, but did not follow through with the recommendations. They were now asking for aid again.

Bruce was the middle child of five, one of whom was moderately retarded. His mother was rather warm and maternalistic, but in a conservative, limited way. She spontaneously criticized the "long hair of boys these days," and the apparent "vogue of permissiveness on the part of many parents." Bruce's father was the constable of a small farming community.

During the initial evaluation the boy acted rather shy and somewhat embarrassed about the whole thing. One gained the impression that the parents had tolerated the symptom for a number of years in the hope that he might outgrow it. Instead, it not only increased in frequency, but also became a problem for everyone else in the family. Bruce began to steal his brothers' and sisters' underwear and to hide his soiled garments behind pieces of furniture instead of throwing them into the laundry where his mother would have noticed them.

Bruce rarely suffered from constipation and almost never had loose or watery stools. His soiling consisted of small amounts of normal feces. The physical examination was within normal limits.

Although at first shy and embarrassed, Bruce turned out to be a rather charming little fellow, who seemed generally unconcerned about his problem. It was very clear that his parents and his siblings were more concerned than he was. He was neither anxious nor depressed. He insisted that he had friends and that they did not tease him. In general, he was a good boy who had never been a disciplinary problem at home or at school.

QUESTION A:
WHAT IS THE DIAGNOSIS?:
1. Conversion reaction
2. Hirschsprung's disease
3. Behavior disorder of childhood
4. Encopresis
5. Improper bowel training

Hirschsprung's disease is the result of a congenital deficiency of certain nerve fibers, and therefore the symptoms should appear in infancy. Although bowel training was carried on in a rather permissive manner and was not completed until he was three years old, this is still within the normal range and should not be considered the cause of his difficulty.

In one sense, this boy does have a behavior disorder, because the encopresis is most likely caused by hostility which he can only express in this rather asocial manner. Although he knows what is expected of him in terms of bowel function, he makes no conscious effort to defecate at some regular time of day in order to avoid soiling himself at other times. However, this does not mean that the symptom is caused by a conscious wish to soil. Rather it seems to result from an unconscious conflict created by his inability to express his hostile feelings in a home where a rather rigid mother and an authoritarian father insist that children are to be seen and not heard. Although unconsciously determined, Bruce's symptom enables him to gain a certain amount of conscious control over the members

CASE STUDY #41

of his family, and he is making no efforts to alter the situation. Warson, et al., 1954, suggest there is a conversion element in encopresis, but the best answer is four, a codable, specific diagnosis.

QUESTION B:
WHICH ONE OF THE FOLLOWING IS NOT A TYPE OF ENCOPRESIS?:
1. Paradoxical constipation - holding back of fecal masses with distention of the rectum and "overflow" of a small amount
2. Partial encopresis - staining only of the underclothes
3. Inverse defecation - defecation with reverse peristalsis
4. Continuous encopresis
5. Discontinuous encopresis
6. Retentive encopresis

Encopresis denotes involuntary defecation not directly attributable to a physical disease. The third answer is the only one which has not been described as a variant of the disorder.

The reader is advised to read James B. Anthony's classic paper (1957) on the subject. He describes three prototypic children and their families:

> "The 'continuous' child is a dirty child coming from a dirty family, burdened with every conceivable sort of social problem. The child's messiness forms an integral part of the general messiness and is, to some extent, camouflaged by it. Symptom tolerance in these families is surprisingly high and the parents are usually driven to the clinic, reluctantly and resentfully, by social agencies." The adjective "continuous" is meant to indicate that the child was never trained. This is analogous to "primary" enuresis (see case 37 for discussion; also see case 16).

> "The 'discontinuous' child is the compulsive child of a compulsive family. He is overcontrolled and inhibited in his emotional life and scrupulous with regard to his habits. The toilet "leakage" is his dark secret and towards it he manifests a mixture of shame and anxiety."

> "The 'retentive' child really belongs to a subgrouping of both the main clinical categories, since either of them may, at times, include elements of retentiveness. He undergoes a severe toilet training, and responds to it not with soiling or precarious continence, but with stubborn constipation which later gives way to encopresis (obstipatio paradoxa)."

QUESTION C:
WHAT WOULD BE A LOGICAL METHOD OF TREATMENT IN THIS CASE:
1. Behavioral modification program aimed at teaching him other ways of behavior
2. Frequent enemas to clean out his colon
3. Discussions with the parents in hopes of helping them to teach their children other ways of expressing hostility rather than holding it in and letting it come out in the manner described in this case
4. Severe punishment whenever he soils himself
5. Individual psychotherapy aimed at gaining an understanding of the underlying conflict

CASE STUDY #41

Enemata and punishment do shape the behavior of children but not often along the lines we like to see. In deciding upon the most logical form of treatment, one must consider the child's environment, as well as the child. In this case, the parents are rather rigid and authoritarian and might distort answer three into answer four. Likewise, they would probably not have patience for answer five. Therefore, answers three and five, though good in themselves, are not likely to succeed here. On the other hand, the parents' compulsiveness can be used as an asset if we involve them in a concrete method of reshaping the boy's behavior. Therefore, the first alternative would be the most efficacious in this case.

In order to establish a behavior modification program, the therapist visited the home at a time when every member of the family could be there. Since everyone was suffering directly or indirectly from Bruce's disorder, it was felt that the program should involve every family member, including the retarded child. From Bruce's past history we had learned that he had sometimes remained clean for two or three hours at a time. We also found out that during school hours his sister could check his pants every other class period, i.e., every 1-1/2 hours. Therefore, we decided that he would receive a poker chip for every 1-1/2 hour period in which he did not soil himself. By selecting such a short time period, we made it possible for Bruce to succeed at least a few times a day and to avoid discouragement. Since Bruce enjoyed eating more than anything else, we decided that he would have to buy all of his food with poker chips. We then set the price for breakfast, lunch, and supper in such a way that he would only be able to eat three meals a day if he were symptom-free during the entire day. We made sure that he could not cheat by stealing food. Since we could not lock up everything securely in the kitchen and pantry, we had to rely upon the cooperation of every member to prevent stealing.

On this regimen, Bruce became symptom-free within two days and remained so for a week. After that we made it more difficult for him to earn his meals by lengthening the time period, but he continued to remain clean. (See case 37 for an enuresis "cure.")

QUESTION D:
WHICH OF THE FOLLOWING IS NOT A COMMON CAUSE OF BEHAVIOR MODI-FICIATION FAILURES?:
1. Failure to find the right reinforcer for a particular child
2. Starting with too difficult a behavioral requirement to get the reward
3. Starting with too easy a behavioral requirement
4. Raising the behavioral requirement too fast or by too large jumps
5. Raising the behavioral requirement too slowly or by too small steps
6. Failing to raise the required behavior at all
7. Allowing the reinforcer without the required behavior

Though some children will work for jelly beans, others abhor them. No assumption should be made about what will reinforce a given child. See case 52 or an example of difficulty finding the right reinforcer, a very unusual one. In researching this matter for a given case, non-tangible social reinforcers should not be overlooked; if they work, the child is already one step on his way to the ultimate goal of self-perpetuating improvement. The behavior initially required must be in the child's repertoire, so that he will have a chance to be reinforced. If this child had initially been required to remain clean all day to be rewarded, he might have given up. Too quick or too large a jump in the behavioral requirement soon enough may bore or satiate the child, reducing motivation. Starting with too easy a requirement is hardly ever a problem, as long as it is promptly raised. Three is the best answer.

CASE STUDY #41

QUESTION E:
THE PROGNOSIS FOLLOWING SUCH TREATMENT PROGRAMS IS:
1. Guarded, because the simple relief of symptoms usually means a shift to new symptoms
2. Poor, because one cannot keep giving poker chips forever
3. Good, because the patient gets constant social reinforcement, e.g. through more and better friendships
4. Poor, because the symptom indicates severe ego impairment
5. Guarded; the symptom will probably return whenever the parents get angry at him

The third answer is best. Stronger friendships and maturity will help prevent return of this particular symptom. This is not to say that it is consciously determined; it is probably a neurotic symptom. If new symptoms occur (answer one), they could be treated appropriately at a later date. On the other hand, by relieving this symptom at age eight, we may prevent a secondary psychoneurosis around the self-image of "stinker."

REFERENCES:
1. Agras, W. S. (Ed.), 1972: Behavior Modification: Principles and Clinical Applications, Little-Brown, Mass., Pub.

2. Anthony, E. J., 1957: An Experimental Approach to the Psychopathology of Childhood: Encopresis. Br J Med Psychol 30:156-162, 172-174. Reprinted in: Harrison, S. I., McDermott, J. F. (Eds.) Childhood Psychopathology, An Anthology of Basic Readings, New York, Int. Univ. Press, 1972, pp. 610-625

3. Graziano, A. M. (Ed.), 1971: Behavior Therapy With Children. Aldine-Atherton, (Pub.), Chicago, Ill.

4. Kanner, L., 1972: Child Psychiatry, 4th Ed. Springfield, Charles C Thomas

5. Patterson, G. R. and M. E. Gullion, 1968: Living With Children. Res. Press Co., Pub., Champaign, Ill.

6. Shane, M., 1967: Encopresis in a Latency Boy; An Arrest Along a Developmental Line. Psa St of the Child 22:296-314

7. Warson, S. R., et al., 1954: The Dynamics of Encopresis. Am J of Orthopsych 24:402-415

CASE STUDY #42

Susan, a Troubled Sleepwalker

A shy, slightly built, nine year-old girl was referred by her parents because of sleepwalking since age four. Recently this had increased from weekly to 3-4 times a week. She had become quarrelsome and excitable and was often afraid to go to the bathroom by herself, even during the day.

Her pattern of sleepwalking was always the same. She whimpered and trembled with her eyes open while running up and down stairs, turning on all the lights. She awakened yawning with no recollection of her dreams or of her behavior.

There were three other children: a twelve year-old sister who suffered mild cerebral palsy, and five year-old twin brothers in good health. The parents were in their late thirties.

The mother presented as a fussy, tense woman who was overdemanding in her relationship with the patient, while the father appeared casual and detached. He was in an exporting business which necessitated his being away for months at a time. He left the raising of the children to his wife and his only concern seemed to be that they didn't disturb him. The parents had never found a home in which they felt comfortable; they had moved at least once every year since their marriage.

The child's developmental milestones were normal and her early history was without incident, with the exception of a short period of time at about four years when the parents suspected deafness. This was ruled out by an otologist. The parents had taken Susan for a neurological consultation before referring her to the clinic. A normal EEG was obtained and the consultant ruled out a seizure disorder.

In the recent past the family dog had been killed by a car while the child was playing with it, and her closest playmate had moved away.

The school reported that the child was doing well in the fourth grade, but that she was sometimes pensive.

A psychological evaluation included intelligence and projective tests. The outstanding feature in her relationship with the psychologist was her physical and emotional immobility. Her only movements were facial gestures; she never touched any of the test materials, and even when she told about the "scary things" she thought about, she spoke in an inappropriately flat voice. She seemed to want the psychologist to like her; she was taking all precautions against arousing displeasure by trying to remain unobtrusive and obedient.

She obtained an I.Q. of 120 on the WISC, which contained many unusual answers involving sinister and dangerous content. Neither the WISC nor the Bender-Gestalt contained any organic signs.

In her drawings of people the eyes were large and heavily accented, with the pupils drawn in, suggesting suspiciousness. All of her human figures, with one exception, were stiff and immobilized. The exception was a drawing of one of her friends being threatened with a whipping by an adult male figure. She also drew a picture of her family sitting in a circle with herself missing. In general, her drawings suggested that her environment failed to respond to her needs in that she portrayed it as either remaining unresponsive or openly rejecting and aggressive.

Her Children's Apperception Test (CAT) stories were riddled with free-floating anxiety and a feeling of ubiquitous danger. The child seemed to feel that to be noticed was to be threatened and attacked, which may help to explain her behavior with the psychologist. (See Case 32 for a frankly paranoid 7 year-old.)

The stories also threw some light on the sleepwalking. They suggested that at bedtime she felt particularly vulnerable and deserted. Her fears seemed to be of male figures who were prone to disturb sleep with cruel threats and who humiliated her for insignificant failures. They also suggested the ordinary sexual curiosity of a nine year-old, but contained feelings of guilt about her curiosity as well as fears of punishment.

CASE STUDY #42

The Rorschach produced additional sinister imaginings as well as intense feelings of depression and despair. Again there were feelings of rejection and of being treated as an object rather than as a little girl who desperately needed affection and support. Father was a terrifying figure while mother was seen as ruthless and frightening when in collusion with father. When seen alone, the mother appeared ineffectual.

In both the CAT and the Rorschach, the child was aware of her own dependent needs. However, she feared that these would go unfulfilled because of angry impulses, either her own or those of others directed towards her. She saw herself sometimes as predator, sometimes as prey. She seemed well defended during her waking hours, but at the cost of her own spontaneity and self-assertiveness. At night her defenses were weaker and her fears slipped through.

QUESTION A:
THIS CASE ILLUSTRATES:
1. What happens to a middle child
2. That the attention required by a physically handicapped child causes siblings to be left out and neglected
3. That moving causes sleepwalking in a child
4. Parental rejection of a child
5. That a combination of unavoidable circumstances within a family can be detrimental to a child's feelings of well-being

Not all middle children develop problems. Although these parents may have been sensitive to the feelings of the patient, circumstances may have made it difficult for them to devote the time and energies she required. The best answer is five.

QUESTION B:
ALTHOUGH THE CHILD WAS THE IDENTIFIED PATIENT, THERE WERE SIGNS OF MARITAL PROBLEMS, INCLUDING:
1. The child's fear of the bathroom
2. That an older sister had cerebral palsy
3. The parents were approaching middle age
4. The child turned on the lights while sleepwalking
5. The child's developmental milestones were normal
6. None of the above

The signs of marital discord were the mother's overdemandingness and tenseness, the father's detached attitude and choice of work requiring long periods away from home, and the fact that the family had moved each year. The latter suggests that the parents may have been projecting the blame for the discord on their environment rather than looking for causes withing their own relationship. "None of the above" is correct.

QUESTION C:
APPROPRIATE PSYCHIATRIC INTERVENTION WOULD HAVE BEEN:
1. Group psychotherapy for the parents to help them to work through their problems
2. Individual psychotherapy for the child
3. Family therapy
4. Marital counseling for the parents and a bedtime sedative for the child
5. Individual psychotherapy for the child and psychotherapy for the parents, followed by family therapy
6. Group psychotherapy for the child and individual counselling for the parents, followed by family therapy

CASE STUDY #42

It would seem that all of the children in this family could have benefited if the tensions between the parents and within the family could have been reduced and the family could have started communicating and sharing their concerns.

Susan, who was almost immobilized by her anxiety, certainly needed help. A trial in group psychotherapy with children of her own age might have been appropriate, provided her parents could have had counselling at the same time. If this failed to reduce her anxiety and sleepwalking, individual psychotherapy could have been considered. The best answer is six, but answer five should be given strong consideration.

QUESTION D:
HINTS THAT THE PATIENT'S EMOTIONAL PROBLEMS MAY HAVE STARTED LONG BEFORE THE REFERRAL WERE:
1. That Susan appeared deaf at age four, with no otological findings
2. That the sleepwalking began at about age four, when the twins were born
3. The family's many moves
4. The mother's tensions and fussiness
5. Susan's sinister projections on the Rorschach, which indicated fear

Occasionally apparent deafness is a sign of withdrawal behavior in a child, i.e., that the outside world is too painful and the child finds more comfort in his inner world of fantasy. Sleepwalking in a young child is often a search for the mother when the child feels he isn't getting enough from her. One and two are correct.

QUESTION E:
THE EXPRESSION "WORKING THROUGH" AS USED IN QUESTION C, MEANS:
1. Being in psychotherapy
2. Attending psychotherapy sessions regularly
3. Gradually coming to understand the implications of an insight into one's behavior
4. Getting a job in order to pay for one's psychotherapy
5. Going as fast as one can in psychotherapy in order to terminate

According to Rycroft (1968) "working through" was originally a psychoanalytic term for the process by which a patient discovers piece by piece, over a period of time, the implications of an insight or interpretation. He gives as an example the mourning process which involves the gradual awareness and acceptance of the fact that the lost object will never be available again. The best answer is three.

REFERENCES:
1. Ames, L. B., Learned, J., et al., 1952: Child Rorschach Responses: Developmental Trends from Two to Ten Years. New York, Hoeber

2. Bellak, L., 1954: The Thematic Apperception Test and the Children's Apperception Test and the Children's Apperception Test in Clinical Use. New York, Grune & Stratton

3. Bender, L., 1938: A visual motor gestalt test and its clinical use. Am Orthopsychiat Assn Monogr. Series No. 3

CASE STUDY #42

4. Burns, R. C. and S. H. Kauffman, 1970: Kinetic Family Drawings (K-F-D) and Introduction to Understanding Children Through Kinetic Drawings, Brunner-Mazel, New York

5. Cobb, S. and A. Butler, 1949: Clinic on psychosomatic problems: psychogenic deafness in a disturbed boy. Am J Med 7:221-227

6. English, O. S. and G. H. J. Pearson, 1972: Irrational fears and phobias. In: Childhood Psychopathology., ed. S. Harrison and J. F. McDermott, New York, International Universities Press, pp. 375-381

7. Frank, G., 1965: The role of the family in the development of psychopathology. Psychol Bull 64:191-205

8. Halpern, F. 1953, A Clinical Approach to Children's Rorschachs. Grune & Stratton, New York

9. Harms, E. E., 1963: Problems of Sleep and Dreams in Children. New York, Pergamon Press

10. Haworth, M. A., 1966: The CAT: Facts about Fantasy. New York, Grune & Stratton

11. Plotsky, H. and Shereshefsky, M., 1960: An isolation pattern in fathers of emotionally disturbed children. Am J Orthopsychiat 30:780-787

12. Rowe, M., 1963: The Bender-Gestalt as a screening technique for psychiatric disorders in children. Unpublished dissertation, U. of London

13. Rycroft, C., 1968: A Critical Dictionary of Psychoanalysis. Basic Books, Inc., New York, p. 179

14. Wechsler, D. Manual: Wechsler Intelligence Scale for Children. The Psych. Corp., New York, 1949

CASE STUDY #43

Too Bad You're Mad, Dad - Your Visits Make Me Sad

A 10-1/2-year-old, white, Protestant, middle-class boy was brought by his divorced parents because of his desire to stay constantly with his mother and his "negative attitude" towards such activities as school trips, vacations with his father, visits with his father, and playing organized baseball.

The trouble dated to about six months previously, when he vomited (apparently because of gastroenteritis) while on a visit with his father. Prior to that time he had seemed to enjoy such visits and had been engaging in the usual activities for a boy his age, including Little League Baseball. However, since that incident he had resisted playing on the organized team even when his mother dropped him off at the practice area. He preferred to play ball with friends in his backyard. He also refused field trips with his class because the lunch on the trip induced nausea. For a few days he even resisted going to school, claiming nausea in the cafeteria. He settled for having lunch at home when his mother firmly insisted on school attendance. His parents' main concern however, was his refusal to visit his father, with complaints of abdominal distress and nausea each time the father arrived to pick him up. He even refused to answer the father's telephone messages.

He had passed the fifth grade with a consistent B average, which had not changed since the onset of symptoms. He had refused to attend school in the first grade for a few weeks but eventually adapted to it.

His father was a 44 year-old aggressive executive who completely dominated the mother even since their divorce three years previously. When the mother mentioned that the boy had been accidentally hit on the head with a golf club, the father interjected the assurance that he was not the one who had hit the boy. He went out of his way to insist that he loved his son.

The boy's mother was a slim, anxious, dependent woman who was just beginning to show her 41 years. She admitted privately that she was afraid to speak up against the boy's father for fear that he would stop support payments. She did some volunteer work and went out approximately once a week with friends.

The boy himself was an intelligent, likable, verbal lad who did not wish to come to the clinic and tended to deny his problems. For example, he explained away his running in front of a car as "I just went for a walk." (His mother felt he was attempting suicide.) In several indirect ways he indicated a wish for his parents to be reconciled, even though he knew his father had already remarried another woman. When asked to draw a person, he drew a character from Sesame Street who lives in a garbage can (see Fig. 43)

QUESTION A:
THIS BOY'S DRAWING OF A "PERSON" SHOWN IN FIGURE 43 SHOWS:
1. That he feels like garbage
2. That he would like to put his father in the garbage
3. That he would like to put his younger sib in the garbage
4. Defensive guardedness
5. An interest in cartoon characters which reflects an impairment of reality orientation

Inclusion of a garbage can in drawings by children with younger sibs usually indicates a fantasied repository for the rival (Burns and Kaufman, 1972), but this boy is an only child. Hence we can suspect that the picture may be more indicative of his feelings about himself: the no-good garbage boy, rejected by his father because of his inability to fulfill his father's expectations. It should be recalled that the term "can" is also a slang expression for toilet. The dog food by the side of the can may also be an expression of the boy's feelings of "being in the doghouse," again a target of the father's scorn. The size and sturdy

CASE STUDY #43

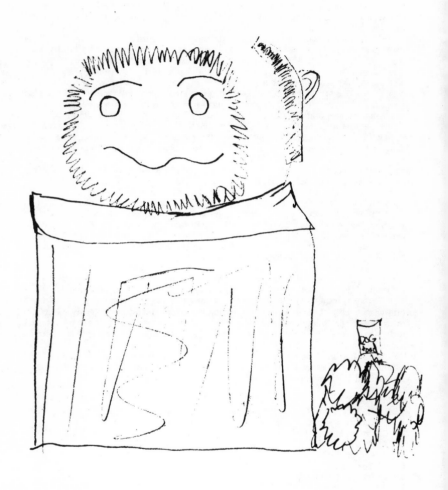

FIGURE 43

CASE STUDY #43

appearance of the garbage can may express the boy's needs for a strong, protected retreat, a place to which he could withdraw when he sensed his father's disappointment and anger with him. The drawing is probably "overdetermined." One and four are the best answers. Nothing in the clinical picture corroborates the possibility of reality orientation impairment.

He and his parents were seen seven times over a period of two months. The treatment modalities used were play therapy, parent counseling, and family therapy. Though initially resistant, he soon developed rapport with his play therapist. The mother revealed more of the depths of her own insecurity. She was particularly upset by such incidents as his saying, "I hate you" or posting a sign on his door to that effect. Neither parent could psychologically tolerate such an expression from him. The parents agreed that the only reason he didn't say it to his father was that the father would "swat him" for it. Both parents tended to blame each other, the father overtly, the mother secretly because she feared the father, her ex-husband. The father felt the mother should have forced the boy to answer his phone calls. The mother claimed privately that the father never took much interest in the boy till after the divorce.

With empathic support, the mother arrived at the conclusion that she would rather have her son behave right and hate her than to have him love her and be bad. At first she was very unsure of this, but after assurance that this was a reasonable position for a parent who really cared about the child, she was able to tell the boy. Much to her surprise, he showed visible relief. After thus learning that his mother could accept his hate feelings as well as his love, he improved dramatically. He and his mother worked out compromises on minor points, such as agreement that he would return home for lunch for the coming school year but eat at school in junior high the following year.

At each step the mother seemed unsure of her own judgment, and would check it with the therapist. As she gradually gained more confidence in her own good judgment, she was able to be both more firm and more reasonable with the boy. For instance, whenever he entered a new situation for the first time, she allowed him one of the pills which the pediatrician had prescribed to "settle his stomach," even though the father objected to such a "crutch." She noted that after successfully negotiating the first experience with the pill's help, he was able to negotiate the same situation subsequently without a pill.

When last seen he had been going on visits with his father and other, and was happier, more spontaneous, and more confident of his ability to deal with people. He decided to terminate treatment with the agreement of the therapist.

QUESTION B:
THE BEST DIAGNOSTIC DESCRIPTION OF THIS CASE WOULD BE:
1. Psychophysiologic gastrointestinal reaction
2. Conversion reaction
3. Phobic neurosis
4. School phobia
5. Father phobia
6. Symbiotic psychosis
7. Agoraphobia
8. Hypochondriacal neurosis
9. Adjustment reaction of childhood

Three, four, five and seven are all defensible answers, but the best is seven, with five a close second. Phobic neurosis would be the official codable nomenclature, but one of the other three would impart more specific information about this case as a diagnostic impression and should at least be added in parentheses. The somatizing childhood agoraphobia which usually presents as school phobia presented in this case as more of a "father phobia," probably because: 1. This mother was able to be confidently firm about the boy's school attendance, but was for unconscious reasons not able to be equally as confident and firm about other

CASE STUDY #43

activities. This nipped the "school phobic" manifestations of the syndrome in the bud, but allowed other manifestations. 2. The father's aggressive, pushy, "scary" manner set him up as a suitable magnet for phobic feelings. 3. The away-from-home bout of gastroenteritis which seems to have precipitated the agoraphobia occurred during a visit with his father, rather than while at school.

Though there is a symbiotic element present in most such childhood agoraphobias, with the child acting out the mother's anxiety, the symbiosis is not of psychotic proportions. Therefore, this should not be confused with symbiotic psychosis (Mahler & Gosliner, 1955), in which the egos of the mother and child blend. Though the situation-dependent gastrointestinal symptoms suggest a psychophysiological phenomenon, and though the converting of anxiety to abdominal distress and the obvious secondary gain involved suggest a conversion reaction, neither of these seems to be the best diagnosis. The focal point is the phobic manifestation, and the secondary gain from the abdominal symptoms is in the service of the phobia.

QUESTION C:
IN ADDITION TO THE MATERNAL INSECURITY, ANXIETY, AND FEELING OF INADEQUACY USUALLY INVOLVED IN THIS TYPE OF PROBLEM, WHICH OF THE FOLLOWING IS A LESS USUAL FACTOR FOUND IN THIS PARTICULAR CASE?:
1. The mother's resentment against her ex-husband's continuing aggressive, critical overcontrol of her and the boy and her inability to do anything overt about it because of her fear of him
2. The mother's resentment about her ex-husband's withdrawal of love from her
3. The mother's inability to tolerate any hint from the boy that he did not think she was a good, loving mother
4. The relative poverty in which the family of an important executive was forced to live
5. The father's brutality
6. The father's lack of interest in the boy

Paternal brutality, at least physical, appears unlikely in this case. The father did not appear uninterested at the time of therapy, though we could not rule this out as a problem in the past. Despite the mother's worries, he did continue to support the family. Three is a usual part of this problem. The mother did indeed resent the father's withdrawal of love from her and was still psychologically married, but we have no solid evidence that this caused the presenting symptoms. Of course, it is possible that this resentment led her to sabotage the father-son relationship by unconsciously sanctioning the boy's refusal to visit the father. However, a better explanation for this unconscious sanction resides in answer one, the best answer.

QUESTION D:
TREATMENT EFFORTS IN SUCH CASES SHOULD BE DIRECTED TOWARDS:
1. Long-term individual psychotherapy of the child, guarding confidentiality by avoiding the parents
2. Concentrating on supportive or nondirective psychotherapy for the mother
3. Desensitization
4. An accepting therapeutic atmosphere for both the child and his parents
5. Group therapy
6. Tranquilization
7. A stimulant drug to help the child feel more like breaking away from his mother

Any therapeutic approach which fails to consider the family dynamics, particularly the mother-child relationship as influenced by the mother's anxiety and

CASE STUDY #43

insecurity, would not likely succeed in treating somatizing childhood agoraphobia. The best answer is four, with two an important supplementary answer. Occasionally such family-oriented therapy may be inadvisable, or the parents may refuse. When family therapy is unfeasible, group therapy may have some value, by re-creating the family problem within the artificial family of the group. However, it would not ordinarily be the therapy of choice for this type of case. Stimulants are not indicated. In fact, drugs of any kind are usually not necessary, but benefit has been reported for tricyclic antidepressants in school phobia (Gittelman-Klein & Klein, 1971). Temporary tranquilization may sometimes help when the level of anxiety interferes with psychotherapy and family therapy, but in a case like this it may be more appropriate to tranquilize the mother than the child. Desensitization works best where the phobia is egodystonic; this case does not seem to meet that criterion.

REFERENCES:
1. Agras, S., 1959: The relationship of school phobia to childhood depression, Amer J Psychiat 116:533-536, 1959

2. Axline, V., 1947: Play Therapy, Ballentine Books, New York

3. Burns, R.C. and S.H. Kaufman, 1972: Actions, Styles, and Symbols in Kinetic Family Drawings, Brunner-Mazel, New York

4. Gardner, R.A., 1970: Boy's and Girl's Book About Divorce, Science House, Scranton, Pa.

5. Gittleman-Klein, R. and D.F. Klein, 1971: Controlled Imiprimine Treatment of School Phobia, Archives of Gen Psychiatry 25:204-207

6. Johnson, A., 1941: School Phobia, Amer J of Orthopsychiatry, 11:702-711

7. Mahler, M.S., 1965: On early infantile psychosis: The symbiotic and autistic syndromes, J Amer Acad of Child Psychiatry 4:554-568

8. Mahler, M.S. and B. Gosliner: On symbiotic child psychosis: Genetic, Dynamic and Restitutive aspects. Psychoanal Study of the Child 10:195-211

9. Missildine, H., 1963: Your Inner Child of the Past, Simon & Schuster, N.Y.

CASE STUDY #44

A 12-Year-Old Hangs Himself

Jim was 12 years old when admitted as an emergency to a psychiatric in-patient unit following a serious suicide attempt. He had tied one end of a bathrobe cord around his neck and the other end to a railing in an attempt to hang himself in the stairwell of his home. When discovered by his mother, he was in such a position that he could not have saved himself.

Jim had previously made other attempts at hanging himself which were much less effective. In those cases he usually sat on the floor of a closet in his home, tied a rope from his neck up over the bar and attempted to pull the rope tight enough to strangle himself. These instances had occurred over a period of ap-proximately six months and often seemed to be attempts to avoid doing something such as delivering the papers on his paper route. Therefore, they had been con-sidered suicide gestures rather than suicide attempts. The mother had been advised to be as casual as she could about such gestures, but the particular in-cident preceding his admission appeared distinctly more serious to everyone.

During the six months prior to admission, the patient's father had become seriously ill with abdominal symptoms and had finally died of carcinoma of the stomach at age 45. For approximately a year prior to admission the boy had become more despondent and disobedient. Thus the mother had three concurrent worries: her husband's health, the boy's suicide gestures, and the boy's dis-obedience. In the belief that the latter represented a behavior disorder rather than a depressive reaction, the child was referred to a neurologist. On Jim's first examination, which took place one month after the father's death, the neurologist discovered café-au-lait spots, which had been present since birth, and which had also been present on the father and a college-aged sister. How-ever, none of the three had displayed any symptoms of neurofibromatosis (von Recklinghausen's disease). The father had not had any neurological findings during his life, but when the child's neurologist heard that the father had recently died of cancer, he took the mother aside and asked her if the father might also have had cancer of the brain. He wondered, of course, if the father might not actually have died of a brain stem neurofibroma. Despite a normal neurological examination and a normal electroencephalogram the physician felt that the be-havior could be related to the cafe-au-lait spots and started Jim on a therapeutic trial of diphenylhydantoin (Dilantin). The medication caused no apparent change in the boy's behavior, but he was still on the anticonvulsant at the time of admis-sion to the psychiatric unit.

QUESTION A:
THE MOST LIKELY DIAGNOSIS IS:
1. Depression over the loss of the father five months earlier
2. Depressive phase of a manic-depressive psychosis
3. Behavior disorder with suicidal gestures as manipulative devices, this par-ticular incident accidentally becoming more serious
4. Depression secondary to an organic process, CNS neurofibromatosis
5. None of the above

Although children do use suicide gestures as a means of manipulating parents, it is difficult to make such a judgment. It would be safer to begin by presuming the act to be a bona fide suicide attempt and to disprove the presumption later if possible. (See discussion of Question C.) The doctor might consider the sort of person the patient is and why it became necessary for him to use this particular way of communicating with his parents or other people. Generally speaking, chil-dren should not be classed with histrionic adults who make many empty suicide threats and gestures and finally kill themselves accidentally. In contrast with adults, children often do not leave suicide notes, although they will frequently tell their friends that they have taken a lot of pills, and thus gain medical attention.

CASE STUDY #44

Jim's use of suicide threats had apparently been a means of avoiding onerous chores. Possibly he had become more depressed during his father's illness and we saw only a continuation of this depression after the death. There was no evidence of a psychotic or organic process, so the first answer is the best working diagnosis.

Jim's behavior in the hospital changed during his 3-month stay. In the beginning he mischievously misbehaved. Then followed a period of considerable resistance to therapy and to his medication. During the final period he was the model patient. The change was brought about when the therapy dealt with two important issues: Jim's resistance to individual psychotherapy and his resistance to taking his anticonvulsant. Jim liked his middle-aged, male therapist and particularly liked to spend time with him informally, but he did not like to come to psychotherapeutic sessions and chose to avoid them as often as he could. He finally explained that the therapist reminded him of his father, because they were the same age and the therapist's desk and desk set were very similar to his father's. Therefore he found it difficult to talk during his therapy sessions. He found it easier to talk with women, particularly his mother, who was very warm and rather wise, although she tended to be somewhat formal, in the customary middle-class manner. Consequently we enlisted his mother as his therapist. Under the supervision of the previous therapist, she carried out regularly scheduled psychotherapeutic sessions. She also made the less formal visits to the ward.

During one of these sessions, which were observed by the supervisor via one-way glass, the boy described how he felt about his anticonvulsant medication. It meant to him that he had a disease of a rather mysterious nature. He was aware that his father and his sister also had cafe-au-lait spots, but neither one of them ever had to take this medicine; in some way he had a disease that they did not have. Also, he knew that his father had died of a tumor, and that this had been of special importance to the neurologist, who, upon hearing about it, had taken the mother aside to talk to her. This made the boy wonder if he, too, had the disease that had been fatal to his father. After consultation with his pediatrician, the medication was discontinued, a move which was followed by dramatic improvement. He was discharged with a final diagnosis of psychoneurosis, depressive type. See case 5 for an example of successful diphenylhydantoin treatment of a behavioral problem.

The physician and the parent must be very careful how they explain diagnoses, medications, surgical procedures, diagnostic tests, and even decisions about no treatment whatsoever to a youngster. When a young child hears that his tonsils are inflamed, he very often becomes anxious that someone is thinking of removing his tonsils. Such associations are learned during his everyday life. One child, a 10 year-old boy, limped for two years after an uncomplicated recovery from a fractured femur, because he knew his grandmother had limped for seven years after a fractured hip; he thought that it takes many years for a bone to regain its full strength. By itself this is not sufficient evidence for a diagnosis of psychoneurosis, and such distortions can be prevented by careful, age-appropriate explanations by the physician.

QUESTION B:
JIM'S MISCONCEPTION REGARDING THE PRESCRIBED MEDICATION (DILANTIN) WAS PROBABLY DUE TO HIS:
1. Limited understanding of the pharmacology involved
2. Being unaware that it was just a therapeutic trial
3. Obstinate refusal to listen to the initial and subsequent explanations, a sign of his behavior disorder
4. Natural anxiety over the meaning of the medicine and his own health
5. Exaggerated anxiety associated with deep-seated fears of death.

CASE STUDY #44

When a child is provided with new information, he associates it with experiences and knowledge, sometimes instantly and sometimes only after he has given the subject considerable thought. Twelve-year old children are often quite logical in their thinking processes, but they are prone to make quantum jumps on occasion. Jim's thinking was perfectly logical, as far as we can tell, and his misunderstanding was due to a natural degree of anxiety; the fourth answer is correct.

QUESTION C:
SUICIDE IN ADOLESCENTS IN THE UNITED STATES IS:
1. Less common in late as compared to young adolescents
2. The leading cause of death
3. Not a serious health problem
4. A significant cause of death and increases with age
5. A rare occurrence and most often accidental

Suicide is the fifth leading cause of death in the 15-19 year age range, and the 18th in the 10-14 year olds. The fourth answer is correct. Twelve percent of all reported attempted suicides in this country are made by the 15-19 year old population who represent only 8.5% of the total population.

Adolescents usually give warnings before attempting suicide. Communication of intent is given in two-thirds of both adult and adolescent psychiatric patients, but 43% of the teenagers go on to an attempt as compared to only 14% of adults. It would appear that adolescent threats should be taken seriously.

REFERENCES:
1. Balser, B. H. and J. F. Masterson, 1959: Suicide in Adolescents. Amer J of Psychiatry 116:400-404

2. Gurney, B. G., Gurney, L. F. and M. P. Andronico, 1970: New Directions in Client Centered Therapy. Hart & Tomlinson, Eds. Houghton-Mifflin Co., Boston, Mass.

3. Hornsby, L. E., 1969: Filial Therapy. Personal Communication

4. Mattson, A., et al., 1969: Suicidal Behavior as a Child Psychiatric Emergency. Arch of Gen Psychiatry 20:100-109

5. Sabbath, J. C., 1969: The Suicidal Adolescent - The Expendable Child. J Am Acad Child Psychiatry 8:272-289

6. Schneer, H., et al., 1961: Events and Conscious Ideation Leading to Suicidal Behavior. Psychiat Quart 35:507-515

7. Seiden, R. H., 1971: Suicide Among Youth. Supplement to the Bull of Suicidology. USPHS Pub. Nov. 1971

8. Shrut, A., 1964: Suicidal Adolescents and Children. JAMA 188:1103-1107

9. Stevenson, E. K., et al., 1972: Suicidal Communication by Adolescents, Study of Two Matched Groups of Sixty Teenagers. Dis of the Nerv Sys 33:112-122

10. Toolan, J., 1962: Suicide and Suicidal Attempts in Children and Adolescents. Am J Psychiat 118:719-724

11. White, J. H., Hornsby, L. G. and R. Gordon, 1972: Treating Infantile Autism with Parent Therapists. Int J of Child Psychotherapy 1:83-95

CASE STUDY #45

"Ann Didn't Get a Fair Shake"

Ann was a 3-1/2 year-old brought to the Child Psychiatry Clinic by her step-grandmother (Mrs. H.) because of her "rebellion, destructiveness, shaking spells, and temper tantrums." Ann's grandfather had taken her and her sister a few months earlier because of her 23 year-old mother's transience and irresponsibility. Her sister, Nettie, was 20 months old and always accompanied Ann and Mrs. H. She was developmentally delayed, with a waddling gait.

Ann's grandfather had recently remarried, partially because of his grand-daughters' needs. The step-grandmother, previously a widow employed as a child care worker in an institution for the retarded, was in her mid-sixties. She had raised her own children and was beginning a second life as mother to these two girls.

On many occasions the children's mother had abandoned them to leave the state with various boyfriends. A history of physical abuse by both mother and father was documented. When abandoned to the grandfather, the girls' weighed less than normal, had no clothes, and were almost mute with fear.

Mrs. H. was concerned because the girls fought with each other and could not share toys. They had recurrent upper respiratory infections from which they recovered very slowly. They either talked back to Mrs. H. or else shrank away in fear whenever approached about misconduct.

Ann's most prominent behavioral feature was shaking after the slightest amount of stress. This was not improved by an antihistamine sedative which Mrs. H. obtained from her local general physician prior to his referral.

QUESTION A:
THE MOST LIKELY REASON FOR ANN'S SHAKING IS:
1. Anxiety, rage, or fear, resulting from inconsistent, abusive, inadequate parenting by mother
2. Incorporation of the mother's rage reactions
3. Inconsistent mothering
4. Starvation, with resultant hypoglycemia
5. A phase which Ann is going through related to her previous bowel training. It will pass in time
6. A disturbance in the mother-child relationship
7. Mirroring of her elderly grandparents' Parkinson-like shakiness

Shaking, waddling gait, and a dull, listless expression are often found in neglected toddlers. These are thought to arise from anxiety, rage, or fear. Therefore answer one is the best. The second answer inaccurately uses the term, "incorporation"; it also seems unlikely that Ann would imitate her mother's rage reactions. Inconsistent mothering is correct but incomplete. Children with hypo-glycemia can shake but starvation would have to be severe to cause hypoglycemia, and these girls had been fed by the grandparents for several months. Answer five is incorrect and overly optimitsic. Answer six is too general and seven is unlikely.

Ann's mother visited on a drop-in basis at the grandparents' house. She sometimes overwhelmed the girls with gifts. During one of the clinic visits, the step-grandmother suggested that the psychiatric social worker interview the mother. After two missed appointments, the mother came for the interview. She stated that the children's father was abusive to them and denied that her own comings and goings were destructive to the children. She seemed very angry that the children had been brought to the clinic and threatened to take them back, although she had no money to raise them.

CASE STUDY #45

QUESTION B:
IT IS LIKELY THAT IN THE NEAR FUTURE ANN'S MOTHER WILL:
1. Be able to explain in detail John Bowlby's theories on separation
2. Continue to be transient in her relationships with the children
3. Pull herself together, remarry, and become an excellent mother
4. Drop in on the girls from time to time
5. Be jealous of the attention her two daughters are receiving in the clinic. She will act out her resentment of the newlywed stepgrandmother by becoming a child herself and demanding to be taken care of
6. Continue to provoke the children's anxieties by inconsistent mothering and by unstable relationships with her father and other men
7. Develop early cirrhosis and become infertile due to gonorrhea

To predict the future of a neglecting parent is very difficult, but answer one appears very unlikely. The second answer is too general. The third answer is possible but overly optimistic with the information given. The mother did drop in on the girls, but answer four is not complete enough. The fifth answer, although possible, is unlikely and did not happen in this case. The mother did continue inconsistent mothering and broke off several relationships with boyfriends. The last answer implies that the mother is a promiscuous alcoholic for which there is not sufficient evidence.

By the sixth visit Ann's shaking had improved a great deal and both girls were gaining weight. As therapy continued, Mrs. H. developed bronchitis and had great difficulty in bringing Ann for therapy. Her health was a concern since both grandparents were in their mid-sixties. When the grandfather had to bring Ann for therapy, he lost half a day's salary, creating an additional burden. During this time, the mother returned and married a rather rigid, demanding minister.

QUESTION C:
AT THIS POINT THE PSYCHIATRIC SOCIAL WORKER AND THERAPIST SHOULD:
1. Arrange for foster home placement because the new marriage shows no prom- ise and the grandparents are getting too old
2. Realize that these girls need a good home
3. Assure the mother and the grandparents that Ann's shaking and weight loss had been temporary problems. Since she appeared healthy now, there should be no future concern
4. Tell the grandparents and mother that Ann's shakiness, although in remission, may return whenever she again gets a strep throat
5. Suggest that her newlywed husband accompany mother on her next visit to the clinic
6. Remind the mother and stepgrandparents that because the new oedipal situa- tion has been formed, extreme caution must be taken in order that the girls will not be frightened of their new stepfather. A graduated introduction in which he gets to know them should be programmed over the next few weeks, with a five-minute increase each time
7. Without alienating the grandparents, the psychiatric social worker should attempt to relate to the new stepfather and continue cautious interviews with the mother. Ann and her sister should be told by their grandparents that mother has remarried and that when the situation is stable, they might be able to return to their mother

Answer one is judgmental and fails to utilize the available resources in the family. The second answer is too general. The third answer does not speak directly to the question and fails to provide adequate follow-up or follow-through. The fourth answer is incorrect because it implies an organic etiology. The fifth answer is a good idea and was done, but is incomplete. The sixth answer is over- cautious and impractical. In fact, the mother and stepfather were to be given the

CASE STUDY #45

children quite soon. Rather than mechanistically structuring the time the children spend with their stepfather, it might be better to talk with the mother and grand-parents about flexibility and sensitivity to children's needs. The last answer is the best - if it can be accomplished.

When Ann arrived for the clinic visit, she would run gleefully to the thera-pist's room, tear the toys out of the toychest, and spread them over the floor. Frequently she had temper tantrums, remained mute, and destroyed any tower built by her or the therapist. Even on the coldest days, she demanded to be taken outside for a walk. In one session, following a drop-in visit by mother, she took an empty baby bottle, curled up in the corner, and sucked vigorously.

QUESTION D:
THE BEST INTERPRETATION OF THIS BEHAVIOR WOULD BE:
1. Ann is hungry and desires nourishment. The therapist should take her to the snack bar
2. Any 3-1/2 year-old brought to the therapist's office should be expected to suck on the bottle
3. During times of stress Ann would be expected to regress to more infantile behavior
4. The sucking on the bottle is a sign of autistic withdrawal. Ann should be given a major tranquilizer and play therapy five days a week
5. Ann's withdrawal into the corner means that memories of previous imper-manence have been stirred up
6. Ann is disturbed by mother's recent drop-in visit
7. Ann's sucking on the nipple in the corner is a sign of severe autistic behavior. Her course will be downhill from here on

Sucking behavior has been found to last longer in little girls than little boys. The first answer ignores the psychological need of the child. Most three-and-one-half-year-old children do not suck on the nipple when brought to the clinic. Furthermore, even Ann had not used the bottle on previous visits although it had been available. It was only at this visit she felt the need for this regressive be-havior. It is unlikely that this was a sign of autistic withdrawal. By itself it certainly is not an indication for medicating any child. The fifth answer is pos-sible, but is only part of the answer. The sixth answer is not specific enough. Answer three is best.

QUESTION E:
THE THERAPIST NOTICED THAT ANN LIKED TO PLAY WITH BLOCKS. FRE-QUENTLY SHE BUILT MANY INTRICATE DESIGNS, INCLUDING WALLS AROUND DOLLS. THEN SHE STOOD UP AND KICKED THEM INTO CORNERS OF THE ROOM. THE THERAPIST COULD:
1. Join her in kicking the blocks into the corners of the room
2. Be aware that she is angry and tell her so
3. Help her place the blocks back in the middle of the room to facilitate her play
4. Watch for staring spells since it is likely that she has petit mal and will need anticonvulsants
5. Suggest that Ann is dissatisfied with what she has built
6. Interpret to Ann that her destructive behavior indicates her wish to kill her mother and her sister, who remind her of her unstable life. Tell her that even though she would like to have grandfather for her own, this is impossible.
7. With short statements try to clarify the meaning of her behavior. For ex-ample, say, "You've torn up what you built."

The first answer would not promote therapy even though at times it might make the therapist feel better. Telling the child she is angry may clarify some, but may not be accepted and is not specific. This child, who constantly gave the

CASE STUDY #45

message "please, mother, I'd rather do it myself," would have seen the therapist's block-moving as interfering. Seizures did not seem likely. Ann's disatisfaction may not be about what she has built but about what she feels about herself. The authors do not feel that the strong interpretation made in answer six would be helpful. Answer seven, the best, may set the stage for the child to show the therapist in the future why she seemed upset.

QUESTION F:
AT THE NEXT VISIT, ANN'S MOTHER SAID THAT AT THE END OF ONE MONTH THE GIRLS WOULD BEGIN LIVING WITH HER AND HER NEW HUSBAND. THE PSYCHIATRIC SOCIAL WORKER AND THE THERAPIST MIGHT BEST HELP ANN AND HER SISTER BY:

1. Preparing both girls for the move as soon as possible by encouraging them to talk with their grandparents and mother about what it will be like to live in their new home. Encourage the new stepfather to meet his stepdaughters at the grandparents' before they move to his house
2. Stating that the children will need intensive preparation therapy, including four-day-a-week visits, for two months. Encourage mother to delay the move for at least an extra month
3. Discussing the move with Ann and her sister. Encourage the girls to speak freely with their grandmother about the move
4. Telling the mother that if the shakiness ever returns, the child needs hospitalization on the neurology service to rule out a degenerative muscular dystrophy
5. Telling mother to bring the children into her new home sooner than planned because the girls will do well as soon as they are in a stable environment
6. Suggesting that the girls be allowed as much information about the move as possible
7. Suggesting the girls be taken to church with their mother and new stepfather in order to see what his occupation is

It seems to the authors that most children respond best when anticipated changes in their lives are mentioned to them early rather than late. Answer one is the best because it includes having the children meet their new stepfather in territory that they feel comfortable in. Some child therapists might say that intensive preparation would be necessary for these two abused girls, but this was not feasible, since the grandparents were obviously very willing to allow the mother and her new husband to take the children. The third answer is incorrect because it was not the therapist's or the social worker's role to inform the children of the change in their lives. It would be inappropriate to tell the mother that the shaking was of an organic nature. It would take several months to determine whether the new environment would become a stable one for these children. The sixth answer is correct as far as it goes, but is not very comprehensive. The seventh answer misses the point about the children's feelings regarding their change. Although they will certainly be interested in what their stepfather does for a living, this would not be the most important suggestion for the therapist and the social worker to make.

The next several years proved difficult for Ann and Nettie. Their mother separated, divorced and remarried her second husband. Shifts into and out of the grandparents' home were frequent. Through all this, mother was able to bring the girls to the clinic intermittently, but had difficulty establishing enough trust to discuss her own behavior. Ann continued to have shaking spells, which caused difficulty in elementary school. Treatment continues.

REFERENCES:
1. Adams, P., et al., 1971: Children's Rights, Praeger Publishers, Inc., New York
2. Axline, V., 1964: Dibs: In Search of Self, Houghton-Mifflin, Boston

CASE STUDY #45

3. Bowlby, J., 1965: Child Care and the Growth of Love, Penguin Books, Baltimore

4. Dollard, J. and N. E. Miller, 1950: Personality and Psychotherapy: An Analysis of Terms of Learning, Thinking and Culture, McGraw-Hill, N. Y.

5. Galdston, R., 1971: Chapter 21 from Modern Perspectives in International Child Psychiatry Ed. by J. G. Howells, Brunner-Mazel, New York

6. Galdston, R., 1971: Violence begins at home, J Amer Acad of Child Psychiatry 10:336-350

7. Holter, J. D. and S. B. Friedman, 1968: Principles of management in child abuse. Amer J Orthopsychiatry 38:127-136

8. Leaverton, D. R., 1968: The pediatrician's role in maternal deprivation Clinical Pediatrics 7:340-343

9. Yarrow, L. H., 1961: Maternal deprivation: Toward an empirical and conceptual re-evaluation. Psychol Bull 58:459-490

CASE STUDY #46

The Trick Knee

An orthopedist referred a 15 year-old, Caucasian girl, to the Psychiatry Clinic with the chief complaint of quadriceps muscle weakness for an eleven-month period, with a resultant two inch thigh atrophy. She and her parents indicated that she had injured her left knee in a fall when running across the street. This injury had not been considered a serious one. No medical attention had been sought until she re-injured it in a minor surfing incident three days later and had noticed weakness the next morning. The referring physician, who had examined her at this time, discovered no objective signs, and the electromyograms (EMG) were normal. He recommended physical therapy, but no improvement occurred. After several months, atrophy became apparent, but the rest of the physcial examination, including a neurological evaluation, remained normal. The patient was now walking on crutches. Her physician decided to explore the knee surgically. An "insignificant tear of the cruciate ligament" was repaired, but neither this procedure nor further conservative treatment brought any improvement. Deep tendon reflexes (DTR) and EMG's remained normal, and no other diagnostic signs developed. Hence the girl was referred to a psychiatrist.

The initial psychiatric examination revealed a rather thin, shy girl, who walked with a cane in her left hand while "locking" her left knee. She was of average intelligence and cooperative, and revealed no evidence of a thought disorder. She spoke in a rather relaxed but shy manner and expressed the opinion that a psychiatric appraisal was not necessary. She related that she was doing satisfactory work in school and had several close friends. Neither she nor her parents mentioned any family problems. She seemed to be concerned about her leg, but more or less resigned to a slow healing process that might take another year or so. Despite her difficulty in walking, she played a trumpet in her school marching band, holding the trumpet in her right hand and the cane in her left.

Although no distinct psychopathology was found, the therapist began individual psychotherapy because of his confidence in the referring physician's judgment. The girl steadfastly presented herself as mentally healthy, but as she developed rapport with the therapist, she indicated that there was something on her mind that she thought ought to be discussed. During the next two visits she was still unable to discuss it. However, on her twelfth visit she finally admitted that she had lied all along. She had not fallen while running across the street, but had fallen down the stairs while drunk. She continued to explain that she had begun drinking at home when she was eleven years old and had gradually increased the frequency until, by age thirteen, she was drinking daily. She used to go to a girl friend's home after school and drink one or two highballs of blended whiskey, and at times she would drink as much as a pint a day. Her parents were unaware of this behavior. The therapist felt that the girl's parents should be told about her drinking and encouraged the patient to take the responsibility of informing them.

For several more weeks the alcoholsim and quadriceps paralysis continued unabated. Then she was hospitalized, and a complete reevaluation was carried out. The physical examination was not helpful. The atrophy was still present in this rather slight but otherwise normal adolescent girl. No abnormal neurological signs were present. The EMG's remained normal, and so did the X-rays of her skull and spine.

The patient's parents were informed of the negative findings. They were also told of her alcoholism despite her objections. The therapist felt that he had given the girl adequate time to inform the parents herself and that he could no longer take the responsibility of withholding the information. Moreover, he needed their help in the treatment, since the lack of alcohol during this hospitalization had resulted in significant withdrawal symptoms. She was started on (Disulfiram) Antabuse and was referred to another psychiatrist, because her current therapist was preparing to move to another state. She never accepted this referral, however, and discontinued psychotherapy.

CASE STUDY #46

QUESTION A:
WHAT IS THE DIAGNOSIS:
1. Peripheral neuritis due to alcoholism
2. Peripheral neuritis resulting from vitamin deficiencies secondary to alcoholism
3. Hysterical neurosis with a conversion reaction resulting in disuse atrophy
4. Behavior disorder resulting in disuse atrophy, alcoholism and refusal to cooperate in treatment
5. a. Personality disorder, passive-dependent type, needing the "paralysis" as an attention-getting device, and b. alcoholism because of her dependency needs

Answers one and two are incorrect for these reasons. First, it is very unlikely that a person would develop toxic or deficiency neuritis in only a single nerve with the other nerves never involved. Secondly, the patient never really exhibited enough evidence to warrant a diagnosis of neuritis; the DTR's as well as the EMG's were always normal.

Answer three, by definition, indicates the presence of an unconscious conflict, answer four a conscious uncooperative attitude, and five a long standing problem in psychological development. Only a long-term follow-up can determine which one of these answers is correct.

Five years after the termination of therapy, the therapist received a letter from the orthopedist who had referred the patient originally. The girl had returned to the orthopedist to inform him that she was now able to move her leg. While working as a telephone operator, she had been required to sit on a high stool. Dangling her feet, she had suddenly discovered that she was able to move her paretic leg.

In the interim, she had continued to play in the marching band and had graduated from high school, but her academic work had depended on the help of others: she had cheated on tests and copied homework assignments, receiving average to marginal grades.

She had continued to drink and had become involved with other drugs. She had received help from a minister who used to be an alcoholic. She had moved out of her home and had lived with friends in a concerted effort to get her into Alcoholics Anonymous and off the drugs. This process had taken two to three years, but she had been dry for about seven months before she discovered that she could move her leg.

QUESTION B:
WHICH OF THE FOLLOWING IS THE CORRECT DIAGNOSIS?:
1. Hysterical neurosis with a conversion reaction resulting in disuse atrophy
2. Behavior disorder resulting in disuse atrophy, alcoholism, and refusal to cooperate in treatment
3. Personality disorder, passive-dependent type
4. One and three
5. Two and three

In the data obtained at the five-year follow-up, we discovered many bits of evidence regarding the dependency needs of this young person. She depended upon friends to get her through high school, depended on alcohol and other drugs to achieve and maintain the mental state she desired, depended on a clergyman and another family to provide her with living space, and depended on friends and Alcoholics Anonymous to get her off alcohol. Her dependency needs were further illustrated by her reliance on her cane at this point in her life. She also depended on friends to get jobs for her. Interestingly, it was during the one job which she had obtained by herself that her improvement began. She does have a personality disorder, passive-dependent type, and three is a correct answer.

CASE STUDY #46

Is one or two also correct? So far we have had no evidence of an unconscious conflict. We have also had no evidence of a lack of cooperation or behavior problems either in school or in the various homes in which she had lived. In fact, there was considerable evidence that she wanted to help herself but was unable to do so. On a follow-up visit, the therapist had an opportunity to gather more background information.

He found that the patient's relationship with her father had never been satisfactory. The girl described an experience at the age of five or six. She had been playing with some neighborhood friends, and when her friends' fathers came home, they all dropped their toys and ran to embrace them. Our patient remembered how she wished that she would feel like doing that to her father. Moreover, the patient related that between the ages of nine and twelve she was sexually molested by her father on several occasions. This made her feel very angry towards him, and at times she even wished that he would be killed in an automobile accident. Just prior to the onset of the weakness in her knee, she had considered taking a course in Karate to learn how to defend herself by kicking.

This patient's relationship with men might be considerably affected by her experiences with her father, and this internalized conflict might well prevent her psychosexual development from progressing to a stage in which she could be truly independent and able to run her own life. Therefore, the <u>most</u> correct answer is four; she has a psychoneurosis (conversion reaction) which was superimposed upon a passive-dependent personality disorder.

Shortly after this therapeutic follow-up evaluation, she discarded her cane, re-established some old friendships, and began playing tennis. Her thigh has increased by one inch in circumference at the time of this writing.

QUESTION C:
THE QUESTION OF CONFIDENTIALITY BECAME AN IMPORTANT ISSUE IN THIS CASE, WHEN THE PATIENT WAS UNABLE TO TELL HER PARENTS ABOUT HER ALCOHOLISM. IT IS ADVISABLE TO MAINTAIN CONFIDENTIALITY WITH ADOLESCENT PATIENTS BECAUSE:
1. They are naturally suspicious anyway
2. They will never forgive you
3. You have a legal responsibility to your patients under House Bill 16-478
4. The parents expect it
5. They will spread the word that you can't be trusted

Whatever House Bill 16-478 is, it isn't this. Actually, you have a real responsibility to parents too, and this compound relationship should be clarified at the outset or very early in the treatment. Therapists must also respond to parents' needs, not only because the parents pay the bill, but because they too are asking for help and are expected to make some changes. As a general rule, though, it is good practice to avoid seeing the parents alone, for miscommunication is minimized if the patient is present. The first answer is the only correct one: you must respect your patients' confidence in order to build a trusting rapport. Without this trust the therapist's skill and knowledge are useless; even prescribing medication and giving advice are much less effective than they could be.

QUESTION D:
IN THIS CASE, WHAT IS THE SYMBOLIC MEANING OF THE PARALYSIS?:
1. The unconscious mind's way of getting attention
2. The unconscious mind's way of avoiding kicking her father
3. An unconscious attempt to be more dependent
4. A conscious withholding mechanism
5. A conscious attempt to gain attention

CASE STUDY #46

The most common error committed by non-psychiatric physicians is to label puzzling symptoms, which cannot be explained physiologically, conscious acts to gain attention. Occasionally, children do malinger, but one should always give them the benefit of the doubt. It is good practice to ask oneself the question: "What does this symptom accomplish for this patient?" The answer must be more specific than "getting attention," which is a secondary gain. One must go further and ask: "What is the primary gain?" In this case it appears that our patient would have liked to kick her father "in the balls," and this unthinkable act was prevented by a paralysis of the thigh muscles. Therefore, two is the best answer.

QUESTION E:
ALCOHOLISM IN ADOLESCENTS IS:
1. Rare because they prefer other drugs
2. Rare because most parents strictly enforce its prohibition
3. Becoming more common, because other drugs are getting harder to find
4. Rare because children learn to drink early in life nowadays and develop a tolerance
5. More common than we think

It may be more common than we think, but the evidence suggests that the incidence is rare among adolescents, because they prefer other drugs. Therefore, the first answer is correct. According to a study of Ohio youths (Coddington & Jacobsen, 1972) they do learn to drink early; 22% of 12-year-olds have had alcohol from 1-6 times, and 38% have had alcohol more than 6 times. But they do not develop tolerances.

QUESTION F:
THE HISTORY OF FATHER-DAUGHTER INCEST UNCOVERED IN THIS CASE:
1. Proves that the father was psychotic
2. Is very rare
3. Is probably related to the development of a hysterical (conversion) symptom rather than some other psychiatric symptom
4. Should lead to a psychotic adjustment in the girl
5. Occurs in 10-15% of psychiatric patients
6. Is probably related to her alcoholism and dependency

Father-daughter incest, reported in about 4% of psychiatrically referred women, (Weiner, 1964) correlates highly with hysteria. Of course, not all female hysterics have experienced father incest, and some of those who report it probably experienced it only in fantasy. Nevertheless, a sexually tinged disturbance of the father relationship seems a common finding with hysterics. The father is often alcoholic, sometimes psychotic. The daughter may become psychotic, but not as often as the son does in mother-son incest. Three is the best answer.

REFERENCES:
1. Bender, L., 1954: A dynamic Psychopathology of Childhood. Charles C Thomas, Springfield, p. 134

2. Coddington, R. D. and R. Jacobson, 1972: Drug Use by Ohio Adolescents. The Ohio State Medical Journal 68:481-484

3. Cory, W., 1963: Homosexual Incest. In Masters, R. E. L. (Ed.): Patterns of Incest. Basic Books, New York

4. Langsley, D. G., Schwartz, M. N. and R. H. Fairbairn, 1968: Father-Son Incest. Comprehensive Psychiatry 9:218-226

CASE STUDY #46

5. Machotka, P. , Pittman, F. S. , III and K. Flomenhaft, 1967: Incest as a
Family Affair. Family Process 6:98-116

6. Proctor, J. T. , 1958: Hysteria in Childhood. Amer J of Orthopsych 28:394-
403. Reprinted in Harrison, S. I. and McDermott, J. F. : Childhood Psychopathology, An Anthology of Basic Readings. Int. Univ. Press, New York,
1972

7. Rhinehart, J. W. , 1961: Genesis of Overt Incest. Compr Psychiat 2:338-349

8. Weiner, J. B. , 1964: On Incest: A Survey. Excerpta Criminologica 4:137-155

CASE STUDY #47

Little Mother

Sherry, a 10 year-old daughter of working class parents, was referred to the clinic by her pediatrician, who had treated her since early childhood for agammaglobulinemia. This necessitated twice-monthly injections and the occasional home use of a small respirator.

She was a chubby, blonde, curly-haired girl whose emotional problems had become evident approximately ten months prior to the referral, when she had become very fearful, withdrew, and started vomiting after meals. The first instance of the vomiting occurred while eating Sunday dinner at the maternal grandmother's. Sherry suddenly announced that she had eaten a red rose, left the table and vomited. A few days later the patient thought she had a match up her nose which mother had just extinguished after lighting a cigarette.

Her fears became more intense, and when her father attempted to comfort her by putting his arm around her, she pulled away and later asked her mother if this would make her pregnant. One day she announced to father that she knew why he and mother slept in their own room and what they "did." She refused to elaborate further. At another time she complained of feeling "a man's hand on my butt."

During the next few months the vomiting became progressively worse, and she was twice hospitalized because of dehydration. During her second hospitalization a child died on her ward, and Sherry was distraught. She kept repeating "I want to die," and refused food and water for a three-day period, necessitating intravenous feeding. Upon returning home from the hospital, she refused to go to school and complained of stomach pains whenever school was mentioned.

Mother presented as a well-dressed, tired-appearing woman in her middle thirties. Her appearance was startling when she spoke because she was toothless. Mother and father did not get along, and he was out of the home as much as possible. He said he couldn't come to the clinic because he was working "more than 80 hours a week." He trained horses. There were two other daughters, ages 6 and 11.

Mother described her pregnancy as a very difficult one in which she was ill the whole time and in "false" labor the last two months. She went into the hospital at midnight the Saturday before Sherry's birth. She claimed the doctor, a very religious man, held the baby back because he refused to deliver babies on Sunday mornings. Hence, the "baby was born blue" and "got the ether."

Mother described the infant as a "pleasant, sweet baby who never cried or fussed." Although Sherry was hospitalized with pneumonia at four years, and "double pneumonia" plus chicken pox at five years, there were no early separations. In the first instance, mother stayed with the child, and in the second mother and father took turns staying with her. Sherry often had high fevers and vomiting as an infant, but was generally healthy. Her developmental milestones were within the ordinary range.

At the time of the referral, she had not started to menstruate, but had been shown a film about menstruation about six months previously in science class. Mother had not discussed sex with her "for fear of upsetting her." In fact, she suppressed any questions about sex and told Sherry "it is not nice to talk about such things." Sherry had developed an intense dislike for a maternal aunt because she overheard her telling her daughter that "sex is how you become pregnant." She also overheard the aunt say "Sherry is not sick, she just needs a good whipping." Sisters, cousins and aunts made fun of her, telling her she wasn't sick and accusing mother of spoiling and babying her.

She got A's and B's in school until the onset of her emotional disturbance. Then some of her grades dropped. She got an F in science, the course in which the menstruation film was shown.

The child was seen in two evaluation, play sessions. She was very verbal, although she suffered a rather severe stammer. The vomiting seemed to serve an oral impregnation fantasy; it seemed to be a constant effort to get rid of that

CASE STUDY #47

which she felt had impregnated her. She said she knew she had a baby inside her because she vomited and felt dizzy. She also suffered nightmares which were so frightening and "dirty" that she wrote them out rather than tell them. Their content was primarily sexual. She also said that she wasn't ten years old, but was really mother's age, and that they were exactly alike. She illustrated this by taking a crayon and drawing her mother's face, and then superimposing her own over it and blending them into one.

When Sherry's muddles about sex were approached, she became angry and said, "I'm not supposed to know how babies are made or where they come from until teens... late teens, because mother said so. " Yet, she told about an uncle who had had a vasectomy "so he couldn't make any more babies, " and then counted all the penises she had seen, mostly of her boy cousins.

She started the second session by announcing, "I always read the obituaries," and went on to count and to describe in detail all of the deaths that she had known about. She used the term "passed away," because mother said "it wasn't nice to say 'died'. " She had never seen a dead person, but mother had taken her to a funeral, and they were disappointed that the casket was closed.

QUESTION A:
SHERRY'S DIAGNOSIS WOULD HAVE BEEN:
1. Schizophrenia
2. Psychophysiological gastrointestinal reaction
3. Anorexia nervosa
4. Unspecified sexual deviation
5. School phobia

Sherry certainly was school phobic, and had many symptoms of anorexia. However, she was a stockily built child who was possibly overweight. Childhood schizophrenia is suggested by her lack of separation from her mother, her delusion that she was pregnant and had eaten a red rose, and her visual and tactile hallucinations. One is the best answer.

QUESTION B:
THE MOST APPROPRIATE INTERVENTION IN THIS CASE WOULD HAVE BEEN:
1. To have provided a behavior modification program to desensitize the child from her fears and to have provided a course for her in sex education
2. Individual psychotherapy for the child, and psychotherapy for the parents
3. Family therapy
4. Residential treatment providing a therapeutic milieu, and individual psychotherapy for the child as well as psychiatric help for the parents
5. To have forced the child back to school and to have set up a behavior modification program for her both in school and in the home.

Sherry was such a seriously ill child both physically and emotionally that she needed hospital placement. Her family had little empathy for, or insight into, her problems, which made her subject to either suppression from mother or ridicule from relatives. In such circumstances, she remained a very unhappy child, with little opportunity to separate out reality from fantasies. Four is the best answer, although two or three might have been given a trial.

QUESTION C:
THIS CASE ILLUSTRATES THAT THE EFFECT OF SCHOOL SEX EDUCATION CLASSES ON CHILDREN:
1. Can be harmful and cause emotional problems
2. Can occasionally feed the fantasies of a child who already has emotional problems in this area
3. Doesn't affect them one way or the other

CASE STUDY #47

4. Is so harmful that such classes should be made illegal
5. Is enlightening to them and obliterates their curiosity about sex

Although it is impossible to determine the exact date of the onset of this child's illness, in all probability it predated her attendance in sex education classes. It is even questionable that she learned much in these classes since she was already very sophisticated in terms of sexual knowledge. One of her problems seemed to be her guilt about knowing more than her mother wanted her to know and her difficulty in suppressing her information according to mother's demands. The guilt, together with her introjection of mother's feelings that sex is dirty, contributed to her confusion about what was real and what was not real about sex. In such a state of sexual confusion, sex education classes probably led to further confusion and sexual preoccupations. Two is the best answer.

QUESTION D:
SHERRY COUNTED BOTH PENISES AND THE NUMBER OF PEOPLE SHE HAD KNOWN WHO DIED BECAUSE:
1. She was not convinced that murder and sexual intercourse were the same
2. She linked every penis with a death
3. "Penis" and "death" both had five letters, and five was her magic number
4. She was preoccupied with sex and death and thought one led to the other
5. Both sex and death were frightening to her and this was one way of defending against her anxiety: if she could count them she could magically control them

Sherry's "primal scene" was possibly her own fantasy of what occurred between mother and father during sexual intercourse. Her confusion about how impregnation occurred (which is common at some stage in normal children) together with the film about menstruation, may have caused her to weave a violent, destructive fantasy that in some way sexual activities lead to death. Her mother's similar treatment of the two topics must have promoted the confusion: "sex" is dirty and not to be talked about and "it wasn't nice to say 'died'." The best answer is five, while four is also tenable. For more about oral impregnation fantasies and food refusal see Case #13.

REFERENCES:
1. Bender, L., 1947: Childhood schizophrenia. Am J Orthopsychiat 17:40-56

2. English, O.S. and G.H.V. Pearson, 1972: Irrational fears and phobias in childhood psychopathology. ed. S. Harrison, and J.F. McDermott, New York, Internat. Univ. Press pp. 375-381

3. Fraiberg, S., 1959: The Magic Years. New York, Schribners, Sons

4. Freud, A., 1965: Normality and Pathology in Childhood. New York, Internat. Univ. Press

5. Gardner, R.A., 1969: Sexual fantasies in childhood. Med Aspects of Human Sex 3:121-134

6. Goldfarb, W., 1961: Childhood Schizophrenia. Cambridge, Harvard Univ. Press

7. Levy, D.M., Meyers, D. and W. Goldfarb, 1962: Relational behavior of schizophrenic children and their mothers: a methodological study. Read before the Orthopsychiatry Association, March, 1962

CASE STUDY #47

8. Mahler, M., 1958: Autism and symbiosis: two extreme disturbances of identity. Int J Psycho-Anal 39:77-83

9. Odier, C., 1956: Anxiety and magical thinking. New York, Internat. Univ. Press

10. Tilton, J. R., 1966: Annotated Bibliography on Childhood Schizophrenia, 1954-1964. New York, Grune and Stratton

11. Weil, A. P., 1953: Clinical data and dynamic considerations in certain cases of childhood schizophrenia. Amer J Orthopsychiat 23:518-529

CASE STUDY #48

The 12 Year-Old Hellion

Craig was a 12 year-old, white boy, referred for pre-admission psychiatric evaluation by his neurologist, who had been treating him for a convulsive disorder. When Craig and his parents were seen together, they presented a rather striking appearance. Craig, dressed entirely in red, sat back in his chair, looking apparently comfortable and a little triumphant, with a faint smile upon his face. One corner of his mouth was raised a little bit more than the other, so that it formed a definite sneer. His mother and father, both intelligent people who were very much interested in some of the finer, cultural aspects of life, also smiled while they gave the history. But their smiles seemed quite different from Craig's, rather wry smiles that seemed to connote a very tolerant attitude. At the same time they gave the clear-cut message that they were at the end of their rope. When they described the events of the previous 2 years, one could not help but wonder how they had been able to put up with their son's aggressive, thoughtless and hostile behavior. He was certainly playing the role of "devil" for which he was appropriately dressed.

Interestingly, Craig behaved fairly well whenever his father was at home. However, when only his mother and sister were there, he frequently went into rages, during which he threw objects through windows, at his sister, and at his mother, including such dangerous, heavy objects as alabaster bookends. He also destroyed furniture, particularly furniture which his father prized highly, such as an antique wine chest. He repeatedly pulled the telephone from the wall to prevent the mother from communicating with the father at work. On one occasion he struck his mother and lacerated her scalp. These rages usually lasted many minutes and were almost always followed by Craig's asking his mother if she loved him. In recent months the boy's behavior had become much worse, and the parents were asking for his admission to a psychiatric unit, because they did not know what else to do.

Craig had been epileptic since infancy and was experiencing occasional seizures at the age of 12 despite the neurologist's careful management of the anticonvulsive medication, currently primidone (Mysoline) 1250 mg per day. The seizures were of the grand mal variety, often associated with incontinence of urine, and occurred in school, at play and at home. Craig had never taken any responsibility for the medication, and the neurologist had recently been encouraging him to accept more responsibility. In addition to the anticonvulsant medication, the boy had been taking methylphenidate (Ritalin) because of his hyperactive behavior.

The parents' marital history was also significant. During the early years of their marriage, before as well as after Craig's birth, the parents had many serious arguments and fights, which the mother often ended by taking the baby and a few clothes and driving off for one or two days. Once she made a suicide attempt, resulting in a brief hospitalization. From then on she was considered weak and fragile by her husband, who obviously resented this weakness. He indicated that he felt Craig would behave better if his mother were stronger and dealt more firmly with him. It seemed that he might even have encouraged Craig to fight with his mother, thereby gaining much vicarious satisfaction. When his wife had had enough, he would come to her rescue and then sometimes deal with Craig too harshly, almost sadistically.

A physical examination revealed an apparent absence of vibratory, touch and pain sensations throughout Craig's body. There were no other abnormal physical or neurological signs. Craig later explained this hypo-sensitivity to tactile and painful stimuli by saying that his peers often pinched and hit him and he had found that the best way to stop them was to become insensitive to their blows. "If I turned them off and acted like a log," he said, "I figured it would hurt their hands more than it would hurt me."

A private interview with the boy and psychological testing both indicated that he was almost overwhelmed with anxiety and fear regarding his own aggressive

CASE STUDY #48

and hostile impulses and that he was very much afraid of some sort of damage to his genitalia. For instance, he began his first individual therapeutic session by running into the office, talking "a mile a minute," and explaining how he must be careful not to run into the corner of a desk, because such a collision would undoubtedly damage his genitalia. He then went on to explain the normal physiology of the male reproductive system. Craig tried to be very brave despite this anxiety. He also stated that he felt he should keep everybody at a distance at all costs.

QUESTION A:
THE RAGE OUTBURSTS AND OTHER MISBEHAVIOR ARE MOST LIKELY DUE TO:
1. The same process that underlies the convulsions
2. A side effect of Mysoline
3. A psychological process distinct from, but perhaps aggravated by, the seizure disorder
4. A genetic defect, separate from but similar to the genetically determined seizures
5. None of the above

The weight of evidence is in favor of the third answer. The psychodynamics could be formulated in the following way. Ever since the mother's depression twelve years earlier, she had seen herself as weak and fragile, an image which was shared by her husband. When the neurologist found that her son had a convulsive disorder, she felt even more inadequate and depended more and more on physicians and medication to help her control the growing child's behavior. Her husband, on the other hand, enjoyed the child's mischievousness, unconsciously encouraged it, and used it to act out his own anger toward his weak wife. He "reasoned" that she should deal more firmly with Craig, and if she did not, she deserved everything the boy dished out.

In cases like these the reader is advised to consider also the first and second answers. Rage outbursts and other severe behavior problems accompany epilepsy often enough that the old term for "explosive personality" was "epileptic personality." This stereotype has some basis in fact, but not every epileptic has behavior problems, and some of those who do may misbehave mainly because of a third factor, as illustrated in this case. Although a side effect of the medication is not the main cause of this boy's trouble, it might be a more important factor in other cases. Hyperactivity can occur as a side effect of anticonvulsants such as phenobarbital and Mysoline and can cause considerable anxiety. The parents might overreact to their child's hyperactive behavior and become rather inconsistent in their handling of him.

QUESTION B:
FROM THE FOREGOING DISCUSSION IT WOULD SEEM THAT FAMILY THERAPY IS INDICATED. IN ADDITION, CRAIG NEEDS:
1. An individual therapist who is an M. D. to facilitate management of the medication
2. An individual therapist who has nothing to do with medication management in order to separate clearly his medical management from the treatment of his behavior disorder
3. To have his Mysoline dosage lowered
4. To have the methylphenidate changed to dextroamphetamine
5. Nothing more

Initially the Mysoline dose should be maintained, but the staff should be prepared to change the dosage, since the patient's requirements may vary, especially if a major tranquilizer were used. Therefore, answer three is wrong, since it implies an abrupt decrease in his medication upon admission to the hospital, a move which is completely unwarranted. Answer four was actually tried because

CASE STUDY #48

the methylphenidate did not seem to be significantly helping the hyperactivity for which it had been prescribed. Neither stimulant seemed helpful, and both were soon discontinued with no change in clinical state. See cases 1 and 18 for examples of successful stimulant treatment of hyperactivity and case 60 for another failure of stimulant treatment.

The main point of this question is whether or not the same therapist should be in charge of Craig's medication as well as his psychotherapy. In some cases this might be advisable, but for this case we prefer answer two. This is not to say that the first answer is necessarily wrong, but our aim was to teach Craig that he could maintain considerable conscious control over his rage outbursts and that his convulsive disorder need not govern his entire life. This type of problem can be handled in settings without psychiatrists, as long as the neurological management is correlated with the psychotherapy and the patient gets the same message from both professionals.

QUESTION C:
THIS THERAPEUTIC GOAL, I. E. , TEACHING CRAIG THAT HE IS RESPONSIBLE FOR HIS OWN BEHAVIOR, COULD BE FURTHER FACILITATED BY:
1. A behavior modification program
2. Discharging him from the hospital
3. Suggesting he read "I'm O. K. , You're O. K. " by Thomas A. Harris, M. D.
4. The use of haloperidol (Haldol)
5. Intensifying his individual therapy from three times per week to daily sessions

The best answer is the first one; none of the other suggestions would as efficiently facilitate the attainment of this particular therapeutic goal. A reward system was designed by Craig and his therapist. Craig felt certain that he could be good for one and a half or perhaps two hours at a stretch, and so they decided to reinforce him with a poker chip at the end of each one-and-a-half-hour period, during which, in the opinion of the staff, he had been reasonably well behaved. His regular weekly allowance of $2. 50 supplied by his parents was withheld, and instead he could periodically cash in his chips at the rate of 10¢ each. After the allowance was exhausted, the money was supplied by his therapist. Craig entered this program eagerly and made it very clear he valued the money that came from his therapist more highly than that which came from his allowance. He behaved well for several days in a row, even when he was eventually required to control himself for three-hour stretches in order to receive the reward. Once he learned that he could control his own behavior, the program became unnecessary.

For a short time in the hospital Craig was also treated with thioridazine (Mellaril), with good results continuing even after it was discontinued. Craig was successfully returned to his family after four months of intensive multi-modal inpatient treatment. Taking only the Mysoline, he maintained acceptable control over his behavior except for a brief relapse three months post-discharge. The latter return to his original symptoms was successfully aborted by crisis intervention, and he continues satisfactory community adjustment at this writing, seven months after discharge.

REFERENCES:
1. Beres, D. , 1952: Clinical Notes on Aggression in Children. Psa St of the Child 7:241-250

2. Beres, D. , 1952: Clinical Notes on Aggression in Children: II Aggression and Libido. Psa St of the Child 7:250-258

3. Beres, D. , 1952: Clinical Notes on Aggression in Children. Psa St of the Child 7:258-262

CASE STUDY #48

4. Clement, P. W. , 1973: Teaching Children to be Their Own Behavior Therapists. J School Health, in press

5. Eisenber, L. , 1957: Psychiatric Implications of Brain Damage in Children.
   Psychiat Quart 31:72-92, 1957, reprinted in: Harrison, S. I. and McDermott,
   J. F. (Ed.) Childhood Psychopathology, An Anthology of Basic Readings, Int.
   Univ. Press, N. Y. 1972

6. Harris, T. A. , 1967: I'm O. K. , You're O.K. Harper & Row, New York, N. Y.

CASE STUDY #49

"I Knew I Couldn't"

A 14 year-old, white, Protestant, working-class 8th grade boy was seen in consultation because he insisted on dropping out of school. He was interviewed in the presence of his father and the school counselor who had requested the consultation.

He stated that he wanted to drop out of school because he didn't know how to read. On further inquiry, he said that he had been told in the second grade he had a reading disability. He had understood from this that he would never be able to learn how to read. When asked what he had tried to read lately, he replied that he had not bothered trying to read anything because he knew he could not. When handed a popular magazine and asked to demonstrate this incapacitating disability, he began reading aloud fluently. After two sentences he stopped in mouth-gaping amazement that was matched only by that of his father and the counselor. He decided to continue in school on a half-day basis, which the counselor had offered to arrange with the vice-principal's permission.

Follow-up two months later revealed that the boy had begun specializing in looking things up and reporting back to the class. In fact, he was beginning to get into trouble because all he wanted to do was read.

QUESTION A:
THIS ANECDOTE IS BEST EXPLAINED BY THE FACT THAT:
1. The boy actually never had any reading disability, but had merely been "brainwashed" by the label put on him in the second grade
2. There was a mistake in the testing or records sometime in the past which resulted in this boy being confused with another child who actually had a reading disability
3. This boy may very well have had a reading disability in the second grade, but outgrew the problem without realizing it and continued to operate under the assumption that he was unable to learn reading
4. His learning disability was caused by an emotional problem which was dramatically cured by the consultant's supportive confidence in him in the presence of his father
5. The patient was suffering the sequelae of encephalitis in the second grade when he was unable to learn reading, and the natural reparative powers of the body restored him to a normal neurological status by the time of the consultation

Though post-encephalitic or other brain damage might cause a special learning disability, and though we might expect progressive improvement after the initial insult, this hardly appears a satisfactory explanation for the dramatic discovery of reading skills six years later. Likewise, an emotional problem severe enough to result in severe reading retardation would not likely be dispelled during a 15-minute consultation. Though the best answer is three, the self-fulfilling prophecy implied in one is also credible.

For purposes of the following discussion, learning disorder and learning disability will be considered synonymous, though the authors realize the nuances of difference.

QUESTION B:
SPECIFIC OR SPECIAL LEARNING DISORDER OR DISABILITY ("SLD") MAY BE DEFINED AS:
1. Inability to learn at the same rate as age peers
2. A two-year lag in achievement level
3. Inability to learn a given skill at the rate expected for the child's mental age
4. An emotionally-caused failure to learn a specific subject
5. Inability to learn because of brain damage

CASE STUDY #49

Specific learning disability needs to be distinguished from mental retardation, although both may be considered developmental abnormalities, and the same child may suffer both problems. A child with a specific learning disability may have normal or even superior intelligence as shown on standardized intelligence tests and as confirmed by intelligent appearance and interview behavior. The problem seems to be a specific one related to learning one or two subjects, although these may be extremely important ones. Usually such a disability seems to be neurologically based, but is not clearly brain damage. Other causes can be primary emotional problems and privation, including "cultural deprivation", the failure to get appropriate stimulation and practice in the prerequisite skills necessary for certain types of formal instruction to proceed. In certain circumstances, such as the inner city, the latter problem may account for most children who have learning problems. Although two is an acceptable operational definition for some research and survey purposes, three is the best answer.

QUESTION C:
THE APPROPRIATE AGE FOR A CHILD TO BEGIN LEARNING TO READ:
1. Is about the first grade
2. Is in kindergarten
3. Is in the second grade
4. Is in the pre-school years when the child can be taught the letters of the alphabet and possibly their sounds
5. Varies from child to child, even among those with normal intelligence

The majority of children appear ready for formal instruction in reading at the usual age of entering first grade and some children learn much younger. However, other children do not have the prerequisite neurological integration and component skills ("reading readiness") until second or third grade or even later. Some such children will learn to read, but at a later time than their age and intellectual peers, while others will become discouraged and give up after a year or two of futile attempts. They may conclude that they are unable to learn, and they may even develop secondary emotional problems. Such children can often be helped by appropriately directed academic intervention (Silver & Hagin, 1972). However, labeling them as having a reading disability without offering compensatory help may merely confirm their feeling of inadequacy. Five is the correct answer.

QUESTION D:
THE RELATIONSHIP BETWEEN EMOTIONAL PROBLEMS AND SPECIFIC LEARNING DISABILITIES, ESPECIALLY READING DISABILITY, IS:
1. They are two separate and distinct entities with only occasional coincidental overlap in the same child
2. Emotional problems cause most reading disabilities
3. Learning disabilities often result in secondary emotional problems which can aggravate and help perpetuate the learning disability
4. Learning disabilities can result in secondary emotional problems which disappear as soon as help is offered for the learning problem
5. None of the above

The high correlation between educational handicaps and psychiatric problems (Rutter, et al., 1970) often leaves clinicians wondering which came first, the chicken or the egg. By the time the child gets to a clinic, his learning problems and emotional problems are often hopelessly tangled, each aggravating and perpetuating the other. However, the authors believe that in many such cases the learning disability is primary. In some cases it appears that the emotional problems may have partly resulted from a social clumsiness - "social disability" - which may have been a manifestation in the affective sphere of the same problem

CASE STUDY #49

which was manifested in the cognitive sphere as a specific learning disability. Three is the best answer. Helping the learning problem usually helps the emotional problems, but sometimes residual emotional problems require psychotherapy.

REFERENCES:
1. Arnold, L. E., 1973: Is This Label Necessary? J of School Health, in Press (October)

2. Boder, E., 1971: Developmental Dyslexia. J of School Health 40:289-290

3. Eisenberg, L., 1966: Reading Retardation: Psychiatric and Sociologic Aspects. Pediatrics 37:352-365

4. Klein, E., 1949: Psychoanalytic aspects of school problems. Psychoanalytic Study of the Child 3-4, 369-390

5. Makita, K., 1968: The Rarity of Reading Disabilities in Japanese Children. Am J Orthopsychiat 38:599-614

6. Nirk, G., 1973: Observations on the Relationship of Emotional and Cognitive Development: A Psychiatric Contribution to Compensatory Education. J Amer Acad of Child Psychiatry 12:93-107

7. Rutter, M., Lizard, J. and K. Whitmore, 1970: Education, Health and Behavior. Longman Group Limited, Great Britain

8. Silver, A. A. & R. A. Hagin, 1972: The Profile of a First Grade Class. J of Amer Acad of Child Psychiat 11:645-674

9. Uyeda, F., 1972: The Detection of Learning Disabilities in the Early School-aged Child, Specifically the Kindergarten Child. J of School Health 42:214-215

CASE STUDY #50

A Boy Nobody Wanted

Donald, a very large, poorly coordinated, fair-haired, 11-1/2 year-old boy was brought by his social worker at a children's home to the clinic for evaluation regarding residential treatment.

Although he avoided eye contact, he expressed himself quite well verbally. He felt his problems dated back about five years to when his parents had been divorced. At that time he was left, at age seven, with his five younger siblings and a mother who was so severely depressed that she was unable to care for them. She spent her time sitting in a room by herself or sleeping, and the patient had to arouse her when the family was out of food or when it was time to do something for the younger children. The children often had to beg food from the neighbors. After a year of such neglect a court hearing was held, and the children were placed in a children's home. The psychotic mother was committed to a state hospital. She remarried several years later and lives in another state.

The boy then entered upon a series of foster home placements, where for one reason or another, each placement broke down. In between placements, he lived in the children's home. He was sent back to the home from his last foster home placement because he could not get along with other children, had little control over his temper, and started many fights. Nevertheless, Donald always did well in school.

An attempt was then made to have him live with paternal grandparents in another state. However, in this setting he again failed to get along with other children. He seemed to set himself up for teasing.

His peers ridiculed him, called him "fat," and often threw stones at him. Possibly because he was so poorly coordinated, he could only respond with rages and temper tantrums, which in turn only increased the teasing. This placement lasted for about ten months. His grandparents sent him back to the children's home, stating that they could not cope with his behavior, and that he had aggravated the grandmother's blood pressure. Donald's father, who had remarried and was childless by this marriage, refused to take him, saying that his wife "didn't have time for Donald."

By this time he was seriously disturbed, indeed. He was about fifty pounds overweight, shy, withdrawn, and unsure of himself. When other children teased or ridiculed him, he would go into rages and chase them with sticks, rakes, or baseball bats. He was so large that when he became physically violent, house parents at the children's home feared for the safety of the younger children. On one occasion, he killed several kittens with karate chops. More and more he would withdraw to his room where he would spend hours playing war games by himself in which he seemed preoccupied by his destructive fantasies.

During the interview he said that his mother had had a "nervous breakdown" but he wasn't sure what that meant. She had also been in a "funny farm." He thought this institution was a "funny farm" too, but it wasn't exactly as he had imagined it.

Although he spoke readily and spontaneously, he appeared depressed and at times angry when he told of the changes he had been through. He rather summed up his situation when he said "I never know what's coming tomorrow."

QUESTION A:
WHAT DIAGNOSIS WOULD YOU GIVE THIS BOY:
1. Hyperkinetic reaction of childhood
2. Withdrawing reaction of childhood
3. Adjustment reaction of childhood
4. Explosive personality
5. Childhood schizophrenia

CASE STUDY #50

This is a difficult decision to make, since he doesn't fit too well into any category. However, hyperkinetic reaction could be ruled out because rather than being overactive and restless, he was a boy who would often withdraw and occupy himself for hours playing war games. Also, he did well in school work, and there were no complaints of hyperactivity from the school

Although he was certainly having trouble adjusting, Adjustment Reaction of Childhood would be diagnostically inappropriate, because his problems were not due to a transient situational disturbance but were more deeply rooted and internalized.

Although Donald could certainly behave explosively, his outbursts of rage were usually precipitated by teasing which he unconsciously encouraged by his reactions. He suffered neither guilt nor repentance about his outbursts, which seemed to make them an ongoing part of his personality rather than isolated incidents which differed from his usual behavior.

Withdrawing Reaction of Childhood seems the most appropriate diagnostic category based on the increasing amount of time he was withdrawing and isolating himself with his war games. Two is the best answer, but four is also correct.

QUESTION B:
AN APPROPRIATE TREATMENT PLAN FOR THE BOY WOULD HAVE BEEN:
1. To have told the father that he must take Donald to live with him and then involved the boy in once-weekly psychotherapy
2. To have found another foster home for Donald where strong limits would have been set in order to help him control himself
3. To have tried to get help from the community such as involving him in Boy Scout activities, finding a Big Brother for him, arranging for people to invite him to their homes for weekends, where he could get the feeling of being a member of a family
4. Residential treatment in an adolescent therapeutic community where he could have received intensive psychotherapy and learned to get along with his peers by living with them
5. A good military school where he would have been forced to conform and where his temper tantrums and aggressive outbursts would not have been tolerated
6. A behavior modification program whereby he would have been able to learn to control his temper through rewards for good behavior

By the time he arrived for his preadmission evaluation, he was a seriously disturbed boy who had internalized the undependable, unfriendly and sometimes sadistic world around him. He badly needed the continuity of a dependable, concerned environment as well as a therapeutic relationship in which he could feel safe enough to look at himself and attempt to work through his problems. He also needed the continuity of contact with peers with whom he could learn to make relationships.

However, in considering residential treatment for a child from such an unstable background, which he himself best described when he said, "I never know what's coming tomorrow," one has to make plans for after-care in order to provide a stable, on-going home situation to which the child can be discharged. This boy had all he could take of the torment he found in his real world and was already on his way to withdrawing into his own world. Thus, to return him to the constant cycle of foster home placements and rejections would possibly undo the gains made in residential treatment.

QUESTION C:
DONALD SHOULD HAVE BEEN ACCEPTED FOR RESIDENTIAL TREATMENT ONLY ON THE CONDITION THAT UPON DISCHARGE:
1. The referring agency would insist that his father and step-mother would take him to live with them

CASE STUDY #50

2. He would be free to go and find his own way in life
3. The referring agency would find a residential children's home for him which would provide him with a protected environment in which he could live until he became of legal age, while continuing his schooling and possibly learning a trade
4. The referring agency would find a foster home for him, where the foster parents themselves had come from broken homes. This would help them to give Donald the understanding and support he so badly needed.
5. The referring agency would send him to live with his natural mother

This boy had already been rejected by both of his natural parents, and their infrequent contact with him suggested little desire on their part to give him a home.

In some cases, adults who have suffered broken homes in their childhood have problems themselves as a result of their own early experiences of emotional deprivation and rejection. Hence, it would be questionable whether this type of foster parent should be requested. The best answer is three

QUESTION D:
THE PROGNOSIS WOULD BE:
1. Hopeless
2. Poor
3. Guarded
4. Good
5. Excellent

The prognosis in this situation is difficult to determine because little is known about Donald's early emotional relationships, particularly with his mother. It is well documented that between six months and three years of age the infant's future emotional health depends upon continuity of care by a constant mother figure on whom he can depend for love and stimulation. We know that Donald was first born, so we can suspect that he did receive some early mothering in a situation where mother could devote herself entirely to him with no sibling competition. However, we don't know the state of mother's mental health at that time and can only guess that the mother-infant relationship may have been chaotic and undependable, which we are sure it became as the number of children increased and as mother's mental health deteriorated. Nevertheless, the continuing maternal relationship, although a chaotic, undependable one, may have saved him from the threshold that can produce irreversible effects. There is hope that he did not become an "affectionateless character." His concern about the well-being of his siblings when he was seven years old, and his feelings of depression and despair help to support this view. The best answer is three. See Case 24 for a similarly deprived black teen-ager and Case 18 for a deprived six-year-old.

REFERENCES:
1. Bowlby, J., 1969: Attachment and Loss. Vol. 1, Attachment. New York, Basic Books

2. Bowlby, J., 1951: Maternal Care and Mental Health. Geneva: World Health Organization Monograph #2

3. Bowlby, J., 1958: The nature of the child's tie to his mother. Int J Psycho-Anal, 39:350-373

4. Earle, A. M. and B. V. Earle, 1961: Early maternal deprivation and later psychiatric illness. Amer J Orthopsychiat 31:181-186

CASE STUDY #50

5. Fraiberg, S., 1962: A therapeutic approach to reactive ego disturbances in children in placement. Amer J Orthopsychiat 32:18-31

6. Frank, G., 1965: The role of the family in the development of psychopathology Psychol Bull 64:191-205

7. Freud, S., 1917: Mourning and Melancholia. Standard Edition, 14:243-258, London, Hogarth Press, 1957

8. Geleerd, E. R., 1945: Some observations on temper tantrums in children. Amer J Orthopsychiat 15:238-246

9. Glaser, K., 1967: Masked depression in children and adolescents. Amer J Psychother 21:565-574

10. Herzog, E. and E. C. Sudia, 1969: Fatherless homes: A review of research In: Annual Progress in Child Psychiatry and Child Development. edited by S. Chess and A. Thomas, New York: Brunner/Mazel, pp. 341-351

11. McCord, J., McCord, W. and E. Thurber, 1962: The effects of paternal absence on male children. J Abnorm Soc Psychol 64:361-369

12. Redl, F. and D. Wineman, 1952: Controls From Within. Glencoe, Ill., The Free Press

13. Solnit, A., 1960: Hospitalization: an aid to physical and psychological health in children. Amer J Dis Child, 99:155-163

14. Thompson, W. R. and J. E. Grusec, 1970: Studies of early experience. In: L. Carmichael, Manual of Child Psychology, ed., P. H. Mussen, New York, Wiley, pp. 603-624

CASE STUDY #51

Rejections Around Robin Result in Reactions

Robin was a 7 year-old white, second-grade girl, when her mother, Nancy, brought her to the Child Psychiatry Clinic because "she has had diabetes since age 5 and feels she is the only person in the world who has it." Nancy expressed concern about Robin's poor appetite, refusal of food, bedwetting, and her expressed feelings of not being loved.

Robin was the firstborn of Nancy, who was then nineteen. Nancy stated that although she was legally married to a military man between ages 17 and 21, Robin and her 3 year-old brother, Clayton, were fathered by another man. A year after his divorce from Nancy, two years before the onset of Robin's diabetes, Robin's legal father drowned accidentally while intoxicated.

When first seen, Robin's mother looked harried and depressed. She was a short, plump, red-haired, pale-complexioned, 26 year-old woman. Shortly before Robin's first clinic visit, she had enrolled in a two-year nursing program whose costs were being paid by Vocational Rehabilitation. She also received child support from Aid to Dependent Children. Prior to this time she had been employed as a factory worker. She had sought help for herself in the adult psychiatry clinic when Robin was 2 years and 4 years old. Robin's maternal grandfather was an alcoholic who was abusive to Nancy and her younger brother.

Robin, her brother, and her mother lived in an apartment in a metropolitan area with a transient Appalachian population. Nancy's therapist had difficulty maintaining an accurate count and understanding of her lovers.

The maternal grandmother and other relatives were frightened of Robin's diabetes and gave little emotional support. Even when the family came through with material needs, mother felt overwhelmed at her plight of being mother, father, and breadwinner. She indicated she would have welcomed some relief, e. g. , by the relatives providing overnight babysitting.

Nancy stated that Robin had been hospitalized several times for "being out of control." These hospitalizations caused frequent absences from school. On the first visit Nancy warned the therapist that contact "with the school could be dangerous." She mentioned that a neighbor who had told school authorities of her child's psychotherapy found the child scapegoated.

Nancy felt that the school was overconcerned about Robin's diabetes. She had understood the pediatrician to say that Robin must have very regular meals and regular morning urine checks, which interrupted the school schedule. Nancy related repeated examples of miscommunication with the principal. She felt that the school personnel's overreaction to Robin's symptoms or complaints caused difficulty. Nancy felt that Robin manipulated "to get herself out of school, " into the hospital, for attention, and to disrupt Nancy's studies.

Robin readily talked of not liking shots. She called her pediatrician her boyfriend. She called herself "dummy" in individual sessions and mentioned her clumsiness. She had wide mood swings. Whenever Robin's urine sugar was high, mother became extremely anxious and tried to follow her pediatrician's instructions by giving more regular insulin. On one occasion this resulted in hypoglycemic shock, which necessitated emergency hospitalization. At that time mother suddenly became paralyzed on her left side. This subsided after two hours with a visit to her psychotherapist.

QUESTION A:

FROM THE HISTORY GIVEN WE CAN EXPECT THAT ROBIN WOULD:
1. Be an obsessive child with repetitive hand-washing
2. Show difficulty in trusting men, act depressed, and have wide swings in mood
3. Talk readily about being abandoned by her father and rejected by her mother
4. Have very few problems with behavior, so that after evaluation individual psychotherapy would not need to be recommended
5. Demonstrate difficulty in relationships
6. Regress at times in therapy

CASE STUDY #51

7. Need prolonged hospitalization to regulate her diet, insulin, and exercises
8. Show erratic psychologic and physiologic responses to stress. Her need for consistency in relationships will manifest itself in school and in behavior problems

Although Robin seemed slightly obsessive, there was no reason to predict that she would have repetitive handwashing. She did show difficulty in trusting men, as did her mother, and had wide swings in mood with frequent "downs." She did not talk readily about being abandoned and rejected. Individual psychotherapy was strongly recommended, since it was felt that her "brittle diabetes" (necessitating frequent hospitalizations) and her mother's chaotic life were intertwined. The fifth and sixth answers are true but incomplete. Prolonged hospitalization for this child seemed contraindicated. The last answer is the best, though two, five, and six are also correct (Rosen and Lidz 1949).

QUESTION B:
AFTER SEVERAL INTERVIEWS, NANCY'S THERAPIST SUGGESTED FOCUSING ON HER TRANSIENT RELATIONSHIPS WITH MEN. NANCY RELATED, "I DON'T CARE WHAT THEY DO TO ME, AS LONG AS THEY KEEP THEIR PROMISES TO MY KIDS." IT MIGHT BE EXPECTED THAT MOTHER'S MINNESOTA MULTIPHASIC PERSONALITY INVENTORY (MMPI) PATTERN WOULD:
1. Show antisocial tendencies
2. Be within normal limits
3. Show extreme hysteria, paranoia, and depression
4. Show poor impulse control and lack of responsibility for her actions
5. Indicate an impulsive, narcissistic, seductive woman with little insight, poor self-concept, paranoia, and a goal of male rejection
6. Be indicative of a chronic brain syndrome
7. Be abnormal in many areas

The Minnesota Multiphasic Personality Inventory is often used to confirm clinical impressions. Robin's mother, Nancy, had a rather unusual MMPI profile. The personality description in answer five was taken from the "blind" interpretation by a psychologist who did not know her otherwise.

QUESTION C:
ROBIN'S FIRST INTERVIEW STARTED WITH SHYNESS. SOON, HOWEVER, SHE SHARED INFORMATION ABOUT CLAYTON, HER THREE-YEAR-OLD BROTHER. SHE CALLED THE PUPPETS "FATSO," ANGRILY, AND MENTIONED THAT HER FATHER DROWNED, BUT SHE DIDN'T REMEMBER HIM. SHE PLAYED AGGRESSIVELY WITH TOY PISTOLS. SHE BEGAN THE SECOND VISIT BY SHOOTING A DART AT THE THERAPIST, HITTING THE THERAPIST'S EYEGLASSES AND KNOCKING THE LENS OUT OF THE FRAME. AT THIS POINT THE THERAPIST MIGHT:
1. Return Robin to her mother and suggest that she is too angry to be able to use outpatient treatment
2. Lock the door and watch Robin closely through the oneway mirror
3. Remove the toy pistols from the room and suggest that guns should never be pointed at people
4. Tell Robin that the therapist is furious with her for the pain she caused
5. Have Robin given an injection of a major tranquilizer
6. Tell Robin that shooting the pistol at the therapist indicates her fury at the loss of her father
7. Tell Robin that he or she was angry at being hit and understands that she must be very angry at someone about something

CASE STUDY #51

In America, toy guns are commonplace both at home and at child guidance clinics. However, some therapists feel very strongly that they have no place in the therapy room. The ideal response would show the therapist's feelings but not stress a need for the therapist to retaliate against the child. If the therapist is so frightened by the child's behavior that he cannot handle it, then, of course, he must tell the parents. The second answer may be tempting but, of course, would not accomplish anything. The authoritarian answer three, though not wrong, would be less helpful than the last answer, which is the best. Answer four might be appropriate under some circumstances. Answer five would most likely be seen as punishment by Robin (and she would probably be right). The strong interpretation made in answer six might be incorrect and would not likely be helpful at this early stage of treatment.

QUESTION D:
NANCY CALLED ROBIN'S THERAPIST AT HOME IN THE EVENING AND SPOKE FRANTICALLY ABOUT ROBIN'S NOT FINISHING HER LUNCH AT SCHOOL. SHE DISCUSSED THE PRINCIPAL'S DEMAND THAT ROBIN BE SENT HOME WHENEVER SHE COMPLAINS OF ABDOMINAL PAIN AND A SCHOOL NURSE IS NOT AVAILABLE TO CHECK HER. AT THIS POINT NANCY SHOULD BE TOLD THAT:
1. She should always call during clinic hours
2. All contact should be through her own therapist
3. Robin should be transferred to another school
4. Her concern about Robin's eating is misplaced anxiety about her own security
5. She needs tranquilization, as well as Robin
6. Psychotherapy takes time
7. Her concern about Robin's eating should be discussed with her therapist and a school visit might prove helpful

When a parent is frantic about his or her child's behavior it is not helpful to remind that late calls are forbidden. Contact with the child's therapist may be helpful if firm limits are set on the relationship without rejection. In this case, it was felt that mother's controlling, dependent behavior needed some response; she was impulsive and might stop therapy or inappropriately transfer Robin to another school. The fourth answer, although correct, would be an overly interpretive response which this mother would not likely understand. Though the mother may need tranquilization, this is not a transaction best handled over the telephone. The sixth answer, although true, would not calm down most mothers' panic. The last answer proved helpful: it set limits on the mother calling the child's therapist while indicating that mother's feelings were not being disregarded.

Robin painted with watercolors in a subdued manner for the first fifteen minutes of the fifth session. She then painted her fingernails, her face, and the doll with red paint. She began to paint the blonde hair of the doll red and asked, "I wonder if they'll be mad at me?"

QUESTION E:
WE CAN BEST INTERPRET THIS TO MEAN THAT ROBIN:
1. Is worried that her mother will scold her if she finds paint on anything but the paper
2. Is concerned that she won't be able to return for individual psychotherapy sessions
3. Wonders if anyone will set limits
4. Is wondering if the therapist is like her mother who would scold her
5. Wants the doll to take home
6. Is asking indirectly about her therapists's feelings of countertransference
7. Wishes no one will be mad at her

CASE STUDY #51

Robin was worried that her mother would scold her. It is also likely that she was concerned about whether her therapist would continue a consistent relationship with her. She frequently asked for limits and also seemed to ask if she seemed lovable. She did ask to take the dolls home on several occasions. The sixth answer would seem incorrect since very few children understand transference and countertransference. The last answer is rather general. The best answers would seem to be two and four, but one, three, and seven are also correct.

QUESTION F:
DURING THE TENTH INDIVIDUAL PSYCHOTHERAPY SESSION ROBIN ASKED TO FILL A BABY BOTTLE WITH WATER AND VIGOROUSLY BIT AND SUCKED ON THE NIPPLE. ALTERNATELY, SHE OFFERED THE BOTTLE TO THE DOLL. HER THERAPIST COULD SAY:
1. "You want to be a baby again"
2. "You are finding that you can act much younger here with me, and I will still accept you"
3. "Sucking on the nipple is fun"
4. "The bottle probably wasn't clean. Why don't we get a new one for your next visit"
5. "When you bite on the nipple, I wonder if you are angry at someone"
6. "Why do you feel you have to be a baby here?"
7. "I saw a little girl once who sucked on her bottle whenever she was afraid"

Though a young child may have ambivalent feelings about wanting to be a baby again, it would be rare that the child could use this interpretation directly the first time around. The second response, although somewhat long, is probably the best. The usefulness of the third answer would depend on how the therapist said it. The fourth answer would indicate that the therapist needs therapy. The fifth answer may be true depending on other contextual cues, and some children might be able to accept it. The sixth answer is accusatory with the red-flag word "why." The last answer does not help clarify the therapist's acceptance of the regression.

Robin's mother continued to scapegoat Robin in the hall on the way to therapy. Mother related to her therapist that the new "suitor" was treating her more fairly and that Robin's behavior had improved at home. She mentioned that Robin's teacher characterized her school performance as very erratic, with excellent work some days and rebellious failure other days.

QUESTION G:
AFTER TEN SESSIONS, PLANS FOR ROBIN AND HER MOTHER SHOULD INCLUDE:
1. Frequent visits to Robin's pediatrician to keep her within the best limits of diabetic control
2. Termination, with a final interpretive session stating that unless mother begins to trust men, Robin will have lifelong difficulties in male-female relationships
3. Recommendation of foster placement for Robin in order to allow mother to finish her education, get a job, and become self-supporting
4. Bringing Robin and her mother together in several interviews to change mother's scapegoating of Robin into positive reinforcement for sharing behavior
5. A change of schools so that Robin's "scapegoating" by the school authorities will cease
6. Continued individual psychotherapy for mother in order to decrease her paranoia and failure set with men

CASE STUDY #51

7. Continued individual psychotherapy for Robin and her mother until Robin accepts her diabetes
8. Group therapy for Robin with other physically handicapped children so that she can learn how other children adapt

Children with "brittle diabetes" are frequently overcontrolled (by parents and pediatrician) concerning urine sugar and acetone. Frequent visits to establish a trust relationship make much more sense than a mechanistic concern about "control." Termination at this point seemed inappropriate for Robin. The third answer sacrifices the child's feelings (and possibly the mother's) for the utopian idea of giving mother a break. The fourth answer is correct but incomplete. Changes in schools do not usually solve problems like Robin's. Continued individual psychotherapy for mother was planned, but answer six is incomplete. Frequently parents and physicians force responsibility for management of diabetes at too early an age. Group therapy for Robin would probably be helpful but it does not need to be with other physically handicapped children. Most important, of course, would be the quality of the therapy given. The best answer is seven.

REFERENCES:
1. Bennett, E. M. and D. E. Johannsen, 1954: Psychodynamics of the diabetic child. Psychological Monographs: General and Applied 68:1-23

2. Bruch, H., 1949: Physiologic and psychologic interrelationships in diabetes in children. Psychosom Med 11:200-210

3. Falstein, E. I. and I. Judas, 1955: Juvenile diabetes and its psychiatric implications. Am J Orthopsychiatry 25:330-342

4. Leaverton, D. R., 1971: The disturbed child with diabetes. The J of the Florida Med Assn 58:47-49

5. Leaverton, D. R., 1970: The Child with Diabetes who is Difficult to Manage. Presented at the Second Annual Birth Defects Symposium, University of Florida College of Medicine, October 30, 1970

6. Rosen, H. and T. Lidz, 1949: Emotional factors in the precipitation of recurrent diabetic acidosis. Psychosom Med 11:211-215

7. Stein, S. P. and E. Charles, 1971: Emotional factors in juvenile diabetes mellitus: A study of early life experience of adolescent diabetics. Am J Psychiat 128:56-60

8. Swift, C. R. and F. L. Seidman, 1964: Adjustment problems of juvenile diabetes. J Am Acad Child Psychiatry 3:500-515

9. Winnicott, D. W., 1958: Collected Papers, Through Paediatrics to Psychoanalysis. Tavistock Publications, London

CASE STUDY #52

The Silent Treatment: A Therapeutic Challenge

A 12-year-old electively mute 7th-grade girl was hospitalized because of increasing misbehavior and falling school marks. For the previous seven years she had not spoken to anyone except her mother, brother, sister, and two cousins. Even her father was left out of the favored group of intimates.

She was the oldest of three children in a middle-class black family. The brother and sister appeared normal. Her mother was overprotective to the point of being paranoid about what the hospital would do to "my little girl." When the chubby "little girl" lost a few pounds, the mother brought in chocolates to fatten her up again. The mother tended to dominate the quiet, hard-working, thrifty father. She predicted that the hospital staff would fail to help the girl. In the past she herself had tried to "trick" the girl into talking to other people, e.g. by means of telephone or having her sell girl scout cookies. These tricks had often seemed to work until the girl "realized what I was doing." Then she would say, "You can't make me talk. I'll do whatever I want."

The parents reported that the girl developed normally the first three years in all respects, including normal speech. After moving from the home of the paternal grandmother, whom she had been calling "Mom" while calling her mother by her first name, she began whispering. About this time she was punished repeatedly for enuresis over a two-year period. The enuresis stopped only after bladder neck surgery at age 5. By the time she started school, she had stopped talking to most people, including her father, who had previously been her favorite.

She passed the sixth grade on the basis of written work, never talking to teacher or classmates. Her work in the 7th grade was adequate until a few months before admission.

She presented as a tense, rigid, hesitant, slow-moving, slightly obese young adolescent. She made eye contact but no attempt to communicate other than by terse, relevant written answers. She would not even nod or shake her head. Her affect was generally flat, but she occasionally flashed an engaging smile which was not always appropriate to the circumstances.

On the ward, she soon made friends. With them she devised a finger signal for "yes," "no," and "I don't know" rather than use more natural nonverbal communication. She controlled by her retentiveness, training people to take care of her.

A multiple therapeutic approach was necessary, including drug, family, behavior, milieu, camp, and group therapies as well as individual psychotherapy. Pharmacologically, an amobarbital (Amytal) interview, a trial of dextroamphetamine (Dexedrine), and a trial of oxazepam (Serax) each resulted in only a slight increase of spontaneity. Trifluoperazine (Stelazine), in doses up to 5 mg. t.i.d., was followed by more definite spontaneity and relaxation and some vocalizations, mostly appropriate giggling.

Individual psychotherapy was by supervised medical students on two-month rotations who provided an atmosphere of patient, optimistic expectation and acceptance. They at first accepted written communication and later provided a practice shelter for emerging verbalization. Continuity was provided by the supervising psychiatrist, the milieu, the social worker, nurses, teachers, and other permanent staff.

QUESTION A:
SUCH FREQUENT CHANGES OF INDIVIDUAL PSYCHOTHERAPISTS:
1. Hindered her progress
2. Helped her progress
3. Made no difference as long as continuity was provided by other staff
4. Was psychologically destructive to the patient
5. Really didn't matter, because everyone understood the students were there to learn, not give service

CASE STUDY #52

The best way to learn how to give good medical care is to give good service under supervision. In our experience, adolescent patients quickly form strong relationships with medical students, and both benefit from the contact. The shortness of the time is usually not destructive if the patient knows from the beginning when the student will leave. Nevertheless, for most long-term patients this frequency of therapist change is probably a disadvantage. In this case, however, it seemed to help: in the first few weeks with each of five students, the patient showed a surge of improvement in socialization and verbalization. Apparently their fresh resources of naive optimism and patience were worth more than experience or acquaintance with this patient. The correct answer is two. For more on therapist rotations, see cases 12 and 32.

Group therapy dissuaded the other patients from cooperating with the patient's passive-aggressive, dependent life-style and elicited peer support for experimenting with new behavior and assuming responsibility for herself.

In family therapy, the father's thrifty hoarding and the mother's perfectionistic feeling of obligation to do right by the girl focussed attention on the "anal" problems in the family. Support of the father's hidden strengths and ventilation of the mother's anger about the girl's passive-aggressive dependency resulted in greater participation by the father in family activities and a diminution of the mother's overprotectiveness, infantilization, and overcoercion. This made home visits feasible as effective reinforcers for a behavior modification program which had previously faltered because no sufficiently rewarding reinforcer could be found. She was able to earn points for home visits at first by giggling, later by words, and later only by complete sentences.

Three intensive one-week group experiences living at camp with hospital staff and patients each resulted in a surge of spontaneity and vocalization. As she improved, she seemed to show depressive side effects of the trifluoperazine, which were relieved by repeated reductions in dosage. Eventually, she asked to stop her point system and continued talking voluntarily.

She was discharged taking 2 mg. trifluoperazine daily, talking to all the staff and patients. She was even talking to her father, who had by that time "loosened up" and treated the family to a day's excursion to an amusement park. On return home, she had two parties at which she thoroughly enjoyed herself, surprising people by talking to them. On returning to the school, she not only talked to classmates and teachers, but also joined the pep club.

QUESTION B:
THIS PATIENT'S BASIC PROBLEM WAS PROBABLY:
1. Schizophrenia
2. Speech disorder
3. Passive-aggressive personality
4. Behavior disorder of childhood or adolescence
5. Father phobia
6. Phobia of talking
7. Depressive neurosis
8. Conversion hysteria (aphonia)

Though this patient in some ways resembled a catatonic schizophrenic, she did not show waxy flexibility or the typical improvement under amobarbital. Neither did she show a clearcut thought disorder. Her written answers were always relevant and logical and those with whom she did talk noted no loosening of association. Though she showed much ambivalence and constriction of affect, schizophrenia hardly seemed the most appropriate diagnosis. Speech disturbance would be technically correct, but hardly implies the gravity of the problem. Answer four and the neurotic diagnoses fail to impart the chronicity of the problem. The best answer is three.

CASE STUDY #52

QUESTION C:
ELECTIVELY MUTE CHILDREN:
1. Are rather rare
2. Are rather common
3. Can usually be treated as outpatients
4. Are usually very difficult to treat and require an intensive long-term program, often needing hospitalization
5. Are equivalent to the slow-to-warm-up children described by Thomas and Chess

The frequency of elective mutism partly depends on the definition. In no event, however, should it be confused with the more common slow-to-warm-up temperament. The slow-to-warm-up child is merely shy and inhibited and tends to withdraw from new situations. Showing little psychopathology, he will with patient encouragement and support eventually talk to most people. Electively mute children, who absolutely refuse to speak to other than a few selected intimates, are comparatively rare. This is fortunate, for treatment of their more serious disturbance is difficult and costly, as shown in this case. One and four are correct.

QUESTION D:
A BEHAVIOR MODIFICATION APPROACH TO TREATMENT OF ELECTIVELY MUTE CHILDREN:
1. Though useful in this case, is not usually a good basis for therapy
2. Was the successful treatment modality in this case
3. Implies control of the patient even over his own objections
4. Is incompatible with a humanistic or psychotherapeutic approach
5. Can work synergistically with other therapeutic modalities, including chemotherapy

Behavior modification need not involve an inhumane control of the patient. In fact, most patients like their program because of the rewards involved and often cooperate in refining their own program, as this patient did. Behavior modification tends to make a useful basis for therapy of elective mutism. In this case it carried a large part of the therapeutic burden, but was only able to do so in the context of a comprehensive therapeutic program where 1. the milieu cooperated in record-keeping, reinforcing, successive approximation, and shifting from tangible reinforcement to social approval, 2. family therapy made feasible the only adequate reinforcer which could be found, home visits, and 3. chemotherapy elicited enough of a behavior (giggling) similar to the desired behavior (talking) to permit a beginning of reinforcement and successive approximations. Five is the correct answer.

QUESTION E:
THE TERM "SUCCESSIVE APPROXIMATION" MENTIONED ABOVE MEANS:
1. The patient's behavior was shaped step-by-step towards the goal of spontaneous speech
2. Therapy was successful in coming close to the goal of spontaneous speech
3. We have to settle for approximate goals in therapy, rather than perfection
4. The steps of therapy were planned, one right after the other
5. None of the above

The correct answer is one. When the desired behavior is not already occasionally emitted, it cannot be reinforced to increase its frequency. In such cases the programmer can reinforce an existing behavior (in this case giggling) which is in the direction of the desired behavior (spontaneous speech). As the

CASE STUDY #52

reinforced behavior (giggling) increases to a high rate, a few behaviors (in this case single words) usually occur which are nearer the goal behavior. When they are reinforced, they increase and the giggling need no longer be reinforced. By such steps the patient's behavior gradually gets closer to - "successively approximates" - the goal behavior. For other behavior modification cases, see cases 13, 37, 39, 41 and 48.

REFERENCES:
1. Blom, G., 1972: A Psychoanalytic Viewpoint of Behavior Modification in Clinical and Educational Settings. J Am Acad Child Psychiatry 11:675-693

2. Browne, E., Wilson, V. and P.S. Laybourne, 1963: Diagnosis and Treatment of Elective Mutism in Children. J Am Acad Child Psychiatry 2:603-617

3. Carrera, F. and P. Adams, 1970: An Ethical Perspective on Operant Conditioning. J Am Acad Child Psychiatry 9:607-623

4. Clement, P.W., 1973: Training Children to be Their Own Behavior Therapists. J School Health, In Press

5. Halpern, W.I., Hannond, J. and R. Cohen, 1971: A Therapeutic Approach to Speech Phobia: Elective Mutism Re-examined. J Am Acad Child Psychiatry 10:94-107

6. Kaplan, S.L. and P. Escoll, 1973: Treatment of Two Silent Adolescent Girls. J Am Acad Child Psychiatry 12:59-72

7. Nolan, J.D. and C. Pence, 1970: Operant Conditioning Principles in the Treatment of a Selectively Mute Child. J of Consulting and Clinical Psychology 35:265-268

8. Norman, A. and H.J. Broman, 1970: Volume Feedback and Generalization Techniques in Shaping Speech of an Electively Mute Boy: A Case Study. Perceptual and Motor Skills 31:463-470

9. Reed, G.F., 1963: Elective Mutism in Children: A Re-Appraisal. J of Child Psychology and Psychiatry 4:99-107

10. Reid, J.B., Hawkins, N., Keutzer, C., McNeal, S.A., Phelps, R.E., Reid, K.M. and H.L. Mees, 1967: A Marathon Behavior Modification of a Selectively Mute Child. J of Child Psychology and Psychiatry and Allied Disciplines 8:27-30

11. Straughan, J.H., Potter, W.K. and S.H. Hamilton, 1965: The Behavioral Treatment of an Elective Mute. J of Child Psychology and Psychiatry 6:125-130

12. Thomas, A., Chess, S. and H.G. Birch, 1968: Temperament and Behavior Disorders in Childhood. New York University Press, New York

13. Thomas, A. and S. Chess, 1970: Origins of Personality. Scientific American 223:102-109

14. Wright, H.J., Jr., 1968: A Clinical Study of Children Who Refuse to Talk in School. J Am Acad Child Psychiatry 7:603-617

CASE STUDY #53

Emily

A young mother brought her two lively children to the clinic because of their uncontrollable behavior. Emily was five years old and Jack was three and a half. Mother complained that when she was around them, their demands for her attention were insatiable. They wouldn't play by themselves; she was unable to get them interested in anything, and they followed her around demanding her undivided attention. The situation became even worse when there was a male visitor. The children would follow him around, climb all over him and smother him with attention. When mother reprimanded or attempted to set limits, the children's behavior only became worse with crying, kicking, spitting and biting. Emily was extremely jealous of Jack and could not tolerate mother giving him any special attention.

They awakened at daybreak and often seemed to find it difficult to let mother sleep in the morning. Ordinarily they played happily and noisily in their room next to hers. However, when they occasionally tried to get her up and she refused, they seemed to lose control and wrecked their room, sometimes flooding it with water.

When Emily was three years old, mother had divorced the children's father after a stormy, sometimes violent relationship. Despite his alcoholism and barbiturate addiction, he had visited the children regularly following the divorce until a year later when he suddenly committed suicide.

When mother told the children about father's death, Jack became very upset and cried. Emily, however, remained very calm and told her mother that she (mother), too, could die if she took too many pills. Emily had not cried about anything since her father's death. Mother said that she often talked with the children about their father and that she often heard the children talking about him to each other.

About a year before the first clinic visit, a male student had moved in with the family. He was very devoted to the children and to mother, but he had graduated and had left the family about six weeks previously. Thus, the children again lost their "father." Emily was also upset because her teacher, of whom she was very fond, had left the school in the middle of the year. However, the school reported that although Emily's new teacher didn't know her very well, she thought that Emily was doing exceptionally well and was popular with the children.

Mother, who was a receptionist at a large restaurant, picked the children up from the nursery school and got their evening meal. She then left home each evening at five-thirty. A baby sitter came in at that time and the children were in bed by the time mother arrived home.

Emily was seen for a psychological evaluation which consisted of the Stanford-Binet (L-M), The Children's Apperception Test (CAT) and a series of drawings. She seemed to enjoy the testing relationship and often interrupted the psychologist to ask questions of her own. "Did you know that boys stand up at the toilet and girls don't?" "Where do babies come from?" There was also constant physical activity and laughter. Although she was anxious and impulsive, she was able to use the situation for her own gratification and seemed to become less anxious when the psychologist didn't become impatient or irritated by her questions. She was found to be functioning at the high average level of intelligence.

The Children's Apperception Test, which consisted of a series of pictures of animals in human situations about which the child makes up stories, portrayed Emily as a very anxious little girl who seemed to have constant fears of imminent disaster which she desperately attempted to allay with a rather manic form of denial. However, this defense wasn't very helpful, and her anxiety generally leaked through.

In one of the stories she seemed to feel responsible for the break-up between mother and father and to feel that nothing could have stopped this from happening. She possibly described it when she said "they didn't hold on very tight." She was apparently preoccupied with the death of her father and seemed to be very confused

CASE STUDY #53

about death. Her stories suggested that her fantasies about death were of a person being "locked in" or so immobilized in some way that he could never escape. In four of the stories, the children were killed or destroyed in some way.

She gave some idea of how she felt about her little brother when she was shown a picture of a mother kangaroo hopping along with a baby in her pouch being followed by a young kangaroo riding on a tricycle. She said that the little girl on the tricycle and her mother were going to get something to eat, but that the baby brother might get eaten up by a fox (rather hopefully). When she was asked how the little girl kangaroo felt about the little baby riding in the pocket she replied, "She feels unhappy because she's never been in the pocket because she is too big and heavy. There wouldn't be enough room to get her whole self in. She would get squeezed."

Her drawings also suggested the manic defense evinced during the intelligence testing. All of the characters had gay smiles and arms outstretched. At the same time, however, they contained strong indications of underlying depression. The drawing of the father, which Emily added without comment, was without arms.

QUESTION A:
EMILY WAS GIVEN A PSYCHOLOGICAL EVALUATION RATHER THAN JACK
BECAUSE:
1. She was older
2. She was the disturbed child and Jack was only copying her behavior
3. She acted unconcerned about her father's death and hadn't cried since
4. Jack was too young to test
5. She behaved like her little brother which suggested she was retarded

In this situation, an intelligence test was used as a diagnostic tool, through observation of her behavior and the content of her responses rather than to obtain an I.Q. She was obviously an intelligent, verbal child who got along well in the nursery class. Retardation was not suspected. However, her lack of concern when she was told about her father's death, her rather inappropriate laughter and her obvious anxiety when mother remained in bed after daybreak were hints that Emily may have been a disturbed child, as was indicated by her fantasies obtained with the CAT. It is also possible that Jack was copying Emily's behavior since children at that age are apt to pattern themselves after an older sibling. However, should Jack have been given projective tests, his fantasies would have been much different from his sister's. The best answer is three, although two is possible.

QUESTION B:
THE PROBABLE CAUSES OF EMILY'S EMOTIONAL DISTURBANCE WERE:
1. She felt guilty about being her mother's favorite
2. Her father had died
3. Mother was too strict
4. She and brother were alone a great part of the time and she didn't have other playmates
5. Her school teacher and the student boarder had left
6. Mother and father didn't get along with each other before the divorce

The child's disturbance was most likely due to a combination of causes. She may have felt rejected by her mother in some ways, and this may have been due to the fact that she saw little of mother during the week and that she had to share her with little brother.

The roots of this child's problems probably started long before father's death. Father's alcoholism and his addiction to barbiturates must have made the relationship between the parents difficult and unpredictable, which could have aroused highly anxious and insecure feelings in Emily.

CASE STUDY #53

As we have seen, the child was unable to express grief over the death of her father. Yet, with each additional loss, earlier feelings of loss were aroused. Hence, psychologically, Emily was suffering all of her losses together, i.e., of father, student and teacher. The best answers are two, five and six.

QUESTION C:
EMILY'S DRAWING OF HER FATHER WITHOUT ARMS SUGGESTS THAT:
1. She got tired and didn't bother to add arms to the figure
2. She was making it impossible for him to fight with mother again
3. She had never liked him
4. She was castrating him
5. Somewhere within herself she was aware that he could no longer hold or support her, i.e., that he was dead

Emily's drawing of her father without arms probably related to her fantasy of him as an immobilized figure who could no longer hold or contain her. In contrast, her other human figure drawings were lively and active. Her father drawing tied in with her CAT stories which suggested that death meant immobilization. It could also be linked with her noisy and destructive behavior when mother failed to get up in the morning. The best answer is five. (For more about death, see case 33.)

QUESTION D:
EMILY'S QUESTIONS ABOUT SEX SUGGESTED THAT:
1. Mother had given her good sex information
2. She was testing the psychologist to see if she knew about sex
3. She was showing off her sexual knowledge
4. She was seeking affirmation and further sexual information
5. She was afraid of sexual information

Emily may have had the undivided attention of an adult for one of the few times in her life when she was evaluated by the psychologist. She found someone who listened to what she was saying and responded appropriately. Hence, she was able to talk about her sexual knowledge, questions and confusion. When she asked the psychologist if she knew "that boys stand up at the toilet and girls don't," she seemed to be seeking affirmation. When a casual response was given, Emily may have felt it safe to ask the more puzzling question,"where do babies come from?"

Emily was an isolated child whose only companionship for a great part of the time was with her little brother. When mother was home, she had to share her with him. Thus, she probably had a very active fantasy life and had reached the age where she needed simple, matter-of-fact answers to her questions. The best answer is four.

REFERENCES:
1. Bellak, L., 1954: The Thematic Apperception Test and The Children's Apperception Test in Clinical Use. New York, Grune and Stratton

2. Bowlby, J., 1960: Grief and mourning in infancy and early childhood. Psychoanal Study Child 15:9-52, New York, International Universities Press

3. Brown, F., 1961: Depression and childhood bereavement. J Ment Sci 107: 754-77

4. Burks, H. and S. Harrison, 1962: Aggressive behavior as a means of avoiding depression. Amer J Orthopsychiat 32:416-422

CASE STUDY #53

5. Burns, R. C. and S. H. Kaufman, 1970: Kinetic Family Drawings (K-F-D) and Introduction to Understanding Children Through Kinetic Drawings, New York, Brunner/Mazel

6. Cain, A. and I. Fast, 1966: Children's disturbed reactions to parent suicide. Amer J Orthopsychiat 36:872-880

7. Deutsch, H., 1937: Absence of grief. Psychoanal Quart 6:12-22

8. DiLeo, J., 1970: Young Children and Their Drawings. New York, Brunner/Mazel

9. Gardner, R. A., 1969: Sexual fantasies in childhood. Med Aspects of Human Sexuality 3:121-134

10. Glaser, K., 1967: Masked depression in children and adolescents. Am J Psychother 21:565-574

11. Haworth, M. A., 1966: The CAT: Facts About Fantasy. New York, Grune and Stratton

12. Hulse, W. C., 1952: Childhood conflict expressed through family drawings. J Proj Tech 16, pp. 66-79

13. Herzog, E. and C. E. Sudia, 1969: Fatherless Homes: a review of research in: Annual Progress in Child Psychiatry and Child Development, ed. S. Chess and A. Thomas. New York, Brunner/Mazel pp. 341-351

14. Klein, M., 1948: Mourning and its relation to manic-depressive states in: Contributions to Psychoanalysis. London: Hogarth Press, pp. 311-338

15. Kogelschatz, J. L., Adams, P. L. and D. M. Tucker, 1972: Family styles of fatherless households. J Child Psychiat 11:365-383

16. Machover, K., 1952: Human figure drawings of children. J Proj Tech 16:85-91

17. Terman, L. H. and M. A. Merrill, 1960: Stanford-Binet Intelligence Scale, Manual for Third Revision, Form L-M, Boston, Houghton Mifflin Co.

18. Winnicott, D. W., 1958: The manic defense. In: Collected Papers Paediatrics to Psycho-analysis. London, Tavistock Publications, Ltd.

CASE STUDY #54

Blindness, Self-Destruction, and Overprotection

Tim was a 9 year-old white boy found to be blind at birth. He had lived alternately with his parents and with his maternal grandmother in a rural setting. He had attended a school for the educable mentally retarded for three years. He progressed very little and stayed in their lowest developmental class. The parents brought him to the psychiatry clinic to obtain therapy for his "emotional block," which they felt prevented him from making any advancement.

Tim, the youngest of four children in the family, was a moderately obese boy with black hair and obvious corneal opacities. He showed many autistic manner-isms, with repetitive movements of objects, and loud, unintelligible utterances. He seemed aware of being in a strange situation. He responded positively to touch or introduction of different toys by momentarily stopping his autistic mannerisms and reaching out to examine his immediate environment. He responded to noise by searching for its source. Tim did not respond to simple verbal commands but showed his awareness of conversation concerning him by becoming increasingly frustrated and more anxious. In these instances he bit his hands viciously. At other times his frustrated behavior would also include temper tantrums.

Tim's mother and father had had many troubles during the previous year. The father's farming efforts had been financially disappointing and mother had worked off and on to support the family. Tim had spent the summers and week-ends at home but at the time of the clinic visit lived with his maternal grand-parents, since their house was "closer to his school." From the first visit it seemed apparent that the grandmother was a strong matriarch.

The family had vacillated between patronizing overprotection of Tim and frustration and guilt over their inability to provide appropriately for him. They saw him as having developed normally until he was about five years old. They even considered him quite bright and verbal until he began kindergarten. But after several weeks it was suggested to the parents that he not continue regular kindergarten; instead, he should seek help from classes for the mentally retarded. The family felt that since that time language development, speech, and coordina-tion had regressed.

Tim was then (age 5) evaluated by the State School for the Blind and was found to be severly retarded, with an IQ less than 40. At that time he exhibited head banging, autistic mannerisms, and thumb sucking. Other diagnostic work done at a children's hospital gave non-specific diagnoses of mental retardation. An electroencephalogram showed minimal, generalized cerebral dysrhythmia.

QUESTION A:
FROM THE INFORMATION GIVEN, THE BEST WORKING EXPLANATION OF TIM'S PROBLEM WOULD BE:
1. Tim's blindness has led to mental retardation with aphasia
2. Tim's diagnoses of blindness and mental retardation are accurate. He exhibits no mental disturbance
3. Tim's autism is related to the chronic brain syndrome which accompanies congenital blindness
4. Tim's responses when he is spoken to or touched probably indicate that his autism is not so severe that he is unreachable
5. Tim's autistic mannerisms result from the ambivalence his parents have shown towards him by allowing his grandmother to help raise him
6. Tim's autistic mannerisms are a cover for an obsessive-compulsive neurosis of a severe degree

The first answer can neither be proven nor disproven from the available data and does not account for the obvious emotional problems, even if it were true as it stands. Answer two does not take into account Tim's obvious anxiety and frustration. Answer three is incorrect since not all congenitally blind

CASE STUDY #54

children have a chronic brain syndrome. Answer four is the best answer. Answer five is not warranted from the data given. Answer six is incorrect since the degree of unrelatedness seems to be of a psychotic nature rather than neurotic.

Tim's parents and his grandmother came regularly to the psychiatry clinic for evaluation and therapy. A psychiatric social worker elicited a fuller picture of the family dynamics. The mother had often sought help from many agencies and individuals in the past. She wrote letters very often to seek help. She seemed to infantilize and overprotect Tim but also seemed sometimes to ignore him. Both the mother and the father seemed to have guilty feelings. During some of the interviews, the grandmother criticized her daughter's inability to cope with Tim.

QUESTION B:
IN REGARD TO THE BIRTH OF A DEFECTIVE CHILD, WE FIND THAT PARENTS:
1. Very rarely have emotional problems
2. Talk over their murderous feelings with each other within the first few days of the discovery
3. Sometimes have problems
4. Come down with psychosomatic illnesses as a result of the stress
5. React with anger and guilt to such degrees that divorce is almost inevitable
6. Have feelings of anger towards the child
7. React unconsciously with guilt and anger towards the child, themselves, and their ancestors

There has been no evidence in the literature to support answer one. The second answer has not been reported and has not been witnessed by the authors. The third answer is correct but too general. Answers four and five are possibilities but not usual. Feelings of anger towards the child are common, though not usually voiced. Answer six is correct, but not as specific as answer seven, the best answer. Just as in the loss of a loved one, denial is one of the first stages in the parents' resolution of feelings. This is probably because the birth of a defective child constitutes also the loss of the expected normal child. Parents must first mourn this loss before they can accept the defective child (Solnit and Stark, 1961).

The parents made efforts towards decreasing their overprotectiveness with Tim. They began to expect more age-appropriate behavior. They learned to interrupt his autistic mannerisms consistently. However, they found initially that his destructive hand-biting increased when they thus frustrated him.

QUESTION C:
WITH CHILDREN WHO APPEAR TO BE SELF-DESTRUCTIVE, THE PROPER COURSE WOULD BE:
1. To sedate them in order to interrupt the process
2. To interrupt their behavior in several ways
3. Not to be overly concerned with their self-destructiveness, since with psychotherapy and changes in the milieu, it usually stops
4. To employ soft restraints and isolation, since these tactics are often effective with children who mutilate themselves
5. To interpret to the child the anger that he is showing towards himself. If necessary, shout at him to get his attention
6. To consider medication, such as a major tranquilizer
7. To consider the possibility of the self-destruction being epileptic in nature. An anticonvulsant could be prescribed

Sedation is often used and may be slightly helpful. The second answer is correct as far as it goes, but gives no specific information. Only occasionally do psychotherapy and changes in the milieu stop self-destructive behavior in the

CASE STUDY #54

severely disturbed. Answer four is an effective means to stop self mutilation but decreases the necessary stimuli which the retarded child needs in order to learn. Answer five has been found to be effective only rarely. Answer six has been commonly used lately as an effective means of decreasing the amount of self destruction, but by no means always completely stops the behavior. Answer seven is not correct; self-destruction is very rarely the result of epileptic seizures, although anticonvulsants are commonly used, sometimes inappropriately, for other behavioral problems. The best answer is a combination of two and six.

Tim was given thioridazine (Mellaril) and was seen weekly in individual psychotherapy. He began pronouncing words more clearly. His self-destruction decreased. He improved in his ability to follow through with directions and requests. He began to relate to people on a much more appropriate level. However, his progress was slow, and he frequently regressed into past behavior patterns during times of frustration.

QUESTION D:

WHILE PLAYING IN THE BATHTUB AT HOME ONE DAY, TIM SAID, "TIM, WHAT'S THE MATTER WITH YOU?" ALSO, WHILE TRAVELING HOME AFTER VISITING THE CIRCUS, HE WAS HEARD TO SAY, "LET'S GO BACK." THESE EXAMPLES OF COMPLEX SENTENCES OCCURRING NOT INFREQUENTLY FROM AN OTHERWISE UNINTELLIGIBLE BOY WOULD INDICATE THAT:

1. Tim tries to frustrate his parents by teasing them with bits of conversation in order to control their behavior
2. His hearing is normal
3. Tim has selective mutism
4. Tim's speech development is progressing, but is chronologically delayed
5. By coincidence, he has brought together words that have meaning
6. On occasions his thinking processes approach normality, but his potential for expressive speech development may not be as great as it appears
7. Tim has correct pronunciation of words at times

The first answer, although possible, cannot be proved. Answer two is irrelevant at this point in therapy. This concern had been previously checked out many, many times. The third answer sounds correct, but does not account for the loud, unintelligible utterances, which are not characteristic of selective mutes. Answer four seems to beg the question. The fifth answer is so extremely unlikely as to be in the realm of the impossible. The best answer is number six. Answer seven merely restates part of the data.

QUESTION E:

WHILE IN INDIVIDUAL PSYCHOTHERAPY, TIM REPEATEDLY REGRESSED INTO AUTOEROTIC BEHAVIOR BY HOLDING A TOY PUPPET TO HIS MOUTH AND TAPPING IT WITH HIS FINGERS. HE SEEMED TO ENJOY THIS, AND LOOKED AS IF HE WERE IN A TRANCE. THE THERAPIST INTERRUPTED THIS BEHAVIOR, SAYING, "YOU WANT TO STAY INSIDE YOURSELF." AT THIS, TIM USUALLY RESPONDED WITH A SMILE AND ATTENDED TO THE THERAPIST. ONCE, FOLLOWING THE THERAPIST'S INTERVENTION, TIM BECAME OVERTLY FRUSTRATED, CRIED, AND SLAPPED AND BIT HIMSELF. THE THERAPIST COULD RESPOND BY:

1. Asking, "Is something bothering you?"
2. Saying, "Let me put a band-aid on your wound." Then check the record to see when he received his last tetanus immunization
3. Stating, "You seem to want to hurt yourself"
4. Asking, "Can I kiss the boo-boo?"
5. Ignoring the behavior to see what develops
6. Stating, "If you bite your hand off, you won't be able to masturbate"
7. Asking, "Would you like a milkshake?"

CASE STUDY #54

Answer three was useful early in the treatment and is the best of the answers given. Later in therapy, it became possible to ask Tim why he seemed to want to hurt himself; with great effort intelligible reasons could sometimes be elicited. The first answer seems very naive and probably would not work. The medical concern in answer two misses the point. Answer five is sometimes appropriate. Answer six, like answer four is thrown in for comic relief, but, of course, would be inappropriate in therapy. Answer seven is irrelevant.

Tim's autistic behavior decreased, as did his self-destructiveness. He became less anxious, less disoriented, and more verbal. He had fewer temper tantrums and developed a regular eating and sleeping pattern. He improved in his ability to follow through with directions and was able to relate to people on a much more appropriate level.

QUESTION F:
FUTURE PLANS FOR TIM SHOULD INCLUDE:
1. Five day/week intensive work to develop insight into his self-destruction
2. Long-term institutionalization at an institute for the retarded
3. Genetic counseling to prevent recurrence of this problem in the family and consideration of sterilization for Tim
4. A residential education program which includes therapeutic programming for Tim's unique needs
5. A suggestion that Tim continue to attend his local school for the trainable retarded. Make appointments to see him every six months
6. Family therapy which will interpret to Tim's parents their ambivalence and conflict so that they will relate to him differently
7. Follow-up in drug maintenance clinic

The first answer given is rarely available for severely handicapped children with deafness and blindness. However, intensive work had been done at camp with Tim and he had shown an improvement. The second answer indicates, unfortunately, where most such children end up. The third answer is an irrelevant one since these parents are past the child-bearing age and there is no known genetic disease to account for Tim's congenital blindness (due to a persistent lens artery). Furthermore, sterilization of the retarded has become a civil rights issue and fortunately has faded from prominence as a procedure done to the retarded. Answer four became a necessity when the local school was unable to help Tim. The sixth answer is partially correct and did occur to some degree. The last answer is incorrect since to give this child drugs without other therapy or a change in his milieu would seem to be inappropriate. The best answer is a combination of four and six.

REFERENCES:
1. Burlingham, D., 1961: Some notes on the development of the blind. Psychoanalytic Study of the Child 16:121-145

2. Burlingham, D., 1965: Some problems of ego development in blind children. Psychoanalytic Study of the Child 20:194-208

3. Burlingham, D., 1967: Developmental considerations in the occupations of the blind. Psychoanalytic Study of the Child 22:187-198

4. Burlingham, D., 1968: The re-education of a retarded blind child. Psychoanalytic Study of the Child 23:369-390

5. Fraiberg, S., 1971: Intervention in infancy. J Amer Acad Child Psychiatry 10:381-405

CASE STUDY #54

6. Menaloscino, F., 1968: Parents of the mentally retarded. J Amer Acad of Child Psychiatry 7:580-602

7. Menaloscino, F., 1970: Psychiatric Approaches to Mental Retardation, Basic Books, New York

8. Solnit, A. J. and M. H. Stark, 1961: Mourning and the birth of a defective child. Psychoanalytic Study of the Child 16:523-537

9. Spitz, R., 1949: Autoerotism. Psychoanalytic Study of the Child 3-4:85-120

10. Spitz, R., 1962: Autoerotism Re-examined. Psychoanalytic Study of the Child 17:283-315

CASE STUDY #55

A Bright 7-Year-Old Gets A Bellyache from School

A 7 year-old white, Protestant, second-grade boy was brought to the clinic by his working-class parents on referral from his school because of refusal to attend. He complained of abdominal pain when it was time for school.

He was the second of four children of a twentyish couple who said that they were trying to make a better home for their children than they themselves had. Both of them had been abandoned by their own parents at a young age, and had spent time with various relatives, in foster homes, and in group homes. The patient's older brother had been doing well in school, with no attendance problems.

The patient was an attractive, likable, very bright, well-behaved lad who had achieved well academically. He was rather passive in the interview situation. He reported feeling sick when it was time to go to school, and worried about his mother when he was at school.

Twice weekly appointments were set up. It was explained to the patient and his parents that no psychiatric reason could be given for excusing the patient from the legal requirement of attending school. Not only would this not be justified, but it would even interfere with therapy, since we "could not teach him how to swim if he were not in the water." It was the parents' responsibility to see that he got to school, and the therapist would help him take care of the anxiety and sick feelings he got about going to school.

Though everyone agreed with this plan, it soon appeared that the parents were not enthusiastically pursuing their part of it. For example, on the days of his clinic appointments, they would not bother sending him to school for the other half of the day, so that essentially he was on a three-day school week. When the patient's mother was confronted with this, she revealed with much anxiety and choking back of tears that she and her husband were both afraid the patient would resent them and feel the same way about them as they felt about their parents rejecting and abandoning them. This fear of the parents seemed to underly their anxious reluctance to make the boy attend school. The parents' anxiety, in turn, appeared to be one of the dynamics behind his fear of leaving for school. Ventilation and interpretation of the mother's feelings began to result in better school attendance.

The patient during his therapy sessions was very constricted and well-behaved, waiting patiently until permission would be granted for any activity he wished to engage in. He would then enthusiastically play with various toys and arrange them neatly on the shelves with obvious pleasure. He agreed that he also liked to keep things neat and clean at home. Even after he had been informed that the toys were there for his use and had played with them in previous sessions, he would still sit indefinitely at each session until again given permission to play with the toys.

QUESTION A:
THIS BOY'S BEHAVIOR IN THERAPY MIGHT BE DESCRIBED AS:
1. Schizoid
2. Autistic
3. Authority-oriented and inhibited
4. Obsessive-compulsive
5. Neurotic

Despite his shy reserve, this boy related appropriately. This makes answers one and two unlikely. Five is correct, but too imprecise to be the best answer. The boy's interest in neatness and cleaning makes the best answer four, which implicitly includes three, also a good answer.

Just as therapeutic results began appearing, the parents terminated therapy because of concern about the clinic charge, which had been set at the $5.00 minimum. At the suggestion of the therapist, they talked with the business office about getting a waiver or getting welfare medical assistance. The mother reported

CASE STUDY #55

with much resentment that they were not able to get any help, even though she saw other people, especially blacks, leaving the office with a big smile as if they had been given assistance. Despite assurances that no legal means would be taken to collect the bill, the parents feared that it would hurt their credit rating to have such a bill outstanding. They felt they could no longer afford to return to the clinic, and terminated.

QUESTION B:
THIS CASE IS TYPICAL OF:
1. Symbiotic psychosis
2. Maternal deprivation
3. School phobia
4. Adjustment reaction of childhood
5. Psychophysiologic gastrointestinal reaction
6. Beginning stages of an anti-social personality
7. Conversion hysteria of childhood

Though this boy does have some trouble separating from his mother, which might be called "symbiotic," there is nothing to warrant the diagnosis of a psychosis. Though the parents may have been maternally deprived, there was no evidence that the patient was thus deprived. A slim case might be made for adjustment reaction of childhood, or for conversion hysteria (abdominal pain), but a much more exact and fitting diagnosis is school "phobia," or "school refusal," which often includes somatic complaints.

QUESTION C:
IN SUCH CASES, THE MAIN PROBLEM USUALLY SEEMS TO BE:
1. Mutual mother-child separation anxiety, with displacement onto school as a phobic object and projection of the fear for one's own safety onto the mother (that is, fear for her safety)
2. Overt maternal rejection
3. Covert maternal rejection with compensatory over-protection
4. Parental need for approval from the child and fear of being considered a bad parent by the child
5. A genetic predisposition
6. Cultural devaluation of school

Maternal rejection is not usually a prominent dynamic in school phobia, though overprotection may be. Subcultural devaluation of school spawns much parent-condoned truancy, but not much school phobia. No genetic predisposition has been seriously considered. The parent's need for approval by the child is often an important consideration, but answer one is the best.

QUESTION D:
THERAPY IN SUCH CASES SHOULD ORDINARILY BE DIRECTED TOWARDS:
1. Helping the parents with their feelings of inadequacy and insecurity as parents, by intensive psychotherapy if necessary
2. Involving the father (especially if the patient is a boy)
3. Returning the child to the school situation as quickly and directly as possible, charging the parents with this responsibility and enlisting the cooperation of the school personnel to keep the child there
4. Long-term psychoanalysis to prepare the child for return to school
5. Intensive, frequent therapy (usually family and community-oriented) at first, followed by longer-term, less frequent therapy as indicated
6. Use of tranquilizers or a tricyclic antidepressant, if necessary, to help the child tolerate school
7. Group therapy

CASE STUDY #55

We have had most success with a combination of one, two, three, five, and sometimes six. Three has chronological priority, but is not of much value without immediate therapeutic follow-up as described in one and five. Some authors might question the value of pushing the child immediately back into school; they might opt for letting him stay at home until, through psychotherapy or analysis, he resolved his phobic neurosis. However, most child therapists feel that such delay runs the risks of 1. seeming to bless a maladaptive behavior (school refusal), 2. allowing the parent-child pathology to settle into a rut rather than capitalizing on the crisis to facilitate change, 3. allowing the child's social skills to atrophy through disuse (out of the natural social situation of the school), 4. allowing the child to be labeled as "different" or "sick" by his peers, who cannot help but notice that he has been excused from school, and 5. depriving the child of the optimum learning situation, which can never be completely compensated for by home tutoring.

REFERENCES:
1. Agras, S., 1959: The relationship of school phobia to childhood depression. Amer J of Psychiatry 116:533-536

2. Gittelman-Klein, R. and D. F. Klein, 1971: Controlled imipramine treatment of school phobia, Archives of Gen Psychiatry 25:204-207

3. Klein, E., 1949: Psychoanalytic aspects of school problems. Psychoanalytic Study of the Child 3-4:369-390

4. Johnson, A., et al., 1941: School Phobia, Amer J Orthopsychiatry 11:702-708

5. Lassers, E., Nordan, R. and S. Bladholm, 1973: Steps in the return to school of children with school phobia. Amer J Psychiat 130:265-268

6. Missildine, H., 1963: Your Inner Child of the Past, Simon and Schuster, N.Y.

CASE STUDY #56

Sugar and Spice and Everything Nice

Beth was a 14 year-old white, Protestant, middle-class girl, referred by a pediatrician with the chief complaint of diabetes mellitus, which got "out of control" so frequently in the previous two years that she required 20 hospitalizations.

Beth's diabetes was diagnosed 4-1/2 years prior to referral. Diabetic control was erratic despite the efforts to teach her the necessity of maintaining the proper insulin-glucose balance. She had been out of school a great deal during the two years prior to referral. She had become more and more involved with girls of whom her parents did not approve and who allegedly used "dope." For approximately three years prior to referral she was seen by another psychiatrist with whom she had steadfastly refused to talk. Consequently, she was being referred for possible inpatient psychiatric care.

She was the youngest of two girls resulting from the mother's first marriage. Diabetes mellitus had been previously diagnosed in the family of Beth's father, and he himself had been diagnosed schizophrenic. A divorce had taken place when Beth was 5 years old. Two additional girls were born after the mother married Beth's stepfather.

QUESTION A:
THE MOST LIKELY PSYCHOLOGICAL PROBLEM OCCURRING IN BETH AND OTHER CHILDREN SUFFERING FROM DIABETES MELLITUS IS:
1. Depression and denial
2. Development of obsessive-compulsive traits
3. Toxic psychosis
4. Hypochondriacal complaints
5. Hysterical manifestations

Beth was admitted to an adolescent unit because of her negative behavior regarding school, family, and diabetic management. She was frequently truant, tended to manipulate people by refusing to control her diabetes, and tended to express aggression through subtle, rather passive means. Psychological testing revealed an IQ of 92 and suggested that she tended to keep people at a distance and was defensive, naive, depressed and anxious. Although many of her answers to the sentence completion test were left blank or merely reflected her dissatisfaction at being hospitalized, many showed dissatisfaction with herself. A few examples follow:

My nerves _____
Much of the time _____
My mind _____
I need _____
There are times _____
My father _____
Eating _____
My greatest worry _____
My dreams _____
My looks _____

Beth seemed to have an intense need to be accepted and loved, but she covered these dependency needs by a facade of independence, aggressiveness and uncooperativeness. She tried to act big and brave when she really wanted to be accepted and cared for. At times she was most delightful, with an attractive yet mischievous glint in her eye, a girl who was liked by most of the staff. However, she was unable to respond appropriately and would rather assume the less attractive but safer posture of defensiveness and keep everybody at a distance.

CASE STUDY #56

The answer to question A is one, depression and denial. There was considerable evidence that she was dissatisfied with herself, more so because she had diabetes. At the same time, she tended to deny the existence of the disease and would not adhere to either dietary or medical regimens. Rosen & Lidz (1949) of Yale University have shown in adults that depression is manifested in subtle suicide attempts: they "lose" control of their diabetes by careless diet or by subcutaneous infection resulting from careless use of contaminated needles. The same things occur in the older children and adolescents.

QUESTION B:
AT WHAT AGE SHOULD THE PHYSICIAN TEACH CHILDREN WITH DIABETES TO MANAGE THEIR OWN TREATMENT, INCLUDING THE GIVING OF INSULIN?:
1. As soon as they are old enough to learn the use of an insulin syringe and the accurate measurement of insulin
2. At any age that they seem to want to control their own insulin
3. Not later than 10 or 11 years of age
4. Mid-adolescence
5. Late adolescence

Pediatric endocrinologists tend to use this rule of thumb: "When they are old enough to learn." They base the decision on the child's intellectual ability to take this responsibility. In the authors' opinion this ignores the question of psychological readiness to assume such control over one's own life. Most children can't psychologically accept this responsibility prior to mid-adolescence. The authors have seen several children who were rebelling against the responsibility which was being unfairly thrust upon them. On one occasion a rather dependent 10 year-old resisted the dietician who was attempting to teach him his diet. He felt that was his mother's task, and he wanted no part of it. In another instance, a child had been taught the importance of rotating the injection site to prevent induration. Unknown to the pediatrician, the child associated the possible induration with the beginning of a process that would require an amputation, such as occurred in a diabetic man who lived down the street. No one would expect the child to make such an association, but it remains his responsibility to check out the child's feelings and understanding in order to prevent such distortions.

QUESTION C:
ONE REASON PEDIATRICIANS FREQUENTLY MISJUDGE THE CHILD'S EMOTIONAL CAPACITY TO TAKE THIS RESPONSIBILITY IS:
1. These children often appear more mature than they really are
2. It has been shown that there is a high correlation between diabetes and superior intellectual capacity
3. The children appear less anxious when they give their own insulin
4. The children seem better able to learn about the disorder than their parents
5. The reported fact that pediatricians are poor judges of cognitive and psychological functioning

The first answer is correct. Many studies, recently Partridge, et al., (1972), have shown that children with diabetes and other chronic diseases defend against their depression and anxiety by development of a pseudomature attitude. They appear capable of responsibility perhaps even suggesting they are old enough. This can easily fool the pediatrician or other adults. Beth, for instance, hung around with girls 2-3 years older and acted very big, brave and worldly-wise. Diabetes does not correlate with superior intelligence. The third and fourth answers are not sufficient reasons. Number five is not true.

CASE STUDY #56

QUESTION D:
THE MOST IMPORTANT ASPECT OF PSYCHOLOGICAL TREATMENT IN A DIABETIC IS:
1. A psychoanalytic approach
2. Accepting the patient as he is
3. A strong positive counter-transference
4. Understanding the metabolic disorder
5. Support of the parents

Each answer is useful in the treatment of a diabetic child, but the second is essential, outweighing the others in importance.

Beth spent several months in the hospital without making much progress. She was considered a "difficult case" by two different therapists and was the proverbial "thorn in the side" of the nursing staff. During a week-long group living experience, camping with five other patients and three staff members, she established a friendship with a physician who accepted her as she was. He had shown his desire to be friends but had been repeatedly rejected. One day he confronted her with this by saying to another staff member in Beth's presence: "She doesn't know what the word friendship means." It was a rather sarcastic comment but Beth responded in a small voice: "Yes, I do." She presently began to cooperate in group activities, dropping her pseudomature facade and acting much more like her real age of 14. The incident seemed to be a turning point in her treatment.

This physician was rather casual about the control of her diabetes. He was, for instance, content to watch her closely on days she refused to take her morning insulin rather than overreacting to this attempt at manipulation. Although he accepted responsibility for her medical care, he was willing also to talk with her about her wish to die and about her anger at her father for giving her this disease and for leaving the family. She was able to work through many of the fundamental problems related to her diabetes, although this was not a formal psychotherapeutic relationship. The physician's casualness depended on his knowledge of the metabolic disorder: he felt confident that he could step in and provide emergency treatment to abort disaster. The most important aspect of the treatment, though, was his affection and acceptance.

Beth was discharged after one year of psychiatric hospitalization. In the ensuing three years she required only one brief hospitalization for diabetic control. She attended school regularly, acquired a job as a counselor in a diabetic camp, and is beginning to think about attending college.

QUESTION E:
WHY WOULD A GIRL WHO IS OBVIOUSLY SUFFERING SO MUCH REPEATEDLY REJECT OFFERS OF FRIENDSHIP AND BEHAVE IN A WAY THAT ENCOURAGES OTHERS TO REJECT HER?:
1. She wants no friends so that she is free to suicide without having to worry about hurting others
2. She is so angry about having diabetes that she wants to hurt others to get even
3. She is attempting to manipulate the staff so they will discharge her
4. She feels damaged and repulsive and expects to be rejected, so she behaves accordingly
5. She is not aware of the way her behavior affects others

Although all the answers are plausible, the fourth is best. Children who acquire chronic diseases or discover inherited disorders in childhood feel they have lost normality, being damaged. They feel "castrated" (in the psychoanalytic sense) and unattractive. They think everyone sees them as repulsive and therefore become anxious and depressed, sometimes seriously depressed. Recognizing the depression, parents and physicians often try to reassure children by telling them

CASE STUDY #56

of some prominent figure like Bill Tilden, the tennis great who made good despite diabetes. In our experience, such attempts at reassurance are rarely effective; it is difficult to treat depression with reassurance. For a younger diabetic see case 51.

REFERENCES:
1. Bruch, H. and I. Hewlett, 1947: Psychologic Aspects of the Medical Management of Diabetes in Children. Psychosom Med 9:205

2. Crain, A. J., Sussman, M. B. and Wm. B. Weil, Jr., 1966: Effects of a Diabetic Child on Marital Integration and Related Measures of Family Functioning. J Health Hum Behav 7:122-127

3. Davis, D. M., Shipp, J. C. and E. G. Pattishall, 1965: Attitudes of Diabetic Boys and Girls Towards Diabetes. Diabetes 14:106-109

4. Hinkle, L. E., Jr., 1956: The Influence of the Patient's Behavior and His Reaction to His Life Situation Upon the Course of Diabetes. Diabetes 5:406-407

5. Koski, Maija-Liisa, 1969: The Coping Processes in Childhood Diabetes. Acta Paediat Scand 198:9-56

6. Parker, J. A., 1968: Camping for Children with Diabetes - a Diet Therapy Section Project. J Amer Diet Assoc 53:486-488

7. Partridge, J. W., Garner, A. M., Thompson, C. W. and T. Cherry, 1972: Attitudes of Adolescents Toward Their Diabetes. Amer J Dis Child 124:226-229

8. Rosen, H. and T. Lidz, 1949: Emotional Factors in the Precipitation of Recurrent Diabetic Acidosis. Psychosom Med 11:211-215

9. Sterans, S., 1959: Self-destructive Behaviour in Young Patients with Diabetes Mellitus. Diabetes 8:379-382

10. Swift, C. R. and F. L. Seidman, 1964: Adjustment Problems of Juvenile Diabetes. J Am Acad Child Psychiatry 3:500-515

CASE STUDY #57

All A's - At What Expense?

Ronnie was a short, nice-looking nine year-old, fourth-grade, Catholic boy of Italian descent. His parents brought him to the Mental Health Center in the fall shortly after they had moved from another state. They complained that Ronnie had developed a facial tic, squinting his eyes very tightly whenever he was under stress. This had lasted for several months with no sign of remission.

Ronnie seemed extremely anxious. His face frequently twitched when he faced the interviewer. He seemed less anxious when he talked about sports, the main theme of his life. During the first interview he obsessively named every player in the American Football League, fourteen recent scores, and the team standings. He also knew many facts about the American Hockey League. He stated that he and his family frequently played together, he and his father "standing off" his older brother and his younger brother. He hated to lose and would go to almost any lengths not to.

At a second interview Ronnie was again terribly "uptight." Ronnie was asked, "Draw your family, including yourself, doing something." (Burns, R.C. and S. H. Kaufman, 1972). The therapist felt that the drawing (Fig. 57.1) exemplified the competitiveness found in the family. Ronnie put himself in the middle of the group as the pitcher controlling the game. When asked about the drawing, he said, "Where we used to live, it was fun. Nobody was being a bad sport." Further evidence of competitiveness emerged during family therapy sessions in which "family sculpture" was used. (Satir, 1972). All of the children seemed to want to be the center of attention and would pout if this was not possible.

The mother and father reported severe marital discord for many years. The mother had suffered depressive episodes five or six years previously, which required a several-week hospitalization. The father had seen a therapist for a year and currently the mother had begun therapy again. The father was a traveling salesman who was usually not home Monday through Friday nights. The parents had been married for thirteen years and had engaged in open arguments about separation and divorce for several years. In psychotherapy, mother's behavior alternated between belittlement and seductiveness.

Ronnie was an "A" student and the parents reported no severe behavior problems other than fighting and squabbling among the brothers. He had wet the bed for years, a problem not helped by shock machines, getting him up in the middle of the night, restricting his fluids, or punishing him. He was a polite boy. He made no sound during the facial twitches.

QUESTION A:
REGARDING RONNIE'S PROBLEMS:
1. This is a classic case of Gilles de la Tourette syndrome, consisting of the triad of nocturnal enuresis, facial twitching, and sadness
2. Ronnie's anger is being expressed through the enuresis which is probably a "wet dream." The facial twitches represent his murderous rage towards his mother for not asserting herself and making his father stay home from his trips
3. The facial twitch is a sign of extreme nervousness
4. The boy has a facial nerve tumor
5. Ronnie's problem is complicated by sibling rivalry and a rejecting mother
6. Ronnie feels abandoned by his father. His mother's rejection on one hand and oversolicitous attitude on the other is confusing to him. He strives to win and shows other obsessive traits
7. The boy's habits and spasms will disappear within a few months, and so will the enuresis

The Gilles de la Tourette syndrome does not consist of the triad given in answer one. It is characterized by facial or wholebody twitching, barking or

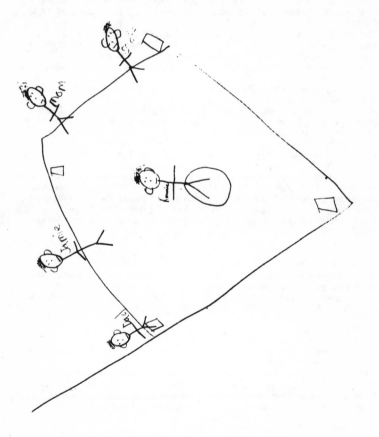

FIGURE 57. 1

CASE STUDY #57

muttering of obscene words and sometimes flinging of arms or legs, and emotional illness. Answer two is overstated, not adequately supported by the data. Answer three is correct but too generalized. A facial nerve tumor, though possible, is rare, and there is much positive psychological evidence in this case to indicate otherwise. There was sibling rivalry and a rejecting mother in Ronnie's case, but answer five is incomplete because it ignores the father's importance. Answer six is the best. Tics and enuresis at Ronnie's age rarely just "disappear."

QUESTION B:
THE MOTHER WAS AN ATTRACTIVE WOMAN WHO VERBALLY ATTACKED HER HUSBAND IN THE FIRST FAMILY SESSION. SHE STATED, "IT IS HOPELESS." SHE CONSTANTLY PUT HERSELF AND THE THREE BOYS DOWN. WHICH OF THE FOLLOWING STATEMENTS BEST DESCRIBES THE MOTHER'S PART IN THIS CASE?:
1. The mother has a great deal of difficulty with male authority figures
2. Although she is a person who talks loudly, the mother shows a great deal of strength. She will be able to support her family in their efforts to work the problem out through family dinner table conversations if left alone with some ground rules
3. The mother's concern for Ronnie should lead her to obtain a full hospital neurological workup for him to rule out an organic disease
4. If the mother were to have a daughter with whom she could fulfill all of her life's ambitions to recreate herself, she would get "off the boys' backs" and get along with her husband normally
5. The mother's anger is a sign of deep-seated paranoid neurosis. Ronnie is acting out her anger through his tics and enuresis. The enuresis signifies the mother's feelings of wanting to murder her husband
6. The mother seems unable to maintain a stable, consistent pattern. Her erratic behavior is very confusing to her family, expecially to Ronnie. Most likely the mother's overwhelming angry reactions have caused Ronnie to suppress his own anger, now manifested through the facial tic and the enuresis
7. The father's absence and the mother's anger cause Ronnie a great deal of difficulty

Answer one is correct but incomplete. Answer two is unrealistically optimistic. A workup is not needed on the basis of present evidence. Answer four is glib and not pertinent. Answer five is overstated and partially incorrect. Answer six seems to carry the best explanation of how the mother's difficulties affect Ronnie. Answer seven is correct but too general.

QUESTION C:
AT THIS POINT THE BEST DISPOSITION WOULD BE:
1. An interpretation that Ronnie's enuresis and facial tic are related to the relationship between the mother and father
2. Telling the father to stop his traveling job and find work locally so that he can attend psychoanalysis every day and serve as a better role model for Ronnie
3. To recommend another more thorough hospitalization, which should include a complete brain scan, EEG, pneumoencephalogram, spinal fluid analysis, and complete genito-urinary workup
4. Have mother continue her psychotherapy
5. Have the mother continue in therapy and Ronnie receive a few counseling sessions, with confidence that the tics and enuresis will disappear within three months
6. Group therapy as well as individual therapy, to allow Ronnie to express some of his unconscious anger. Occasional family consultations are indicated
7. Hospitalization with intensive psychotherapy to allow deeply repressed thoughts to be expressed. While he is undergoing residential treatment, the family should be involved in intensive family therapy for several months

CASE STUDY #57

Answer one, though possibly correct, is incomplete. Answer two might help and it might not, but is certainly impractical. Answer three would not seem indicated. Answer four is obviously correct, but incomplete. Answer five is too optimistic. Ronnie's problems are of several months' duration. Since both symptoms can be from unconscious repressed feelings, often of an angry nature, crisis intervention is not likely to be of immediate benefit to Ronnie or the family. Answer six is the best answer, recognizing that Ronnie's behavior is unconsciously derived. This case does not warrant residential treatment.

QUESTION D:
RONNIE WAS VERY QUIET DURING THE FIRST TWO SESSIONS IN GROUP THERAPY. HOWEVER, HE SEEMED ENTHUSIASTIC AND COOPERATED WITH THE TASK OF MAKING A COLLAGE. HE BEGAN TO SHARE HIS FEELINGS. THIS KIND OF START WOULD MEAN THAT:
1. Ronnie's desire to please is his way of expressing anger. Ronnie's tics are probably hallucinations, and one can expect him to deteriorate unless there is immediate expression of anger
2. Ronnie's cooperativeness at the beginning of the group therapy means that he has a sincere wish to try to rid himself of his symptoms
3. The immediate improvement in Ronnie's mood following initiation of therapy indicates that Ronnie's sadness is workable and that his anger will come out in transference within a few weeks. He will drop the politeness once he becomes aware that expression of angry feelings is permitted
4. Ronnie's symptoms have subsided because he is maturing
5. Ronie will continue to be polite, cooperative, and creative in the group since his IQ is high. Following the evaluation and a few weeks of adequate counseling, his symptoms will disappear
6. When they begin group therapy, all children are cooperative, polite and wait until later to show their symptoms
7. Ronnie's facial tics and enuresis can only be corrected by using haloperidol, a major tranquilizer

Answer one: Tics are usually not hallucinations. Ronnie's cooperativeness is only partly explained by sincerity in wanting to rid himself of the symptoms. Answer three proved to be correct in Ronnie's case. Answer four indicated developmental change over a very short period of time, rather unlikely. Answer five is superficial and overly optimistic, because habit spasms and enuresis rarely quickly disappear. Although answer six may be partially true, it is not specific to this case. Answer seven seems to assume that the diagnosis is Gilles de la Tourette's syndrome (incorrect).

QUESTION E:
AFTER A FEW WEEKS OF GROUP THERAPY, RONNIE BECOMES ANGRY WITH THE MALE CO-THERAPIST AND FREQUENTLY CALLS HIM NAMES IN A SULKY, ANGRY, WHINING VOICE. THE GROUP CO-THERAPISTS SHOULD HANDLE THIS BY:
1. Reflecting the feelings of the group so that the children will feel they are being treated fairly
2. A warm supportive attitude despite Ronnie's verbal attacks
3. Doing nothing, because it is expected that if children are given free rein in a latency group, they will express anger towards authority figures
4. Interpreting that Ronnie's angry outbursts indicated his wish to castrate his father and marry his mother, and he was generalizing the sibling rivalry feelings from the brothers onto the male co-therapist
5. Giving Ronnie a large dose of a major tranquilizer to decrease his anxiety, to stop his bedwetting, and allow his anger to be expressed

CASE STUDY #57

6. Switching to intensive four-day-a-week psychoanalytic therapy. He should not have been in group therapy
7. Accepting, as much as possible, Ronnie's vicious verbal attacks. The female co-therapist could comment on the intensity of Ronnie's feelings. He has developed transference, and his feelings are workable

Answer one has some merit, but can be boring at times and may be too non-specific to be of help. Answer two is correct but incomplete. Though latency children may be expected to express anger towards authority in a group, it does not follow that it should be ignored. The content of answer four may be true, but there is not yet enough evidence for interpretation. Answer five is contradictory since major tranquilizers tend to suppress angry feelings and rarely stop bed-wetting. Ronnie's angry outbursts are no reason to take him out of the group. Answer seven is the most comprehensive and specific.

QUESTION F:
FOLLOWING THE FIRST FEW SESSIONS OF GROUP THERAPY AND INDIVIDUAL THERAPY, ANOTHER FAMILY EVALUATION IS HELD. THE FATHER STATES HIS NEED TO REMOVE RONNIE FROM GROUP THERAPY SO THAT HE CAN PLAY SPORTS IN THE AFTERNOON. THE MOTHER IS CYNICAL AND SAR-CASTIC AND HAS ALMOST DECIDED TO TERMINATE WITH HER PSYCHO-THERAPIST. THE FATHER CONTINUES TO AVOID BECOMING INVOLVED. AT THIS POINT:
1. Ronnie has had an honest trial of group therapy and should be allowed to play baseball as his father wishes
2. Ronnie's problems are of an emotional nature and the parents need to be in-formed of this
3. Ronnie should be seen again for a physical examination, neurology workup, and genito-urinary workup, since his symptoms have not subsided
4. Group therapy for Ronnie will most likely be needed for several more months. The parents should be gently informed of the severity of Ronnie's problems without overwhelming them. A trial of an antidepressant might be in order at this time to try and control the symptom of enuresis
5. Because Ronnie has failed in outpatient treatment to show signs of symptom alleviation, he should be hospitalized, and plans for a foster home should be made
6. The father's desire to win and his need to have Ronnie in sports indicates severe insecurity. The mother's vicious "castrating" battle with her psycho-therapist indicates that additional modes of treatment must be begun. The father should be in individual treatment and the other two boys should be brought in for evaluations. Weekly family therapy should be scheduled
7. Ronnie should continue in group therapy and the mother should be encouraged not to terminate at this point

Since group therapy often shows benefits only after several months, answer one is incorrect. The parents already know that Ronnie's problems are of an emotional nature (answer two). A physical examination at this time is inappro-priately late. Answer four is the best since Ronnie's problems are deep-seated and will require more than individual therapy. The antidepressants have been helpful in enuresis. Hospitalization or a foster home would not be indicated for Ronnie. Answer six over-reacts in a "shotgun" fashion. Answer seven is true, but incomplete.

CASE STUDY #57

REFERENCES:
1. Alessi, S. S. and M. D. Kahn, 1972: Group psychotherapy with latency age boys: Research, training and practice in different settings. Paper presented at the Annual Meeting of the Amer. Assn. of Psychiatric Services for Children, Washington, D. C., Nov. 5, 1972

2. Barcai, A. and E. H. Robinson, 1969: Conventional group therapy with adolescent children. Int J Group Psychotherapy 19:334-345

3. Berger, M. M. , 1968: Nonverbal communications in group psychotherapy. Int J Group Psychotherapy 8:161-178

4. Bindelglas, P. M. , Dee, G. H. and F. A. Enos, 1968: Medical and Psychosocial Factors in Enuretic Children Treated with Imipramine Hydrochloride. Amer J Psychiatry 124:1107-1112

5. Burns, R. C. and S. H. Kaufman, 1972: Actions, Styles and Symbols in Kinetic Family Drawings (K-F-D), Brunner-Maxel, New York

6. Challas, G. , Chapel, J. L. and R. L. Jenkins, 1967: Tourette's Disease: Control of Symptoms and its clinical course. Int J Neuropsychiatry 3:96-109

7. Clement, P. W. and D. C. Milne, 1967: Group play therapy and tangible reinforcers used to modify the behavior of eight-year-old boys. Behavior Res and Therapy 5:301-312

8. Frank, M. G. and J. Zilback, 1968: Current trends in group therapy with children, Int J of Group Psychotherapy 18:447-460

9. Gerard, M. W. , 1946: The psychogenic tic in ego development, Psychoanalytic Study of the Child 2:133-162

10. Godenne, G. D. , 1964: Outpatient adolescent group psychotherapy (Part I) Amer J of Psychotherapy 18:584-593

11. Godenne, G. D. , 1965: Outpatient adolescent group psychotherapy (Part II) American J of Psychotherapy 19:40-53

12. Levy, B. S. and E. Ascher, 1968: Phenothiazines in the treatment of Gilles de la Tourette disease, J Nerv Ment Dis 146:36-40

13. Lucas, A. R. , Kauffman, P. E. and E. M. Morris, 1967: Gilles de la Tourette's disease: A clinical study of 15 cases. J Amer Acad of Child Psychiatry 6:700-722

14. Mahler, M. S. , 1949: A psychoanalytic evaluation of tic in psychopathology of children; Symptomatic and tic syndrome. Psychoanalytic Study of the Child, 3-4:279-310

15. Mesnikoff, A. M. , 1959: Three cases of Gilles de la Tourette's syndrome treated with psychotherapy and chlorpromazine. Archives Neurol Psychiatry 81:710

16. Ritvo, E. E. , et al. , 1969: Arousal and nonarousal enuretic events, Amer J of Psychiatry 126:77-84

17. Satir, V. , 1972: People Making, Science and Behavior Books, Palo Alto

CASE STUDY #57

18. Satir, V., 1967: Conjoint Family Therapy, Science and Behavior Books, Palo Alto

19. Shapiro, A. K. and E. Shapiro, 1968: Treatment of Gilles de la Tourette's syndrome with haloperidol. Br J Psychiatry 114:345-350

20. Sperling, M., 1965: Dynamic considerations and treatment of enuresis, J Amer Acad of Child Psychiatry 4:19-31

CASE STUDY #58*

A 7-Year-Old Who Fought His Way Up

A seven year-old black, second-grade boy at a fringe area school was first seen in August because during the previous year (first grade) he was "violent with other children at school. " He had the same problem in his neighborhood at home, and his mother had resorted to keeping him in the yard in order to prevent his fighting with other children. His pediatrician had diagnosed him hyperkinetic and prescribed d-amphetamine 15 mg. per day. This seemed to help some, but fighting continued to be a problem, and the pediatrician referred him for psychiatric treatment.

His parents were middle class but voluntarily chose to live near the ghetto because of "a sense of responsibility" to their race. His older brother and sister learned to fight just enough to survive in this environment, being generally intelligent, pleasant and well-behaved. He, however, had blossomed into a skilled, impulsive fighter who was feared by other children and their parents. His mother described him as temperamentally different from his sibs, being more erratic, less responsible, more labile, and harder to socialize.

He described himself as the worst boy in his class and said that he had come to the Child Psychiatry Clinic because of being bad in school. He appeared motivated. In fact, he said he would like to be the best in his class. Psychological testing showed a Stanford-Binet I. Q. of 119. Despite evidence of neurological handicaps on human figure drawing and the Bender Gestalt, he achieved satisfactorily in the first grade.

QUESTION A:
THE MOST LOGICAL FIRST INTERVENTION AT THIS POINT WOULD BE:
1. To change the d-amphetamine dose
2. Family therapy
3. Play therapy
4. Group therapy
5. Parent counseling
6. Intensive individual therapy

Obviously, all of these have something to offer, and most therapists would not like to be limited to a single choice. However, when a child carries a well-established diagnosis of hyperkinetic syndrome (minimal brain dysfunction), the most logical priority is to make sure he's optimally medicated. Of course, psychological management, including parent counseling, is also an essential part of treating such a child. See also cases 1, 28, 32, 48 and 60.

QUESTION B:
THE BOY'S MOTHER ALSO MENTIONED THAT SHE AND HIS FATHER DISAGREED ABOUT HOW TO HANDLE HIM. HOW WOULD THIS ADDITIONAL INFORMATION ALTER THE CHOICE ABOVE?:

Sometimes parental disagreements over management of a hyperkinetic child melt away when his behavior improves with medication, so optimizing the medication still retains some importance. However, the addition of parent counseling, previously indicated, now appears mandatory, perhaps supersedes medication in importance.

The d-amphetamine was eventually optimized at 20 mg. a day. With this, his school work and attentiveness improved and he was able to control his be-

*Parts of this case originally appeared in Journal of School Health 42:458-459, 1972, and are reprinted with permission of the American School Health Association.

CASE STUDY #58

havior somewhat better than he had before. It was noted that he partly accomplished the latter by spending his time with the older children on the playground
rather than with his age-mates. He behaved very well with the older children,
but tended to fight with peers, even when medicated.

Conferences with the parents (sometimes with the whole family) showed rapid
gains in insight, adaptation, and partial resolution of sibling rivalry. The mother
was a genteel, refined, perfectionistic daughter of middle-class parents. She
tried to please the father, a self-made, gruff man who grew up in the ghetto. He
wished her to take care of raising the children, but according to his directives.
At first she felt he was giving her the message not to be too affectionate with the
kids so they wouldn't be sissies. He wanted them to be able to "cope." However,
when the patient began having behavior problems, he chided her for not giving the
boy enough affection, and she was confused as to what to do. They were both relieved to learn that children's needs for affection vary and they do not have to be
treated alike. They were able to utilize some behavior modification principles.
The father began taking more interest in the children and the mother relaxed her
perfectionism, worrying less. The family climate improved, but the patient still
had trouble controlling his fighting with age peers.

QUESTION C:
AT THIS POINT (LATE NOVEMBER) THE THERAPIST FELT FURTHER ACTION
WAS ADVISABLE. IT MIGHT BE INTERESTING TO GUESS WHAT HE DID. HE:
1. Intensified family therapy
2. Hospitalized the patient for further study and more intensive treatment
3. Assured the parents that fighting was normal for an urban black boy and that
   they should be proud of his guts and prowess
4. Recommended advancing him a grade in school
5. Switched medication
6. Switched to a combination of individual and group therapy

Family therapy seemed to be accomplishing its goals satisfactorily; nothing
further was likely to be gained by intensifying it. The boy's problems did not
warrant hospitalization. Answer three, besides being inaccurate, is racist in its
stereotyped assigning of the boy to a role because of his color. The current medication seemed definitely helpful, with little to be gained by trying others. Answer
six would have been a reasonable move, but the correct answer here is four. This
bright boy behaved much better with older children than with his classmates, and
was academically successful. It seemed reasonable to try advancing him a grade
so that he could be constantly with slightly older children.

This recommendation was made to his principal, who was hesitant to try it.
He pointed out the realistic problems that 1) it was a difficult time of the year
(December) to make the change, 2) if it didn't work out, the boy would have a
failure experience rather than a success experience, 3) he might not be able to
develop the same rapport with his new teacher as he enjoyed with his current
teacher, and 4) his sister was in the grade to which he would be advanced (in a
different classroom). The principal also stated that he had not heard of this being
done and had never done it himself, considering the procedure highly irregular.
However, he agreed to try the advancement, with the idea that if necessary, the
boy could the following year repeat the grade to which he was being advanced this
year.

His first week in the new class he was baited by the other students. However, his experienced, perceptive teacher asked the class if this was any way to
welcome a new classmate. Thereafter, he was accepted by the other students.
Though he had some trouble with math and cursive handwriting, to which he had
not previously been exposed, he picked these up and progressed steadily in his
work. By May he was surpassing his new classmates in some areas. His new
teacher was questioning his need for medication, but his delighted parents were
unwilling to "rock the boat" by withdrawing it at that time. His fighting ceased

CASE STUDY #58

at school and even diminished in his neighborhood, as he directed more and more of his energy towards the successes he was experiencing in school and the challenging new class to which he had been advanced. For the following year, the amazed principal and teacher both decided to place him in the fourth grade along with his new classmates. Telephone follow-up two years after initial contact revealed that he was continuing peacefully with these new classmates in the fifth-grade.

QUESTION D:
FOR SUCH ADVANCEMENT TO WORK, ALL OF THE FOLLOWING CRITERIA NEED TO BE MET EXCEPT WHICH ONE?:
1. The child's main problem is behavioral rather than academic
2. The behavior problem seems worse in the presence of younger children and better controlled in the presence of older children
3. The child is intelligent and free of learning disorders
4. The child is healthy and free of medical or psychiatric disorders
5. An experienced, flexible teacher is available in the advanced grade
6. The child is willing

Though any medical or psychiatric disorders, such as epilepsy or hyperkinetic syndrome, need to be adequately treated, their presence would not necessarily rule out advancement. Therefore answer four is the only one which is not necessary for successful advancement.

REFERENCES:
1. Arnold, L. E. , 1972: Control of aggression by advanced grade placement, J of School Health 42:458-459

2. Comer, J. P. , 1972: Beyond Black and White, Quadrangle, New York

3. Simonds, J. F. , In Press, 1973: School mental health case consultation: Program description and follow-up study. J of School Health

4. Thomas, A. , Chess, S. and H. G. Birch, 1970: Temperament and Behavior Disorders in Childhood, New York University Press, New York

5. Thomas, A. , 1968: Significance of temperamental individuality for school functioning, Learning Disorders 3:345

6. Wender, P. , 1971: Minimal Brain Dysfunction in Children, John Wiley & Sons, New York

CASE STUDY #59

The Boy Who Was Older Than His Father

Joey, a 13 year-old seventh grade boy of Italian extraction, was referred by the Juvenile Court for evaluation. He had been charged with bullying a younger boy and stealing his bicycle.

QUESTION A:
AT THIS POINT THE BEST DIAGNOSIS TO CONSIDER IS:
1. Unsocialized aggressive reaction of adolescence
2. Adjustment reaction of adolescence
3. Over anxious reaction of adolescence
4. Group delinquent reaction of adolescence
5. Incipient schizophrenia

A diagnosis of unsocialized aggressive reaction of adolescence could be considered because of Joey's bullying and stealing. If he had done this as part of a gang, four would have been a better answer. Solitary delinquency though, is more likely a sign of answer one. We will soon see that first appearances can be deceiving.

Approximately three months prior to the stealing incident his family, which consisted of his parents, sixteen-year-old brother, and three younger siblings, had moved to their own home after having lived with maternal grandmother from the time Joey was an infant. The new home was about a mile away from the grandmother's home. About six weeks after the move, the boy suddenly developed hypochondriacal anxiety attacks, during which he became terrified of dying. These attacks were so frightening that several times he ran from his home in the middle of the night to the emergency rooms of nearby hospitals; the police had to call his parents to let them know his whereabouts. He seemed preoccupied with "kidney trouble," "heart attacks" and "cancer." He was placed on a pediatric unit for observation; his anxiety attacks ceased and he was discharged.

There had been several recent deaths among the boy's acquaintances. A boy in his class had died following a kidney transplant; a former playmate had been killed in an automobile accident; and an uncle had died of a "heart attack."

The mother, a rather somber, heavy-set woman in her thirties, seemed to be quite depressed and verbalized her feelings of loss after moving away from her mother. Father, who owned a plumbing business, had difficulty in relating to his sons, and felt that his only role in the family was to provide financial support. Joey's older brother had been in trouble for stealing cars. Joey had felt very close to him and used him as a father in many ways. However, the brother had quit school and was working with the father. He had also recently acquired a girlfriend, which seemed to leave Joey out.

There was much confusion about roles in the family, possibly because of having lived with maternal grandparents for so long. Father was regarded as the head of the family by mother, but her non-verbal consent had to be obtained for all that went on. Father seemed to take the role of an older brother. For instance, when Joey was in the hospital as a child and begged to be discharged, father told him that he couldn't get him out because he wasn't old enough to sign the papers.

The patient was a full-term baby with an easy birth. Developmental milestones were normal. Mother considered him a "good, quiet child" until he entered the first grade. About that time he seemed to change personalities with his older brother. The older brother became "quiet and good" while Joey suddenly became "mischievous and noisy."

The school reported that the patient had been a troublemaker in school for the past three years, and that he was becoming progressively worse. He was an aggressive bully and had the school terrorized. He was also very clever at mani-

CASE STUDY #59

pulating the teachers; he always had a plausible excuse for any misdemeanor. His grades were average and below.

Joey was given the Wechsler Intelligence Scale for Children (WISC), Bender-Gestalt, Children's Apperception Test (CAT), and the Rorschach. His full scale IQ of 101 on the WISC indicated he was of normal intelligence. The Bender-Gestalt contained no organic signs. Both the Rorschach and the CAT suggested that the boy was in good contact with reality at the time of the testing.

The Rorschach, in particular, suggested that Joey was a "burnt child," who had possibly suffered some form of early rejection experiences. At the time of the testing, he was completely preoccupied with his own egocentric needs; he was overly cautious in his emotional contacts; he found it difficult to involve himself in interpersonal relationships. He was very tense, and any expression of aggression seemed to be followed by regression to a more childish level of functioning. The Rorschach was heavily flavored with anatomical preoccupations, suggesting psychosomatic complaints.

Both projective tests suggested Joey was very dependent on his mother while at the same time afraid of being incorporated by her. Joey saw his father as a rather ineffectual "has-been," i.e., as a figure who was no longer powerful, frightening, nor supportive of him.

Joey was initially apprehensive with the psychologist, but gradually settled down and worked hard. He was able to discuss his fears of being "sent away," and said that when he was away from home he felt frightened, especially at night. He was not afraid of the dark, only of being alone.

QUESTION B:
IN LIGHT OF THIS ADDITIONAL HISTORY AND PSYCHOLOGICAL EVALUATION, THE MOST APPROPRIATE DIAGNOSIS WOULD BE:
1. Hypochondriacal neurosis
2. Schizophrenia
3. Depressive neurosis
4. Anxiety neurosis
5. Hysterical neurosis

Though Joey seems very disturbed, a schizophrenic diagnosis is not warranted at this point. Anxiety and hypochondriasis seem the most prominent features here. The differential diagnosis seems to be between one and four. The panic quality which induced Joey to get up in the night and run to the hospital emergency room suggests an anxiety neurosis rather than a hyopchondriacal neurosis. The latter is more of an ongoing preoccupation with feelings of dysfunction of various organs, while the former places emphasis on the feelings of panic, although hypochondriacal trends could be added. The best diagnosis would be: anxiety neurosis with depressive and hypochondriacal trends.

QUESTION C:
JOEY HAD PROBABLY BEEN EMOTIONALLY DISTURBED SINCE:
1. His birth
2. He exchanged roles with his older brother at about age 6, and became the mischievous, noisy one
3. His brother quit school and got a girlfriend
4. At least three years ago
5. The recent deaths among his acquaintances

It is very difficult to determine at what age this boy's emotional problems set in. His change from a rather "quiet and good" boy to a "mischievous, noisy" child may have been an ordinary developmental experience partially stimulated by his starting school. The earliest solid evidence of emotional problems can be found in the school report which stated that he became a difficult problem in

CASE STUDY #59

the classroom three years prior to the referral, i.e., from the time he was 10. The best answer is four.

QUESTION D:
JOEY BULLIED THE YOUNGER BOY AND TOOK HIS BICYCLE FROM HIM BE-
CAUSE:
1. He was cured of his anxiety neurosis and had shifted to an unsocialized aggressive reaction of adolescence
2. He may have been trying to regain the interest and companionship of his older
brother
3. He was competing with his older brother for father's attention
4. He wanted transportation to visit his grandmother
5. He identified with his lost older brother who stole

Joey's father was never able to assume parental responsibility. Instead, from the time they were young boys, Joey's older brother seemed to offer the support and stability which Joey needed. The act of stealing was probably part of Joey's identification with his older brother who stole. The best answer is five. Two and four may have also contributed.

QUESTION E:
MOTHER'S FEELINGS OF LOSS AND DEPRESSION (ABOUT THE MOVE FROM
HER MOTHER'S HOME) MAY HAVE MADE JOEY FEEL:
1. That he wasn't responsible for her sadness
2. That father was to blame
3. That he would like to run away
4. Even more lonely, and that mother wasn't interested
5. That if he caused enough trouble it would arouse her attention and responsive-
ness

A child often blames himself for his mother's depression and feels that the depressed mother is no longer interested in him. In this case, the effect on the patient may have been even more depriving because his father offered him little and his older brother had recently developed other interests. We occasionally see children who get into trouble at school, clown, or run away in an attempt to rekindle their mother's interest. Therefore, Joey's misbehavior may have been overdetermined. In addition to the psychodynamic determinants discussed in Question D, the stealing and school misbehavior may have been unconscious at-tempts to get into trouble in order to rearouse mother's interest. The best answer is four, but five is also a possibility.

REFERENCES:
1. Bates, L., et al., 1959: Adolescent Rorschach Responses. New York, Hoeber

2. Bellak, L., 1954: The Thematic Apperception Test and the Children's Apperception Test in Clinical Use. New York, Grune & Stratton

3. Bender, L., 1938: A visual motor gestalt test and its clinical use. Am Orthopsychiat Assn Monogr Series No. 3

4. English, O.S. and G.H.J. Pearson, 1972: Irrational fears and phobias in:
Childhood Psychopathology. ed. S. Harrison and J.F. McDermott, New York,
International Universities Press. pp. 375-381

5. Frank, G., 1965: The role of the family in the development of psychopathology.
Psychol Bull 64:191-205

CASE STUDY #59

6. Freud, S., 1917: Mourning and melancholia. Standard Edition. 14:243-258. London: Hogarth Press, 1957

7. Garner, A. and C. Wenar, 1959: The Mother-Child Interaction in Psychosomatic Disorders. Urbana, Ill: Univ of Illinois Press

8. Haworth, M. A., 1966: The CAT: Facts about Fantasy. New York, Grune and Stratton

9. Nagera, H., 1969: Children's reaction to the death of important objects: a developmental approach. The Psychoanalytic Study of the Child. 25:360-400. New York, Int. Univ. Press

10. Plotsky, H. and M. Shereshefsky, 1960: An isolation pattern in father of emotionally disturbed children. Am J of Orthopsychiat 30:780-787

11. Prugh, D. G., 1963: Toward an understanding of psychosomatic concepts in relation to illness in children. In: Modern Perspectives in Child Development. ed. A. Solnit, and S. Province. New York: International Univ. Press pp. 246-367

12. Rorschach, H., 1942: Psychodiagnostics. Bern, Switzerland: Huber

13. Waelder, R., 1930: The principle of multiple function: observations on over-determination. Psychoanal Quart 5:45-62

14. Wechsler, D., Manual: Wechsler Intelligence Scale for Children. The Psych. Corp. New York, 1949

CASE STUDY #60

A Three-Generation Matriarchal Tragedy with a Cast of Four

Amy S.- "the patient"
Mrs. S. - her divorced mother
Mrs. T. - her divorced maternal grandmother
Eloise S. - her younger sister

Amy S., an 11-year-old white, Protestant, sixth-grader, was referred by a court social worker because of rebelliousness, nervousness, and underachievement. She was accompanied to the clinic by her divorced mother, Mrs. S., who added temper tantrums and emotional lability to the list of complaints.

The social worker had become involved when Mrs. T., the maternal grandmother, with whom Amy, her sister Eloise, and Mrs. S. were living, brought court charges against Amy for incorrigibility and against Mrs. S. for neglect. The social worker reported the home to be unkempt and filthy even to the point of animal excrement from dogs and other pets which roamed the house. This description was confirmed independently by a pediatrician who had made a house call (and whose bill had gone unpaid). A casual observer would never have guessed the home conditions from the appearance of Amy and her mother, who always appeared refined, immaculately groomed, and tastefully dressed in the latest fashion. In fact, their expenditure on clothes, horseback riding, and music lessons in preference to paying bills was one example of the "irresponsibility" which Grandmother T. complained about.

QUESTION A:
FROM THE INFORMATION THUS FAR WE MIGHT SUSPECT THAT:
1. Mrs. S. has always aspired to be high society
2. Mrs. S. uses a lot of denial
3. Mrs. S. will always have a filthy home
4. The family has a reaction formation to obsessive-compulsive tendencies
5. Mrs. T. hates Mrs. S. and Amy

Answers one, three, and four are neither indicated nor disproved by the information presented. Five may be true, but Mrs. T.'s complaints need not be motivated by hate. They could just as well be motivated by love - desperate attempts to get help for Mrs. S. and Amy. Two is the best answer. Mrs. S. seems to show denial by spending on luxuries while in debt, by ignoring the filthy home condition while being personally neat and clean, and by not seeking help for Amy's obvious problems until forced to.

Amy herself was an attractive, pleasant, fidgety, anxious girl of obviously superior intelligence who complained of inability to concentrate on her lessons and admitted feeling inadequate and worthless. Her feelings of inadequacy were apparently aggravated by the achievements of her even more talented 9 year-old sister, whom grandmother favored. She seemed most fidgety and anxious in the presence of her mother, but was never able to relax even when seen alone at weekly intervals.

QUESTION B:
CHILDHOOD BEHAVIOR PROBLEMS SUCH AS AMY'S:
1. Never result from family dynamics or parental psychopathology
2. Mostly result from family dynamics and parental psychopathology
3. Are sometimes manifested by "easy" or "good" children who are sincerely trying to do what their parents want but are confused by conflicting messages or subtle messages to act out the parents' unconscious conflicts

CASE STUDY #60

4. Indicate family pathology
5. Should not raise a suspicion of minimal brain dysfunction when a serious disturbance is found in the parent

Family or parental pathology is an important common cause of childhood behavior problems, either because the child is reacting to parental rejection, neglect, overprotection, overcontrol, etc. or because the child is conscientiously acting out a subtle unconscious message of the parent. Three is the best answer. Two, four, and five are not good answers because other important common causes of behavior problems, such as minimal brain dysfunction, need to be considered even in the presence of overt evidence of parental or family pathology, since they sometimes occur together.

Because of Amy's fidgetiness, difficulty concentrating, underachievement with high intelligence, temper tantrums, and lability, some of her problems were suspected to be at least partly a result of minimal brain dysfunction. Therefore she was given an unsuccessful therapeutic trial of dextroamphetamine. Eventually a better explanation for her fidgetiness emerged from the family dynamics. (See cases 1 and 32 for successful stimulant therapy of overactivity and impulsiveness and case 48 for another failure.)

At first the main therapeutic effort was directed towards Amy and Mrs. S., including individual psychotherapy for Amy, supportive counseling for Mrs. S., and some joint sessions. However, Grandmother T. 's role in the problem became increasingly prominent. Mrs. S. resisted inviting her and even claimed Mrs. T. would not come. Eventually the therapist directly invited Mrs. T. to a joint session with Amy, Eloise, and Mrs. S.

QUESTION C:
BRINGING ALL MEMBERS OF THE PATIENT'S HOUSEHOLD TOGETHER IN THE SAME ROOM FOR A CONFERENCE:
1. May endanger rapport with the patient by compromising confidentiality
2. May elicit information, verbal or nonverbal, not accessible individually, even by talking individually with various members of the family
3. Is seldom therapeutic
4. Should be done routinely as a standard therapeutic tactic
5. Is the most efficient way to treat a child

Though such a tactic is often therapeutic and can be useful in many circumstances, it is sometimes contra-indicated. One of the risks is mentioned in answer one. However, the risk to rapport is usually slight if the therapist is clear in his own mind what he is doing and prepares the patient. The possible gains are sometimes dramatic. Two is the best answer. In this case the origins of the child's acting-out behavior and leads for therapeutic intervention emerged from just two family sessions, after months of previous individual contact had been fruitless. It is doubtful that the relation between Mrs. S. 's psychodynamics and the genesis of Amy's problems would ever have been adequately understood without observing Mrs. S. in the presence of her own mother.

In the presence of Mrs. T., a dramatic change took place in Mrs. S. Ordinarily very poised, refined, confident, and verbal, Mrs. S. withered into a nail-picking, foot-shuffling, anxious, unsure little girl, very much resembling Amy in Mrs. S. 's presence. When this was pointed out, she agreed that she felt very inadequate and unsure of herself in the presence of Mrs. T. Mrs. T. seemed unconcerned about these feelings and continued her vindictive castigations of Mrs. S. 's irresponsibility.

CASE STUDY #60

QUESTION D:
MRS. S.'s BEHAVIOR IS AN EXAMPLE OF:
1. Reaction formation
2. Repression
3. Denial
4. Sublimation
5. Regression

Mrs. S. seems to regress in the presence of Mrs. T. in a way which gives us some insight into what her childhood must have been like.

In the heat of two family sessions, the following story was distilled. Mrs. T. had herself suffered a rather traumatic childhood with painful memories of a vindictive father. She experienced an unhappy marriage, eventually divorcing Mrs. S.'s father, Mr. T. She inculcated in Mrs. S. a distrust of men, particularly of Mr. T. Mrs. S. predictably had troubles with her marriage, soon divorcing the girls' father, and had trouble relating to any other man. Mrs. T. had unconsciously encouraged the very irresponsibility and acting out by Mrs. S. which she condemned so vehemently. This included Mrs. S.'s premarital affair, her divorce, and her defrauding Mrs. T. of a savings account to buy a new car. Mrs. S., in turn, tended to encourage acting-out and rebelliousness in Amy, partly as an unintended result of her own inept insecurity as a woman and mother, and partly as a means of retaliation against Mrs. T. Mrs. T. agreed that Amy was very much like Mrs. S., whereas the favored Eloise was like Mrs. T. Thus there was a three-generation circuit of acting out, with grandmother T. subtly encouraging Mrs. S. to act out Mrs. T.'s neurotic conflicts, and Mrs. S. encouraging Amy to act out Mrs. S.'s resentment against Mrs. T.

That both Amy and Eloise were uncomfortable with this situation seemed obvious from their implied plea for firmer limits. They volunteered that they behaved well when they stayed with Grandfather T., who "has a big hand." Even though he apparently resorted to corporal means of enforcing limits, the girls seemed grateful for this. Mrs. S. corroborated their claim of better behavior in his house. She had been taking them to visit him since she had learned that he was a better person than Mrs. T. had led her to believe.

QUESTION E:
WITH THIS INFORMATION, THE THERAPIST:
1. Continued family therapy
2. Started Mrs. T. in individual psychotherapy
3. Gave all three generations appropriate medication
4. Supported Mrs. S. in setting firmer limits and in establishing her own independence from Mrs. T.
5. Gave Mrs. S. a minor tranquilizer

The therapist felt that the total-family meetings had served their purpose and it was a bit late to begin working on Mrs. T.'s problems. She was allowed to opt out of further treatment when she indicated she saw no need for herself. Mrs. S. was advised to emulate her father in setting firm limits. She was also supported in her beginning attempts to establish her own independence. The therapist saw no need for medication. Therefore four is technically correct.

Unfortunately, Mrs. S. was not able to tolerate the anxiety associated with becoming independent of Mrs. T., and she withdrew the family from treatment. In retrospect, a minor tranquilizer for Mrs. S. may have allayed enough of her anxiety to allow her to tolerate both treatment and her increasing independence. The therapist should have combined answers four and five.

When last heard from, Mrs. S. was trying to get Amy into a boarding school with the help of the welfare department. This was a move which Amy herself had indicated earlier she would welcome as a way of getting out of the home.

CASE STUDY #60

QUESTION F:
THE TERM "MATRIARCHAL":
1. As applied to this family means that the senior female controls the other members, who are overly dependent on her, and males are considered either unimportant, expendable, or bad
2. Is not quite appropriate here because this is a middle-class white Protestant family
3. Is an anthropological term describing some primitive tribes with female rulers where the family lines are traced through mothers rather than fathers, in contrast to the patriarchal system of most cultures
4. In this case refers to the fact that both mother and grandmother are divorced
5. Implies a pathological set of family dynamics which can account for much mental illness

A matriarchy in itself does not imply family pathology. However, its occurrence in a patriarchal culture may reflect a disturbed family's inability to function in the culturally acceptable fashion. Poor minorities do not have a monopoly on matriarchy, as this case well demonstrates. Answers three and four may be correct as far as they go, but are incomplete. One is the best answer for this case.

REFERENCES:
1. Arnold, L. E.: October, 1973 (In press): Is This Label Necessary? J of School Health

2. Johnson, A., 1952: The genesis of anti-social acting-out in children and adults. Psychoanalytic Quarterly 21:323-343

3. Minuchin, S., et al., 1967: Families of the Slums Basic Books, New York

4. Sager, C. J. and H. S. Kaplan, 1972: Progress in Group and Family Therapy, Brunner-Mazel, New York

5. Satir, V., 1967: Conjoint Family Therapy. Science and Behavior Books, Palo Alto

CASE STUDY #61

An Adopted Infant and Parents Who Felt They Were "Not O.K."

Joy had just passed her third birthday when she was brought to the clinic by her adoptive parents, Dan and Susie, because of her recurrent fears, head banging, rocking, overfriendliness, impulsivity, and incorrigibility. These symptoms had been present for several months. Dan and Susie had decided to seek psychiatric help only after talking with their pediatrician and their friend in the welfare department who had assisted with Joy's adoption.

Joy was between 5 and 6 weeks when Dan and Susie were allowed to take her home. They had been warned that they might not be able to take her. Three years previously they had adopted 1-week-old Julie through a lawyer. They found the agency procedure much more anxiety-provoking. They recalled that "the adoption worker often seemed upset."

They found Joy almost impossible to feed in the usual manner. She would cry vigorously, arching her back, rocking from side to side, and refuse to suckle. After several days they devised a compromise of holding her on a pillow in their lap and "almost propping" the bottle. They gradually moved her feeding position closer and closer to them over the next several months. They remembered being very anxious and frustrated by Joy's behavior. They even doubted they would be able to make a go of it with Joy, though Julie had given them almost no difficulty.

They felt that she was an irritable child but otherwise normal. At the time of the first child psychiatry visit, the symptom checklist they filled out reflected a concern about behaviors commonly found at age three, such as "does same thing over and over again," "undependable," "misbehaves even after warning," "denies having done wrong," "fidgets," "runs rather than walks," "unable to watch TV for long," "gets overexcited," "acts like driven by motor," "trouble getting to sleep." They feared for Joy's safety when she might suddenly dart away from their hands in a parking lot, in traffic, or in department stores. They also worried about many other areas of control.

Susie, Joy's adoptive mother, was a 28 year-old ex-ice skating performer who taught ice skating for enjoyment and extra income. After four years of marriage and an extensive fertility workup, she and her husband had been told that it was "unlikely they would have children." They therefore adopted Julie. At the time of Joy's adoption, mother found that she was two months pregnant. She stated that "they never even considered not taking Joy" since they had already made up their minds to adopt her. Their biological daughter was born when Joy was eight months old. At that time they felt that Joy and Julie felt feelings of rivalry.

Susie came from a strict, religious family wherein the father was dominant. He was an auto mechanic and worked hard until retirement. Three days prior to the first clinic visit, a diagnosis of colon cancer had been made on him. He had a bowel resection and a long hospitalization. The family did not discuss this "secret" directly with him until after 8 months' psychotherapy with Dan and Susie. Joy's mother, Susie, remembered that her father had had a great deal of bowel trouble and possible precancer symptoms and had put off going to the doctor. Susie herself had suffered "colitis" several years previously when she was adjusting to the marriage.

Susie had travelled with an ice show for over a year. Being a year or two older than the rest of the troupe, she had accepted a great deal of responsibility, including the roles of housemother and bus driver. After months of parent guidance it came out that though she had been a confident driver prior to marriage, she became phobic of driving following her marriage. She had recurrent dreams of her husband abandoning her.

Dan, Joy's adoptive father, was a 40-year-old sales manager and part-time draftsman. He was a tall, heavyset, bald, friendly, talkative man. He also taught ice skating to beginners. He readily expressed his frustrations with Joy. He had felt angry and inadequate because it took two years before Joy would allow

CASE STUDY #61

him to hold her on his lap. During the first interview he was somewhat concerned about his job security, and talked of business failure early in the marriage. He had also had colitis. He considered himself a moderately strict disciplinarian, but a family-oriented man who changed diapers and helped with the children. The family's hobby was trailer camping.

Joy was a pretty, petite, blond, neatly dressed three year-old girl who was friendly and outgoing from the first visit. Her vocabulary was highly developed for her age. She was somewhat demanding and talked in individual psychotherapy about the need for "10 fathers" to control her. Using water paint, she seemed to enjoy getting messy after the therapist gave permission.

QUESTION A:
THE PARENTS' VIEWS ABOUT JOY INDICATED THAT:
1. Joy is a normal child living with obsessive-compulsive parents
2. Joy's parents have not resolved their own ambivalence towards adopting Joy
3. Joy's parents are unable to deal with their own marital discord and are displacing their own anxiety onto Joy
4. Joy's parents do not feel that they are adequate parents
5. Joy's parents would really like to return her to the agency
6. Joy suffered deprivation in the first six weeks of life
7. Joy's impulsivity is the result of congenital minimal brain dysfunction

Joy's parents were obsessive and some of their complaints were about behaviors that could be considered within normal limits for a three-year-old, but her therapist did not consider her normal. It is only partially true that Joy's parents did not resolve their ambivalence about the adoption, which they were able to discuss rather freely. The third answer may be partially correct. The fourth answer is correct, but this is not the main problem. Probably the parents felt many times like returning Joy; they had even talked about it with each other. However, most of the time they considered her a delight; they were not about to give her up. The sixth answer, though very difficult to prove seems likely because of the uncertainty surrounding the adoption and because of Joy's rocking, headbanging, and other behavior. The last answer, though difficult to rule out completely at this point, does not seem as likely as answer six, especially since Joy was not considered distractable by any observers. Furthermore, any minimal brain dysfunction in this case could just as well have resulted from deprivation as from congenital factors (Newton and Levine). Another alternative, not listed, which should be considered in the differential diagnosis, is the "difficult child" constellation of temperamental traits, as described by Thomas and Chess (1969). It may even be that deprivation, constitutional temperament, and minimal brain dysfunction all three contributed to this problem. However, deprivation seems the most prominent and likely with this history.

QUESTION B:
JOY PRESENTED AS A CHILD WITH WIDE SWINGS IN MOOD, A HISTORY OF AUTOEROTIC BEHAVIORS (ROCKING AND HEADBANGING), RECURRENT FEARS, AND PARENTS WHO FELT THAT SHE WAS DIFFICULT TO CONTROL. IN REGARD TO HER ROCKING, WE MIGHT SAY:
1. Rocking is found in children with inconsistent parenting
2. Rocking is found in children of parents with "criminal chromosomal" abnormalities
3. Spitz mentions that such children may be "arrested at the level of primary narcissism"
4. It comes from her parents' ambivalent feelings of rejection because at the time of her adoption they found they were going to have a natural child
5. Joy's rocking behavior is because she is adopted

CASE STUDY #61

6. Rocking behavior is found in almost every child at one time or another and
    will have no effect on Joy's personality later in life
7. When Joy was adopted she was possibly suffering the effects of deprivation.
    Because she was so difficult to manage, her adoptive parents probably treated
    her inconsistently and had many unconscious angry feelings of rejection
8. Joy's rocking is an attempt to punish herself

  The first answer is partially correct. The second is not supported by evidence known to the authors. Rene Spitz (1965) does mention that children with
rocking behaviors are "arrested at the level of primary narcissism." The parents
vigorously denied ambivalence about the adotpion, and it seemed unlikely to be a
major factor to their therapist. Adoption itself is not a cause of rocking. Rocking
behavior is not found in most children. It is usually thought to be a sign of deprivation (an attempt at self-gratification) affecting the personality in later life.
The seventh answer is the best.
  The parents spent less and less time talking about Joy and more and more
time talking about their relationship. Dan began examining his male chauvinistic
attitudes. When Susie expressed her anger towards Dan, she suffered within a
few days from nonspecific dizziness. She sought help from her family physician
and then an otolaryngologist, who could find no organic cause. This also occurred
whenever she discussed her father's cancer. She also related this dizziness to
her menstrual period, with some evidence for pre-menstrual tension. She mentioned that in her family menstrual periods were referred to as "falling off the
roof." She admitted that she had always wanted to be male and aggressive. At
card parties whenever she felt inadequate, she felt dizzy.

QUESTION C:
WITH THIS INFORMATION, WE MIGHT DESCRIBE DAN AND SUSIE IN THE
FOLLOWING MANNER:
1. These parents are extremely eager to solve their child's problems. They
    share feelings easily and have become very insightful. It is likely that they
    will be able to support Joy in ways that markedly decrease her wide swings
    in behavior
2. Dan's obsessive personality, manifested by his occupation and his previous
    colitis, indicated that he likely deals with Joy in demanding, strict ways.
    The mother's poor self-concept, phobias, and rejection of the feminine ma-
    ternal role, will more than likely cause Joy to be a tomboy and have severe
    sexual identification problems
3. Dan's lack of assertiveness and Susie's inability to separate from her parents
    will continue to cause Joy difficulty
4. It is likely that Susie's sense of inadequacy about not becoming pregnant was
    reinforced when she found a very difficult child to deal with. Her identifica-
    tion with her father, and her inability to express angry feelings further com-
    plicated her problems. The father's need to have everything perfect disposed
    him to reject imperfect Joy unconsciously though he did not wish to consciously
5. Susie had a need to show her adequacy as a mother, which was foiled when
    she encountered Joy's feeding difficulty
6. Joy's parents' problems are rather mild and are not related to Joy's tempera-
    mental difficulty
7. The father's perfectionism and the mother's self concept are related to Joy's
    maladaptation

  The first answer will hopefully be true in the future, but at this point does
not answer the question. The second answer overstates the problem. The third
answer is glib and unwarranted by the facts. The fourth answer is comprehensive
and best. The fifth answer only describes the mother. Joy's parents did not feel

CASE STUDY #61

that their problems were mild, and they were able to see how they had begun rejecting Joy. The seventh answer is too general.

Joy frequently would throw water around the therapy room. Occasionally, she would lose control and throw herself into the air, screaming loudly. She was unable to stop this without the therapist's physical intervention. Joy enjoyed this external control and would permit physical closeness for a while, but then would become anxious and pull away. Frequently Joy would roleplay a punitive mother and control the therapist, whom she would cast as an infant-child.

QUESTION D:
WHEN A PRE-SCHOOL CHILD THROWS WATER AT THE THERAPIST, THIS MAY MEAN:
1. That the water is a symbol of love and sharing feelings
2. That the water symbolizes the child's wish to urinate on the therapist
3. That the child is angry and wants to dissolve the therapist
4. A testing maneuver to see if the therapist will retaliate
5. That the child wants to show his skill as an acrobat
6. That the child wants to test the limits of the clinic
7. That the child wants to wash away a visual hallucination

When a child throws water playfully in therapy, this may merely be a way to spread glee. This makes answer one possibly correct. Answers two and three are possible, but very difficult to prove. The fourth answer is the most likely. Many children have learned at home that they can get attention by misbehaving and wonder if the therapist will retaliate as their parents would. With a child as young as this whose verbalizations of anger have been suppressed, it may be the only way she feels safe in testing out an angry thought. The fifth and seventh answers are probable but unlikely. The sixth answer is similar to four but less personal.

Frequently Joy role-played mother, with her female therapist being the child. The repeated theme was the mother's preoccupation with other duties. Joy said: "I'm making your lunch now; don't bother me; go outside and play." Occasionally Joy also role-played father who would say, "You are naughty and nasty. You are going to get spanked."

QUESTION E:
JOY'S CONSTANT LIMIT TESTING IN THE PLAYROOM AND HER INABILITY TO BE COMFORTABLE WITH INTIMACY TELLS US THAT:
1. Joy feels unaccepted and continued to test the therapist to see if she will be rejected
2. Joy's behavior is normal for her age, allowing for the usual variations in children's temperament
3. Joy's tendencies toward controlling behavior are typical of adopted children, whose parents are often ambivalent about their right to parenthood
4. Joy most likely received inconsistent mothering in early infancy and has failed to establish a sense of basic trust
5. Joy feels a great need for attention in order to satisfy her dependency needs. Because she feels that these needs are not met, she feels hostile and unable to accept intimacy
6. Joy is brain-damaged, as shown in her inability to become close after several visits
7. Joy's ego is still incomplete and her superego development has only begun. The Oedipal conflict will soon add to her troubles

The first answer is correct as far as it goes. A great deal of Joy's behavior is normal for her age. However, her continued testing and discomfort with intimacy after several visits is not normal. Studies on adopted children are con-

CASE STUDY #61

flicting; there is no one typical behavior. However, case reports do indicate that adopted children manifest symptoms related to their parents' ambivalence. The fourth answer cannot be proven, but is likely to be true. The fifth answer is the most comprehensive and the most likely. Limit-testing and discomfort with intimacy neither prove nor disprove brain damage. Answer seven, though possibly impressive in its platitudinous jargon, adds little meaning to the case.

REFERENCES:
1. Adams, P. A. , 1972: Family characteristics of obsessive children, Amer J Psychiat 128:98-101

2. Bowlby, J. , 1969: Attachment and Loss, Basic Books, New York

3. Bowlby, J. , 1965: Child Care and the Growth of Love, Penguin Books, Baltimore

4. Chandler, C. A. , Lourie, R. S. and A. D. Peters, 1968: Early Child Care: The New Perspectives. Atherton Press, New York

5. Lewis, H. , 1971: The Psychiatric Aspects of Adoption (Chapter 18) from Modern Perspectives of Child Psychiatry, Brunner-Mazel, New York

6. Newton, G. and S. Levine, 1971: Early Experience and Behavior, Basic Books, New York

7. Spitz, R. and W. G. Cobliner, 1965: The First Year of Life, International Universities Press, New York

8. Thomas, A. , Chess, S. and H. G. Birch, 1968: Temperament and Behavior Disorder, New York University Press, New York

CASE STUDY #62

Failure to Thrive

Joan was 9 months old when a psychiatric consultation was requested by the Pediatric Service. At that time her weight was slightly less than her birth weight, and this was her fifth hosptialization for the same difficulty. She had been vomiting since 4 months of age despite numerous changes in formulae. Many laboratory procedures, X-rays, and an exploratory laporotomy had failed to reveal an adequate cause. The vomiting always ceased shortly after admission to the hospital. Shortly after each discharge (without a definitive diagnosis) the vomiting would recur. On one occasion, the baby vomited while the mother fed her in the car on the way home from the hospital. On several occasions during the hospitalizations, the nurses fed the baby and then watched the mother as she fed her; under these circumstances all the feedings were completed without subsequent vomiting.

The mother had married while she was a student nurse. When she became pregnant, she had to drop out of nursing school one month before graduation in order to deliver the child. However she was not too concerned about this, because according to the rules of the school she knew that she could return and comcplete her education as soon as she was able. Toward the end of her pregnancy, she had felt the baby drop into the lower uterine segment, and had informed her husband that the baby should be delivered in about a week. Actually, though, it took two weeks from that point, and she had reasoned that the increased pressure on the baby's head in the lower uterine segment would result in molding of the head. She had informed her husband about this but at the same time had reassured him that it would revert to normal within two weeks after birth. When the baby was born, its head did, indeed, show some molding, but she again reassured her husband and asked him to reassure the grandparents. The baby and the mother were discharged on the 4th postnatal day, and the molding disappeared, as predicted, within two weeks. The mother kept careful notes of the child's development and consulted with her pediatrician regularly. The baby girl experienced no difficulties for the first four months of life, but then she began vomiting.

QUESTION A:
ASSUME FOR THE MOMENT THAT THE PEDIATRICIANS WERE CORRECT IN THEIR OPINION THAT THIS WAS A PSYCHIATRIC PROBLEM. THEN ASSUME THAT THE PSYCHIATRIC PROBLEM HAD TO DO WITH ANXIETY ON THE PART OF THE MOTHER. WHAT IS THE MOST LIKELY CAUSE OF THE MOTHER'S ANXIETY?
1. Fear of a bowel obstruction
2. Fear of being an inadequate mother
3. Fear of some sort of brain damage
4. Fear that she will never go back to school and complete her education
5. Fear of some marital discord with her husband

The mother was asked what she had feared most when the baby suddenly began to vomit at the age of 4 months. She responded that she had been afraid of bowel obstruction. The therapist, however, was impressed by her apparent concern over the molding of the head, with obsessive reassurances. Therefore he suggested that he thought her greatest concern was not that the baby might have a bowel obstruction, but that the baby might be brain damaged. At this suggestion, the mother, who had been calm and aloof toward the baby, who was crying in a nearby crib, began to cry herself and picked up the baby to comfort her. The mother was so afraid of brain damage that she had suppressed or repressed the idea to the preconscious level. This fear seemed one of the reasons for her careful notes on the child's development.

CASE STUDY #62

QUESTION B:
HOW MIGHT THIS MATERNAL ANXIETY BE ASSOCIATED WITH THE INFANT'S
VOMITING?:
1. The anxiety is secondary to the vomiting
2. The anxiety causes muscular tension which is sensed by the infant and causes
   the vomiting
3. The anxiety causes an increased maternal heart rate which is perceived by
   the infant and causes the vomiting
4. The anxiety is not associated either directly or indirectly with the vomiting
5. The anxiety and the vomiting are both caused by a different, as yet unknown,
   factor

The first answer may be partially correct but doesn't go far enough, giving
only half of the vicious cycle. The fifth answer could be correct, but in this case
no additional factor was ever discovered. The second answer is undoubtedly
correct, at least in part, and the third may be correct, too. The feeding experience should bring pleasure to both mother and infant. The infant obtains both
nutritional satisfaction and two kinds of erotic satisfaction: 1) through stimulation
of the oral mucous membrane, and 2) through the tactile stimulation of being held
in its mother's arms. Maternal anxiety may result in muscular tension which
can be perceived by the infant as unpleasant tactile stimulation. Conceivably
this could reach an intensity that makes feeding experiences distinctly unpleasant
and produces enough tension in the infant to cause vomiting. Such vomiting might
easily increase the mother's anxiety and muscular tension, resulting in a vicious
cycle. In fact, the original episode of vomiting may have resulted from some
other cause, such as gastroenteritis, which initiated a vicious cycle of maternal
anxiety and infantile vomiting.
There is some evidence that the fetus becomes conditioned to the maternal
heart rate during its pleasant intrauterine existence, and therefore responds
most readily in its extrauterine life to a similar rhythm. Presumably maternal
tachycardia, if perceived at all by the infant, would be experienced as unpleasant
and might, therefore, cause vomiting if it occurred during feedings.
Joan's therapist arranged a second visit, this time with both parents, during
which they explored and discussed various difficulties which are common among
young parents. He explained to the mother that her anxiety could be transmitted,
through muscular tension for instance, to the baby's body during the feedings,
and that it might be advisable to let the father take over some of the feedings
when she felt overwrought about one thing or another.
An 18-month follow-up indicated that there had been no further recurrences
of the vomiting. Joan appeared to be a happy 2-year-old.

QUESTION C:
WHICH OF THE FOLLOWING DISEASES OF INFANCY MAY BE PSYCHOGENIC?:
1. Diarrhea
2. Convulsions
3. Eczema
4. Developmental retardation
5. "Failure to thrive" syndrome

Except for convulsions, all of these disorders may be caused by psychological
factors. Diarrhea is commonly psychogenic. One of the authors saw a one-week
old infant that had had six stools within an hour or two following discharge from
the newborn nursery. Another physician had seen him in the hospital and had
given him a small blood transfusion because of a mild anemia. Of all the things
he said to the mother, she recalled only his advice to "...keep up the baby's
blood so he wouldn't need another transfusion..." She interpreted this to mean
that he wanted her to maintain the baby on an adequate iron intake, and she be-

CASE STUDY #62

came very anxious when the infant refused an iron-enriched formula. The diarrhea ensued. When the author explained that the baby had adequate iron stores to last three months, and that her doctor had been thinking of the long term iron maintenance, she relaxed and the diarrhea ceased.

Spitz includes eczema among the psychogenic diseases of infancy. Engel, Reichsman and Segel (1956) and Coddington (1968) have documented the functional retardation and marasmus that can result from disturbed mother-infant relationships.

REFERENCES:
1. Coddington, R. D. , 1968: Study of an infant with a Gastric Fistula and Her Normal Twin. Psychosom Med 30:172-192

2. Engel, G. L. , Reichsman, F. and Segel, H. L. , 1956: A Study of an infant with a Gastric Fistula. Psychosom Med 18:374-398

3. Freud, A. , 1946: The Psychoanalytic Study of Infantile Feeding Disturbances. Psa St of the Child 2:119-132

4. Ribble, M. D. , 1943: The Rights of Infants. New York, Col. Univ. Press

5. Spitz, R. A. , 1965: The First Year of Life, New York, Int. Univ. Press

6. Spitz, R. A. , 1951: The Psychogenic Diseases in Infancy: An Attempt at Their Etiologic Classification. Psa St of the Child 6:255-271

7. Winnicott, D. W. , 1931: Clinical Notes on Disorders of Childhood. London, Heinemann

CASE STUDY #63

The "Floppy" Infant

George was the first-born of a white Catholic middle-class family. There were no pregnancy complications. His neo-natal course was unremarkable, and his health and development were within normal limits for the first three to four months. His father brought him for the regular pediatric evaluations and immunizations. The child was five months old before the pediatrician realized that he had not seen the mother since her discharge from the maternity ward. He explained to the father that he was glad to see fathers interested in their infants' development, but that he wanted the mother to come in on the next visit. She came and did not strike the pediatrician as being unusual in any way.

By this time, around the fifth or sixth month, the pediatrician was becoming concerned about George's poor muscle tone. Nevertheless, the child seemed to be developing well in the emotional and social spheres as well as in his ability to use the finer motor units. There was no apparent paralysis, only the hypotonia. He was a "floppy child."

QUESTION A:
"FLOPPY CHILDREN" MAY RESULT FROM WHICH OF THE FOLLOWING:
1. Myasthenia gravis
2. Child battering
3. Affective deprivation
4. Early infantile autism
5. Lead poisoning secondary to pica

The symptom of the "floppy child" can be seen in a number of situations, resulting either from organic or psychogenic factors. Myasthenia gravis and lead poisoning due to pica, however, will not be seen at this age. A battered child may manifest poor muscle tone but will probably exhibit other signs such as tender areas and eccymoses, and will rarely be described as "floppy."

Children that are retarded will sometimes show this sign. Those suffering from early infantile autism will not. The third answer is correct. Engel, Reichsman and Segal (1954), and later Coddington (1964), demonstrated clearly the profound psychological and physiological effects that affective deprivation can have on the infant. Hypotonia may result from the mother's inability to give of herself to her baby. This can result from serious maternal depression or psychosis or from the mother's inability to relate to her child because of some defect in the child which has an unpleasant connotation.

In this case we have a hint that the mother was suffering some sort of emotional disturbance. She did not assume the usual role of a mother taking her infant to a pediatrician, despite the fact that she did not seem emotionally disturbed to the pediatrician when she did come. As it turned out, a thorough evaluation in a children's hospital failed to discover any specific cause for the symptom. The child, without any specific treatment, finally began to develop more normally at around eighteen months of age. No psychiatric evaluation was ever obtained.

When the child was three years old, the pediatrician made a house call because of an acute febrile illness. Upon entering this middle-class home in a nice residential community, he was dismayed at the condition of the living room. It was dirty; large crumbs of food were lying about the floor and on the furniture, and the room was in serious disarray. Conditions were so filthy the pediatrician felt quite uncomfortable sitting down to examine the child. The mother showed no concern over the condition of the house; she made only one half-hearted apology about how they were attempting to fix up a game room and had not worried much about the living room. The pediatrician, still filled with consternation at the situation, felt it might be due to the suddenness of his visit and the mother's concern about her sick child. Therefore, he arranged a second visit three days later

CASE STUDY #63

to check on the child (and the house). He found the living room in exactly the same condition.

There was no telephone in the home because the mother had made extended long distance calls to her mother, running up huge bills which necessitated the removal of the phone.

QUESTION B:
THE MOTHER'S MOST LIKELY DIAGNOSIS, GIVEN ONLY THIS SKETCHY IN-FORMATION ABOUT HER, IS:
1. Anti-social personality disorder
2. Psychoneurosis, depressive type
3. Schizophrenia
4. Mental retardation, mild to moderate
5. Psychotic depression

It is risky to make even a working diagnosis from such sketchy information, but this woman showed a rather distant and peculiar sort of interest in her child, a very strong relationship with her mother (perhaps even a symbiotic relationship) poor relationship with peers in her community and with the pediatrician, and a lack of reality testing regarding the condition of her living room and the effect that it had upon the pediatrician. Was she really unaware of the way her behavior affected other people? Was she unable to cut down the length of her phone calls to her mother prior to her husband's having the phone removed? Did she feel no shame regarding the condition of her living room in the presence of the pediatrician? In light of these things, the most likely diagnosis is schizophrenia. Depression must be considered, but a depression of such long standing is unlikely, and she did not appear depressed.

QUESTION C:
WHEN THIS INFANT WAS TEN TO TWELVE MONTHS OF AGE THE PEDIA-TRICIAN SHOULD HAVE:
1. Referred the mother to a psychiatrist because he had a vague but unpleasant feeling about his relationship with her
2. Referred the mother to a psychiatrist because she had a floppy child
3. Talked to the father about the wife's difficulties and let the father take the responsibility for seeking psychiatric care, or obtaining a divorce and custody of the boy
4. Taught the mother how to stimulate her child through specific neuro-motor exercises
5. None of the above

Exercises alone for a child with a mother who is not able to give affectively would be foolish. Similarly, it would seem a shame for the father to divorce this wife who needs him. Psychiatric consultation would seem most appropriate, and the pediatrician needs no other reason than his own feelings about this woman. He has considerable experience with mothers of infants, and can rely on his ability to relate to them and to identify with their problems. He should be very concerned when one of his patients' mothers does not relate to him in a meaningful way. Such a lack of rapport is as scientific and valid a reason for referral as any other specific symptom. The second answer would have been right in this case, but the pediatrician should investigate the causes of the hypotonia rather than simply refer the parents of all such children to a psychiatrist. So answer two is correct, but for the wrong reason. Answer one is entirely correct.

CASE STUDY #63

QUESTION D:
ASSUMING THE MOTHER REMAINS PRETTY MUCH AS SHE IS, THE PROGNO-
SIS FOR THE CHILD IS:
1. Good, since his development will probably accelerate after he gets over this
   critical period
2. Good, because his father can make up for his mother's inadequacies
3. Guarded, because he may develop problems in the expression of affect even
   though able to function in school and society
4. Guarded, because he will probably become psychotic as a result of his relationship with his mother, a folie-a-deux
5. Poor, because he has probably inherited schizophrenia

If a child is deprived of a healthy relationship with a mother or surrogate
mother for 4-5 years, some of the damage may be irreparable. George's father
may be his saving grace, but one would be doing the family a disservice if the
situation were ignored or passed off as a temporary thing with a good prognosis;
the first two answers are wrong. The genetic component in the etiology of schizophrenia is certainly a significant one, but not so much so that we can predict the
development of this disorder in all the children of schizophrenic parents. (An
excellent review of this subject was written by Offord and Cross 1969). The
prognosis is definitely guarded. Three is the best. George may develop a folie-
a-deux, but this is not a "probable" outcome. It is much more likely that he will
have poor object relations with difficulty expressing warmth, love, and affection.
He may become sociopathic (Robins 1966) or delinquent due to a lack of concern
for other people. (See Case 21)

REFERENCES:
1. Bowlby, J., 1965: Child Care and the Growth of Love. Penguin Books,
   Baltimore, Md.

2. Coddington, R. D., 1968: A Study of an Infant with a Gastric Fistula and Her
   Normal Twin. Psychosom Med 30:172-192

3. Engel, G. L., Reichsman, F. and H. L. Segal, 1956: A Study of an Infant
   With a Gastric Fistula. Psychosom Med 18:374-398

4. Offord, D. R. and L. A. Cross, 1969: Behavioral Antecedents of Adult Schizophrenia: A Review. Archives of Gen Psychiatry 21:267-283

5. Robins, L. N., 1966: Deviant Children Grown Up. Williams & Wilkins,
   Baltimore, Md.

6. Yarrow, L. J., 1961: Maternal Deprivation: Toward an Empirical and Conceptual Re-evaluation. Psychol Bull 58:459-490

CASE STUDY #64

A 6-1/2-Year-Old Who Hid Her Feces

A 6-1/2 year-old white girl was brought by her working class parents because she was becoming more and more difficult to manage. They described her as having "fierce" temper tantrums, being a clever mischief maker and being secretive and often very unhappy.

Sandy was a pretty girl with blonde curly hair and smiling brown eyes. She was dainty, feminine, and spoke in a soft, confidential manner. Although she related easily, she seemed superficial.

Mother suffered morning sickness during the first five months of her full-term, otherwise uneventful pregnancy. Mother breastfed for the first month, but the child didn't gain weight, and her pediatrician shifted the infant to bottle feeding. However, despite many formula changes, the child vomited after every feeding and screamed incessantly for the next six months. Then, in desperation, mother gave the infant a cup of cow's milk. The child retained it and slept through the night for the first time. From that moment, she seemed a contented baby with only occasional stomach upsets and diarrhea. When the child was about 2-1/2 years old she developed asthma and eczema, while at the same time the stomach upsets and diarrhea disappeared. At the age of 3-1/2 the child was rushed to the hospital with an asthma attack. She stayed for two weeks, and upon discharge the family immediately moved to a village in the country. The whole family was unhappy in this new situation, and the child's asthma worsened. After about a year, the family returned to the city, and moved into a basement apartment in the paternal grandparents' house. There was tension in the family because parents and grandparents disagreed on "everything." However, the grandparents adored Sandy and gave her everything she wished and believed that anything she said was wonderful. There were no limits placed upon her activities.

Mother started toilet training Sandy when she was 3 months old, without much success. However, by the time she was age 2 she was dry both day and night. A brother was born when she was 2-1/2 years-old. Mother had prepared her for the new baby and Sandy seemed very interested when he was born and loved to hold him. Yet, at that time, she entered a long phase of defecating behind chairs, under tables and in closets. She also reverted to constantly sucking her pacifier, which she did not give up until she was age 4.

When Sandy was age 5, her 2-1/2 year-old brother pulled a bowl of scalding soup over himself and suffered severe burns. Although he was not hospitalized, his burns necessitated daily trips with mother to the hospital for many weeks, while grandparents looked after Sandy. Sandy didn't seem bothered by this. She started school and the school reported she was no trouble and that her work was excellent. However, she seemed unhappy each day when she returned from school. After about six months, she started quarreling with the other school children and became very anxious about her lessons. She began to tell lies, constantly picked her nose, scratched her eczema, or pinched the skin on the back of her hands. She also carried tales and played parents off against grandparents.

Although Sandy was very careful of her own possessions, she became very destructive of mother's. When mother was busy, Sandy would sneak into her room where she would unscrew tubes of creams and smear them on the walls or mirrors, would pull things out of the drawers and scatter them, or would break things. Although she was distressed when punished or scolded, she would repeat the misbehavior within a very short time as though she were unable to control her behavior.

Psychological testing indicated that Sandy was of average intelligence, but that she felt shut off from her family.

QUESTION A:
SANDY DESTROYED MOTHER'S POSSESSIONS BECAUSE:
1. She was envious of mother who had more things than she did

CASE STUDY #64

2. She thought if mother didn't have make-up and beauty creams, she would then be a little girl like herself
3. She was angry with mother and her attacks on mother's possessions may have been a substitute for an attack on mother
4. She was able to gain attention by destroying mother's possessions
5. She felt that if she couldn't have these things, mother shouldn't be allowed to have them.

It is possible that Sandy harbored angry feelings towards her mother because of the attention her little brother received due to his burns. It is also possible that the early infant-mother relationship didn't offer mother gratification or a good concept of herself as a mother. An infant who vomits mother's milk after each feed, who doesn't gain weight and who cries incessantly can cause misgivings in a woman about her adequacy as a mother. (See cases 26, 37 and 61 for more about mothering.) In contrast, the little brother may have been an easier baby and perhaps mother felt closer to him, which Sandy may have sensed. The fact that she clung to her pacifier until four years of age may have been partially due to feelings of being left out and having to comfort herself. The best answer is three.

QUESTION B:
SANDY'S DEFECATIONS UNDER TABLES, BEHIND CHAIRS AND IN CLOSETS SUGGESTS THAT SHE:
1. Was not toilet trained
2. Wanted to surprise mother
3. Was in an anal aggressive stage
4. Was retarded
5. Was acting out her anger and hostility towards mother

Defecating in closets, under tables and behind chairs suggests that Sandy had good bowel control. However, she was using her feces, which we can assume she felt were "bad" in an aggressive way, i.e., leaving these "bad" parts of herself around as an attack on mother. At this age, Sandy may have also had many fantasies about her feces, such as that they could have been a part of herself with magic properties which she could leave behind in order to find out what was going on between mother and brother. Since we don't know, this can only be used as an illustration of a child's "magic." The best answer is five, but three is also correct.

QUESTION C:
THE PROPER TIME TO START A CHILD'S TOILET TRAINING IS:
1. When he is three to six months old
2. Before he is old enough to crawl around so that mother can be sure he stays on the pot
3. When he is too old to wear diapers
4. Six months to a year old
5. When mother gets tired of changing diapers
6. None of the above

Rather than an exact age, the indications that an infant is ready for toilet training are sphincter control, the ability to sit on the pot and the ability to understand what is wanted from him. There are variations in the ages when these milestones are achieved, but they ordinarily occur around age two.

Although training may be started around this time, the child of three or even four may have an occasional accident. Parents who treat toilet training rather casually will find that the ordinary child will cooperate and take pride in becoming clean and dry. Six is the best answer.

CASE STUDY #64

QUESTION D:
THIS CHILD COULD HAVE BEEN DIAGNOSED AS:
1. Unsocialized aggressive reaction of childhood
2. Anxiety neurosis
3. Encopresis
4. Psychophysiologic disorder
5. Reactive disorder

The symptoms suggested that this little girl initially suffered a psychophysiologic disorder which may have been augmented by the early, stressful mothering relationship. Of course, the possibility of allergy must also be considered for the eczema and asthma. Most likely the symptoms resulted from the interaction of organic and psychosocial factors. The overlay of a reactive disorder is suggested by the child's aggressive behavior, nose picking, skin pinching and her hidden defecations. The latter may have also been augmented by the attention her brother received following his accident. The best answers are a combination of four and five, a psychophysiologic disorder with an unsocialized aggressive reaction of childhood.

REFERENCES:
1. Abramson, H. A., 1954: Evaluation of maternal rejection theory in allergy. Ann Allergy, 12:129-140

2. Dare, C., 1969: Your 6 Year Old. London, Corgi

3. Fraiberg, Selma, 1959: The Magic Years. New York, Charles Schribner's Sons

4. Freud, Anna, 1972: The psychoanalytic study of infantile feeding disturbances. Childhood Psychopathology. eds. S. Harrison & J. F. McDermott, New York, Int. Univ. Press, pp. 296-309

5. Garner, A. and C. Wenar, 1959: The Mother-Child Interaction in Psychosomatic Disorders. Urbana, Ill.: Univ. of Illinois Press

6. Geleerd, E. R., 1945: Some observations on temper tantrums in children. Am J Orthopsychiat 15:238-246

7. Jessner, L., Lamont, J., Long, R., Rollins, N., Whipple, B., and N. Prentice, 1955: Emotional impact of nearness and separation of the asthmatic child and his mother. Psychoanal Study Child 10:353-375, New York, International Univ. Press

8. Knapp, P. H., 1972: The asthmatic child and the psychosomatic problem of asthma: toward a general theory in Childhood Psychopathology, eds. S. Harrison and J. F. McDermott, New York, International Univ. Press pp. 591-609

9. Lipton, E. L. and J. Richmond, 1966: Psychophysiologic disorders in children. Review of Child Development Research, eds. L. Hoffman and M. Hoffman, 2:169-220. New York: Russell Sage Foundation

10. McLean, J. A., Ching, A. T. Y., et al., 1961: A study of relationships between family situation, bronchial asthma, and personal adjustment in children. J Pediat 59:402-414

CASE STUDY #64

11. McLean, J. A. and A. Y. T. Ching, 1973: Follow-up study of relationships between family situation and bronchial asthma in children. J Am Acad Child Psychiat 12:142-161

12. Rutter, M., Birch, H. G., Thomas, A. and S. Chess, 1964: Temperamental characteristics in infancy and the later development of behavioral disorders. Brit J Psychiat 110:651-661

13. Winnicott, D. W., 1958: The antisocial tendency. Collected Papers Through Paediatrics to Psycho-analysis. London, Tavistock pp. 306-315

INDEX

The numbers shown after each topic are the numbers of the case studies.

INDEX

INDEX

INDEX

INDEX

INDEX

INDEX

INDEX

INDEX

INDEX